DORLAND'S

Radiology/ Oncology Word Book

for Medical Transcriptionists

DORLAND'S

Radiology WORD BOOK

for Medical Transcriptionists

Series Editor
SHARON B. RHODES, CMT, RHIT

Edited & Reviewed by:
Janet Christie Pugh, CMT

W.B. SAUNDERS COMPANY
A Harcourt Health Sciences Company

Philadelphia   London   New York   St. Louis   Sydney   Toronto

W.B. Saunders Company
A Harcourt Health Sciences Company

The Curtis Center
Independence Square West
Philadelphia, Pennsylvania 19106

Library of Congress Cataloging-in-Publication Data

Dorland's radiology/oncology word book : for medical transcriptionists / Sharon Rhodes, editor.

p. cm.

ISBN 0-7216-9150-1

1. Radiology, Medical—Terminology.   2. Oncology—Terminology.   3. Medical transcription.   I. Title: Radiology/oncology word book.   II. Rhodes, Sharon.

R895.A3 D67 2001

616.07′57′014—dc21   00-059569

Dorland's Radiology/Oncology Word Book for
Medical Transcriptionists   ISBN 0-7216-9150-1

Printed in the United States of America.

Last digit is the print number: 9 8 7 6 5 4 3 2 1

I am proud to present the *Dorland's Radiology/Oncology Word Book for Medical Transcriptionists*—part of a series of word books compiled for the professional medical transcriptionist. For one hundred years, W.B. Saunders has published the *Dorland's Illustrated Medical Dictionary*. With the advent of medical transcription, it became the dictionary of choice for medical transcriptionists.

When approached last year to help develop a new series of word books for W.B. Saunders, I have to admit the thought absolutely overwhelmed me. The *Dorland's Illustrated Medical Dictionary* was one of my first book purchases when I began my transcription career over thirty years ago. To be invited to participate in this project is an honor I could never have imagined for myself!

Transcriptionists need and will continue to need trusted up-to-date resources to help them research difficult terms quickly. In developing the *Dorland's Radiology/Oncology Word Book for Medical Transcriptionists,* I had access to the entire *Dorland's* terminology database for the book's foundation. In addition to this immense database, a context editor, Janet Christie Pugh, CMT, a recognized expert in the field of radiology transcription, was selected to review the material from the database, to contribute new and unique terms, and to remove outdated and obsolete ones. With Janet's extensive research and diligent work, I believe this to be the most up-to-date word book for the field of radiology.

In developing the radiology word book, I wanted the size to be manageable so the book would be easy to handle, with a durable, long-lasting binding, and using a type font large enough to read while providing extensive terminology. Illustrations of radiographic orientation were added as well as a listing of positions and planes utilized in performing radiographic procedures.

Although I have tried to produce the most thorough word book for radiology available to medical transcriptionists, it is difficult to include every term as the field of radiology is constantly evolving. As you discover new terms, please feel free to share them with me for inclusion in the next edition of the *Dorland's Radiology/Oncology Word Book for Medical Transcriptionists.*

I may be reached at the following e-mail address: Sharon@TheRhodes.com.

SHARON B. RHODES, CMT, RHIT
Brentwood, Tennessee

abarticulation

Abbe-Zeiss counting chamber

ABCD
Adriamycin (doxorubicin),bleomycin, CCNU (lomustine), and dacarbazine

abdomen
pendulous a.

abdominal

abdominogenital

abdominoscrotal

abdominothoracic

abdominovaginal

abdominovesical

abduct

abductio

abduction

abductor
a. pollicis longus

aberrant vessel or band

ablation of thyroid gland function

abluminal

abnormal
a. attenuation
a. fluid collection
a. staining
a. vascularization

ABO blood group

aborad

aboral

abrasion

abrasor

Abrikosov's (Abrikossoff's) tumor

abruptio placentae

absence of haustral markings

absence of vascular markings

abscess
acute a.
Brodie's a.
a. formation
iliopsoas a.
ischiorectal a.
Munro a.
paracolic a.
Pautrier's a.
perinephric a.
perinephritic a.
perirectal a.
peritoneal a.
peritonsillar a.
phlegmonous a.
psoas a.
pulp a.
pulpal a.
pyogenic a.
splenic a.
subphrenic a.
sudoriparous a.
walled-off a.

absconsio

abscopal

absorbance

absorptiometry
dual photon a.

absorption
external a.
interstitial a.

abuts

abutting

ABVD
Adriamycin (doxorubicin), bleomycin, vinblastine, and dacarbazine

1

AC
    Adriamycin (doxorubicin)
      and cyclophosphamide

acanthocytosis

acantholysis

acantholytic

acanthoma
    a. adenoides cysticum
    clear cell a.
    Degos a.
    pilar sheath a.

acanthopelvis

acanthopelyx

acanthosis
    a. nigricans

acanthotic

acanthrocytosis

acarodermatitis
    a. urticarioides

acaroid

ACBE
    air contrast barium enema

accelerator
    linear a.
    particle a.
    serum prothrombin con-
      version a.
    serum thrombotic a.

accelerin

access
    vascular a.

accessorius

accident
    cerebrovascular a. (CVA)

acervuline

acetabular

acetabulum *pl.* acetabula

acetowhite

acetowhitening

acetrizoate

achalasia

Achilles tendon

achlorhydria

achondroplasia

achoresis

achrestic

achromasia

achromatosis

achromia
    a. parasitica

achromic

achromotrichia

acicular

acinar

acini (plural of acinus)

acinic

aciniform

acinose

acinotubular

acinous

acinus *pl.* acini
    pancreatic acini

acladiosis

aclasis
    diaphyseal a.

acne
    a. atrophica
    bromide a.
    chlorine a.
    common a.
    a. conglobata
    conglobate a.
    contact a.
    a. cosmetica

acne *(continued)*
    cystic a.
    a. detergicans
    epidemic a.
    a. estivalis
    excoriated a.
    a. excoriée des filles
    a. excoriée des jeunes filles
    a. frontalis
    a. fulminans
    halogen a.
    a. indurata
    infantile a.
    iodide a.
    a. keloid
    Mallorca a.
    a. mechanica
    mechanical a.
    a. necrotica miliaris
    occupational a.
    oil a.
    a. papulosa
    picker's a.
    pomade a.
    premenstrual a.
    a. pustulosa
    a. rosacea
    a. scrofulosorum
    tropical a.
    a. tropicalis
    a. urticata
    a. varioliformis
    a. venenata
    a. vulgaris

acneform

acnegen

acnegenic

acneiform

acnitis

acoustic
    acoustic canal
    acoustic nerve
    acoustic nerve tumor
    acoustic neurilemoma
    acoustic neurinoma
    acoustic neuroma

acoustic *(continued)*
    acoustic schwannoma

acoustical shadowing

ACR
    American College of Radiology
        ACR category

acral

acrochordon

acrodermatitis
    a. continua
    Hallopeau's a.
    infantile a.
    papular a. of childhood
    a. papulosa infantum
    a. perstans

acrodermatosis

acrokeratosis
    paraneoplastic a.
    a. verruciformis

acromelic

acromial

acromioclavicular joint separation

acromion
    a. process

acromphalus

acropachyderma
    a. with pachyperiostitis

acropustulosis
    infantile a.

acroscleroderma

acrosclerosis

acrospiroma
    eccrine a.

acroteric

acrylonitrile

actinodermatitis

actinomycosis

actinotherapy

activation
   contact a.

activator
   plasminogen a.
   prothrombin a.
   single chain urokinase-type
      plasminogen a.
   tissue plasminogen a.
   t-plasminogen a.
   u-plasminogen a.
   urinary plasminogen a.

activity
   increased a.
   leukemia-associated inhibi-
      tory a.
   osseous a.
   specific a.
   peristaltic a.
   seizure a.
   tracer a.

acus

Acuson (sonographic equipment)

ACX coronary artery balloon

adamantinoma
   a. of long bones
   pituitary a.
   pituitary a.

adamantoblastoma

adamantoma

adaxial

ADC
   apparent diffuse coefficient

adenomatosis
   malignant pulmonary a.

Addison
   A's disease
   A's planes
   A's point

adducin

adduct

adductio

adduction

adductor
   a. pollicis longus

adenia

adenic

adeniform

adenitis
   cervical a.
   cervical a., tuberculous
   mesenteric a.
   sclerosing a.

adenoacanthoma

adenoameloblastoma

adenocarcinoma
   acinar a.
   acinic cell a.
   acinous a.
   alveolar a.
   bronchioalveolar a.
   bronchiolar a.
   bronchioloalveolar a.
   bronchoalveolar a.
   bronchogenic a.
   clear cell a.
   ductal a. of the prostate
   endometrioid a.
   follicular a.
   gastric a.
   a. of kidney
   a. of the lung
   mucinous a.
   papillary a.
   polypoid a.
   polymorphous low-grade a.
   a. of the prostate
   renal a.
   a. of the stomach
   terminal duct a.
   urachal a.

adenocele

adenocystoma
  papillary a. lymphomatosum

adenoepithelioma

adenofibroma
  a. edematodes

adenographic

adenography

adenohypophysis

adenoids

adenolipoma

adenolymphitis

adenolymphocele

adenolymphoma

adenoma *pl.* adenomas, adenomata
  acidophil stem-cell a.
  acidophilic a.
  ACTH-secreting a.
  adrenal a.
  a. of the adrenal cortex
  adrenocortical a.
  adrenocorticotropic hormone–secreting a.
  aldosterone-producing a.
  aldosterone-secreting a.
  alpha subunit a.
  a. alveolare
  basal cell a.
  basophil a.
  basophilic a.
  bile duct a.
  bronchial a's
  canalicular a.
  carcinoid a. of bronchus
  carcinoma ex pleomorphic a.
  chief cell a.
  chromophobe a.
  chromophobic a.
  colloid a.
  cortical a's
  corticotrope a.

adenoma *(continued)*
  corticotrope cell a.
  corticotroph a.
  corticotroph cell a.
  cortisol-producing a.
  embryonal a.
  endocrine-active a.
  endocrine-inactive a.
  eosinophil a.
  eosinophilic a.
  fetal a.
  follicular a.
  a. fibrosum
  functional a.
  functioning a.
  gastric a.
  glycoprotein a.
  glycoprotein hormone a.
  gonadotrope a.
  gonadotroph a.
  gonadotroph cell a.
  growth hormone cell a.
  growth hormone–secreting a.
  hepatocellular a.
  hilar a.
  Hürthle cell a.
  hyperfunctional a.
  hyperfunctioning a.
  islet cell a.
  a's of kidney
  lactotrope a.
  lactotroph a.
  langerhansian a.
  liver cell a.
  macrofollicular a.
  mammosomatotroph a.
  membranous a.
  microfollicular a.
  mixed somatotroph-lactotroph a.
  mixed-cell a.
  monomorphic a.
  mucinous a.
  nephrogenic a.
  nonfunctional a.
  nonfunctioning a.
  nonsecreting a.
  nonsecretory a.

adenoma *(continued)*
  null-cell a.
  oncocytic a.
  a. ovarii testiculare
  oxyphilic a.
  oxyphilic granular cell a.
  papillary cystic a.
  parathyroid a.
  pineal a.
  pituitary a.
  pleomorphic a.
  pleomorphic a., malignant
  plurihormonal a.
  prolactin cell a.
  prolactin-secreting a.
  sebaceous a.
  a. sebaceum
  somatotrope a.
  somatotroph a.
  thyroid stimulating hormone–secreting a.
  thyrotrope a.
  thyrotroph a.
  thyrotroph cell a.
  trabecular a.
  trabecular-tubular a.
  TSH-secreting a.
  tubular a.
  a. tubulare testiculare ovarii
  villous a.

adenomatoid

adenomatosis
  multiple endocrine a.
  pluriglandular a.
  polyendocrine a.
  pulmonary a.

adenomatous

adenomyofibroma

adenomyoma

adenomyomatosis

adenomyomatous

adenomyosarcoma
  embryonal a.

adenopathy
  mediastinal a.
  periaortic a.

adenosarcoma
  embryonal a.

adenosis
  sclerosing a.

adermia

adermogenesis

adhesio
  a. interthalamica

adhesion
  pleurodiaphragmatic a's
  pleuropericardial a's

adherent

adhesiveness
  platelet a.

adiposalgia

adiposis
  a. dolorosa
  a. tuberosa simplex

aditus
  a. ad antrum mastoideum
  a. laryngis
  a. orbitalis
  a. orbitae
  a. ad pelvem

admedial

admedian

adminicula

adminiculum
  a. lineae albae

adnexa *(always a plural noun)*

adnexal

adnexus *(rarely used)*

adoral

Adrenalin

adrenogram

Adriamycin

Adrucil

Adson's maneuver

adsternal

adumbration

adventitia

adventitial

adynamic

Aeby's plane

aequator

aeration

aerocystography

aerodermectasia

aerodigestive

aerophagia

AFBG
    aortofemoral bypass graft

afebrile

afibrinogenemia
    congenital a.

aflatoxin

African lymphoma

age
    anatomical a.
    bone a.
    chronologic a.
    gestational a.

agenesis
    a. of the corpus callosum

agent
    alkylating a.

agent *(continued)*
    neuromuscular blocking a.
    neuromuscular blocking a.,
      depolarizing
    neuromuscular blocking a.,
      nondepolarizing

agger *pl.* aggeres
    a. nasi

agglutination
    intravascular a.
    platelet a.

aggregation
    nuclear a's
    platelet a.

aggregometer

aggregometry

agranulocyte

agranulocytosis
    infantile genetic a.

AIDS
    acquired autoimmune defi-
      ciency syndrome

air
    a.-fluid level
    free a. under the dia-
      phragm
    intraperitoneal a.
    liquid a.
    a.-swallowing
    a.-trapping

air contrast views of the stom-
    ach

airway

AKA
    above-knee amputation

akinesia, akinesis

akinetic

ala *pl.* alae
    a. cristae galli
    a. lobuli centralis

ala *(continued)*
    a. major ossis sphenoidalis
    a. minor ossis sphenoidalis
    a. nasi
    a. ossis ilii
    a. ossis ilium
    a. ossis sacri
    a. of vomer
    a. vomeris

alae (plural of ala)

alar

alate

Albert's position

albinism
    a. I
    a. II
    Amish a.
    autosomal dominant oculo-
        cutaneous a.
    brown a.
    complete imperfect a.
    complete perfect a.
    localized a.
    ocular a.
    ocular a., autosomal reces-
        sive
    ocular a., Forsius-Eriksson
        type
    ocular a., Nettleship-Falls
        type
    ocular a., X-linked (Nettle-
        ship)
    oculocutaneous a.
    partial a.
    red a.
    rufous a.
    tyrosinase-negative (ty-neg)
        oculocutaneous a.
    tyrosinase-positive (ty-pos)
        oculocutaneous a.
    xanthous a.
    yellow mutant (ym) oculo-
        cutaneous a.

albinismus
    a. circumscriptus

albino

albinoidism
    oculocutaneous a.
    punctate oculocutaneous a.

albinotic

Albl's ring

albuginea

albugineous

albumin
    a. A
    aggregated a.
    aggregated a.
    blood a.
    iodinated I 125 a.
    iodinated I 131 a.
    macroaggregated a.
    serum a.

Alcock's canal

aldehyde
    formic a.

Alder
    A's anomaly
    A's constitutional granula-
        tion anomaly
    A-Reilly anomaly

aldesleukin

aldosteronoma

aleukemia

aleukemic

aleukia
    a. hemorrhagica

aleukocytic

aleukocytosis

Alexander view

Alezzandrini's syndrome

Alfenta

aliasing

alienia

aliform

alignment
  bony a.

Alkaban

alkaline phosphatase
  leukocyte a. p.

alkaloid
  vinca a's

Alkeran

alkyl
  a. sulfonate

allergy
  contact a.

alleviate

allochromasia

allocortex

allophore

alopecia
  drug a.
  drug-induced a.
  radiation a.
  radiation-induced a.
  x-ray a.

alopecic

alpha$_2$-antiplasmin

alpha fetoprotein

alvei (plural of alveus)

alveolar

alveolarization

alveolate

alveolus *pl.* alveoli
  alveoli pulmonis

alveus *pl.* alvei
  a. hippocampi

alymphia

alymphoplasia

Alzheimer's disease

ambient wing of the quadrigeminal cistern

ambilateral

ambustion

amebiasis
  a. cutis

amebocyte

amelanosis

ameloblastoma
  acanthomatous a.
  basal cell a.
  cystic a.
  extraosseous a.
  follicular a.
  granular cell a.
  malignant a.
  melanotic a.
  multicystic a.
  peripheral a.
  pigmented a.
  pituitary a.
  pituitary a.
  plexiform a.
  plexiform unicystic a.
  solid a.
  unicystic a.

Americaine

amethocaine hydrochloride

amethopterin

amiculum *pl.* amicula
  a. olivare
  a. of olive

amidobenzene

amifostine

aminobenzene

p-aminoazobenzene

o-aminoazotoluene

p-aminobiphenyl

p-aminodiphenyl

aminoglutethimide

3-aminotriazole

Amiodarone lung disease

Amipaque

Amish albinism

amitrole

ammonia
    a. N 13

amniocentesis

amniography

amosite

amphileukemic

amphiregulin

Amplatz
    A. coronary catheter
    A. dilator
    A. technique

amplification
    gene a.
    image a.

ampulla *pl.* ampullae
    a. biliaropancreatica
    a. canaliculi lacrimalis
    a. chyli
    a. ductus deferentis
    duodenal a.
    a. duodeni
    hepatopancreatic a.
    a. hepatopancreatica
    a. membranacea anterior
    a. membranacea lateralis
    a. membranacea posterior
    a. ossea anterior
    a. ossea lateralis
    a. ossea posterior
    phrenic a.
    rectal a.
    a. recti

ampulla *(continued)*
    a. tubae uterinae
    a. of Vater

ampullae (plural of ampulla)

ampullar

ampullary

ampullate

ampullotomy

ampullula

amputation
    above-knee a. (AKA)
    below-knee a. (BKA)
    Guyon's a.
    traumatic a.

amsacrine

amygdala

amygdaline

amyloidosis
    immunocytic a.

anagen

anakmesis

analgesia
    continuous epidural a.
    epidural a.
    infiltration a.
    patient controlled a.
    patient controlled epidur-
        al a.
    spinal a.

analgesic

analyzer
    pulse height a.

anaplasia

anaplastic

anasarca

anastomosis
    a. arteriolovenularis
    a. arteriolovenularis glo-
        meriformis

anastomosis *(continued)*
    a. arteriolovenularis simplex
    a. arteriovenosa
    end-to-end a.
    Roux-en-Y a.

anastrozole

anatomic
    a. landmarks
    a. pattern
    a. position
    a. position and alignment
    a. snuffbox

anatomical

anatomicomedical

anatomicophysiological

anatomist

anatomy
    applied a.
    artificial a.
    artistic a.
    clastic a.
    clinical a.
    comparative a.
    corrosion a.
    descriptive a.
    developmental a.
    general a.
    gross a.
    homologic a.
    macroscopic a.
    medical a.
    physiognomonic a.
    physiological a.
    plastic a.
    practical a.
    radiological a.
    regional a.
    special a.
    surface a.
    systematic a.
    topographic a.
    transcendental a.
    x-ray a.

ancipital

ancistroid

Ancure Endograft System

ancyroid

Andernach's ossicles

Anders' disease

androblastoma

AN-DTPA

anechoic

anemia
    achrestic a.
    achylic a.
    anhematopoietic a.
    aplastic a.
    Arctic a.
    aregenerative a.
    aregenerative a., congenital
    Bartonella a.
    Blackfan-Diamond a.
    cameloid a.
    a. of chronic disease
    a. of chronic disorders
    congenital a. of newborn
    Cooley's a.
    cow's milk a.
    deficiency a.
    Diamond-Blackfan a.
    dilution a.
    dimorphic a.
    dyserythropoietic a., congenital
    elliptocytary a.
    elliptocytic a.
    elliptocytotic a.
    Fanconi's a.
    folic acid deficiency a.
    goat's milk a.
    Heinz body a's
    hemolytic a.
    hemolytic a. of newborn
    hemolytic a., autoimmune
    hemolytic a., congenital
    hemolytic a., congenital nonspherocytic
    hemolytic a., drug-induced immune

anemia *(continued)*
    hemolytic a., immune
    hemolytic a., infectious
    hemolytic a., microangio-
      pathic
    hemolytic a., nonsphero-
      cytic
    hemolytic a., toxic
    hemorrhagic a.
    hereditary iron-loading a.
    hypochromic a.
    a. hypochromica sid-
      eroachrestica hereditaria
    hypochromic microcytic a.
    hypoplastic a.
    hypoplastic a., congenital
    immunohemolytic a.
    iron deficiency a.
    leukoerythroblastic a.
    macrocytic a.
    macrocytic a., nutritional
    macrocytic a., tropical
    Mediterranean a.
    megaloblastic a.
    megalocytic a.
    microangiopathic a.
    microcytic a.
    milk a.
    myelopathic a.
    myelophthisic a.
    a. neonatorum
    normoblastic a., refractory
    normochromic a.
    normocytic a.
    nutritional a.
    osteosclerotic a.
    pernicious a.
    pernicious a., congenital
    pernicious a., juvenile
    physiologic a.
    polar a.
    posthemorrhagic a. of new-
      born
    posthemorrhagic a., acute
    pure red cell a.
    pyridoxine-responsive a.
    a. refractoria sideroblastica
    refractory a.
    scorbutic a.

anemia *(continued)*
    sickle cell a.
    sideroachrestic a.
    sideroachrestic a., ac-
      quired
    sideroachrestic a., congeni-
      tal
    sideroachrestic a., heredi-
      tary
    sideroblastic a.
    sideroblastic a., acquired
    sideroblastic a., hereditary
    sideroblastic a., primary
      acquired
    sideroblastic a., refractory
    sideroblastic a., X-linked
    sideropenic a.
    spherocytic a.
    splenic a.
    spur cell a.

anemic

anencephalic

anerythroplasia

anerythroplastic

anerythropoiesis

anerythroregenerative

anesthesia
    acupuncture a.
    ambulatory a.
    balanced a.
    basal a.
    Bier's local a.
    block a.
    brachial plexus a.
    caudal a.
    closed circuit a.
    conduction a.
    electric a.
    endotracheal a.
    epidural a.
    frost a.
    general a.
    high pressure a.
    hypnosis a.
    hypotensive a.
    hypothermic a.

anesthesia *(continued)*
    infiltration a.
    inhalation a.
    insufflation a.
    intercostal a.
    intraspinal a.
    intravenous a.
    intravenous regional a.
    local a.
    lumbar epidural a.
    open a.
    paraneural a.
    paravertebral a.
    peridural a.
    perineural a.
    plexus a.
    rectal a.
    refrigeration a.
    regional a.
    sacral a.
    saddle block a.
    semiclosed a.
    semiopen a.
    spinal a.
    subarachnoid a.
    surgical a.
    topical a.
    transsacral a.

anesthesiologist

anesthesiology

anesthesiophore

anesthetic
    general a.
    local a.
    topical a.

anesthetist

anesthetization

anesthetize

anetoderma
    Jadassohn's a.
    Jadassohn-Pellizari a.
    perifollicular a.
    postinflammatory a.
    Schweninger-Buzzi a.

aneurysm
    anencephaly a's
    aortic a.
    berry a.
    dissecting a.
    false a.
    fusiform a.
    leaking a.
    pulsating a.
    saccular a.

aneurysmal

aneutrocytosis

Angelchik antireflux prosthesis

Anger camera

angina
    agranulocytic a.
    neutropenic a.
    a. pectoris
    Schultz's a.

angioblastoma

angiocardiogram

angiocardiography
    equilibrium radionuclide a.
    first pass radionuclide a.
    gated equilibrium radionu-
        clide a.
    radionuclide a.

Angiocath

angiodermatitis
    disseminated pruritic a.

angiodysplasia
    papular a.

angioedema
    hereditary a.
    vibratory a.

angioedematous

angioendothelioma

angioendotheliomatosis
    systemic proliferating a.

angiofibroma
    juvenile nasopharyngeal a.

angiofibroma *(continued)*
    nasopharyngeal a.

angiofollicular

angiogenesis
    tumor a.

angiogram
    vertebral a.

angiograph

angiography
    aortic a.
    cerebral a.
    coronary a.
    digital subtraction a. (DSA)
    digital subtraction a., intra-
        arterial
    digital subtraction a., intra-
        venous
    magnetic resonance a.
        (MRA)
    nuclear a.
    pulmonary a.
    retinal a.

angiohemophilia

angiokeratoma
    a. of Fordyce
    a. of Mibelli
    a. of scrotum
    solitary a.

angiokeratosis

angioleiomyoma

angioleucitis

angioleukitis

angiolipoleiomyoma

angiolipoma

angiologia

angiology

angiolupoid

angiolymphangioma

angiolymphitis

angioma
    a. arteriale racemosum
    capillary a's
    cherry a's
    hypertrophic a.
    a. lymphaticum
    senile a's
    a. serpiginosum
    spider a.
    venous a. of brain

angiomatoid

angiomatosis
    cerebroretinal a.
    retinocerebral a.

angiomatous

angiomyolipoma

angiomyoma

angiomyosarcoma

angiomyxoma

angiophakomatosis

angioplasty
    balloon a.
    laser a.
    laser thermal a.
    percutaneous translumin-
        al a.
    transluminal a.
    transluminal coronary a.

angioreticuloendothelioma

angioreticuloma

angiosarcoma
    hepatic a.

angiosteosis

angle
    anterior a. of petrous por-
        tion of temporal bone
    Baumann's a.
    beta a. of the acetabulum
    Böhler's a.
    cardiodiaphragmatic a.
    cardiophrenic a.

angle *(continued)*
    carrying a.
    cephalic a.
    cerebellopontine a. (CPA)
    Cobb a.
    coronary a.
    costal a.
    costophrenic a.
    costovertebral a.
    epigastric a.
    Ferguson's a.
    flip a. images
    frontal a. of parietal bone
    inferior a. of parietal bone, anterior
    inferior a. of parietal bone, posterior
    inferior a. of scapula
    inner a. of humerus
    Louis' a.
    Ludwig's a.
    a. of the mandible
    mastoid a. of parietal bone
    occipital a. of parietal bone
    phrenopericardial a.
    posterior a. of petrous portion of temporal bone
    a. of pubis
    radiocarpal a.
    Ranke's a.
    a. of rib
    sternal a.
    a. of sternum
    subcostal a.
    subpubic a.
    substernal a.
    superior a. of parietal bone, anterior
    superior a. of parietal bone, posterior
    superior a. of petrous portion of temporal bone
    superior a. of scapula
    Welcker's a.
    xiphoid a's
angled
angulation
    volar a.

angulus *pl.* anguli
    a. acromii
    a. anterior pyramidis ossis temporalis
    a. costae
    a. frontalis ossis parietalis
    a. inferior scapulae
    a. infrasternalis
    a. iridis
    a. iridocornealis
    a. lateralis scapulae
    a. Ludovici
    a. mastoideus ossis parietalis
    a. occipitalis ossis parietalis
    a. oculi lateralis
    a. oculi medialis
    a. posterior pyramidis ossis temporalis
    a. pubis
    a. sphenoidalis ossis parietalis
    a. sternalis
    a. sterni
    a. subpubicus
    a. superior pyramidis ossis temporalis
    a. superior scapulae

anhidrosis

anhidrotic

anidrosis

anidrotic

aniline

o-anisidine

anisochromasia

anisochromia

anisocytosis

anisopoikilocytosis

ankylosis

ankyrin

ankyroid

anlage

AN-MAA

AN-MDP

annectent

annular

annulus *pl.* annuli
    bulging a.
    mitral a.

anochromasia

anociassociation

anociated

anociation

anococcygeal

anode
    hooded a.
    rotating a.

anomaly
    Alder's a.
    Alder's constitutional gran-
        ulation a.
    Alder-Reilly a.
    congenital a.
    Hegglin's a.
    Jordans' a.
    May-Hegglin a.
    Pelger's nuclear a.
    Pelger-Huët a.
    Pelger-Huët nuclear a.

anonychia

anoperineal

anorectal

anorexia
    a. nervosa

anospinal

anovesical

anoxia
    anemic a.

anoxic

ansa *pl.* ansae
    a. cervicalis
    a. peduncularis
    a. subclavia

ansae (plural of ansa)

ansate

anserine

anserinus

ansiform

AN-Sulfur Colloid

antalgic

antebrachium

antecardium

antecedent
    plasma thromboplastin a.

antecubital

antecurvature

anteflect

anteflexed

antegrade

anteriad

anterior
    a. communicating artery
        (*sometimes dictated*
        "acom")
    a. spinal ligament calcifica-
        tion

anteroexternal

anterograde

anteroinferior

anterointernal

anterolateral

anteromedial

anteromedian

anteroposterior

anteroseptal

anterosuperior

anteroventral

anthracenedione

anthracosilicosis

antibody
    indium-111 antimyosin a.

antibrachium

anticardium

anticlinal

anticoagulant
    circulating a.
    lupus a.

anticoagulation

anticoagulative

anticus

antieczematic

antiepithelial

antifibrinolysin

antifibrinolytic

antigen
    blood group a's
    cancer a. 125
    carcinoembryonic a. (CEA)
    common acute lymphoblas-
      tic leukemia a.
    D a.
    E a.
    H a.
    high frequency a's
    high incidence a's
    low frequency a's
    low incidence a's
    oncofetal a.
    pancreatic oncofetal a.
    private a's
    prostate-specific a.
    prostate-specific membra-
      ne a.

antigen *(continued)*
    public a's
    Rh a.
    T a.
    tumor a.
    tumor-associated a.
    tumor-specific a.
    tumor-specific transplanta-
      tion a.

antihelix

antihemolytic

antihemophilic

antileukocytic

antineoplastic

antineutrino

antineutron

antiniad

antinial

antinion

antioncogene

antiparticle

antiplasmin
    α_2-a.

antiplastic

antiplatelet

antiprothrombin

antipruritic

antipsoriatic

antithenar

antithrombin
    a. I
    a. III

antithromboplastin

antithrombotic

antitragicus

antitragus

antitrope

antitropic

antitumorigenic

antra (plural of antrum)

antral

antrum *pl.* antra
    a. mastoideum
    a. pylori
    a. pyloricum

anulus *pl.* anuli
    a. conjunctivae
    a. femoralis
    a. fibrocartilagineus membranae tympani
    a. fibrosus dexter/sinister cordis
    a. fibrosus disci intervertebralis
    a. inguinalis profundus
    a. inguinalis superficialis
    a. iridis major
    a. iridis minor
    a. lymphaticus cardiae
    a. tendineus communis
    a. tympanicus
    a. umbilicalis

anus
    imperforate a.

aorta *pl.* aortae
    abdominal a.
    a. abdominalis
    a. ascendens
    ascending a.
    coarctation of the a.
    descending a.
    dissection of the a.
    native a.
    a. thoracica
    uncoiling of the a.

aortae (plural of aorta)

aorticomediastinal

aorticopulmonary window (*not* aortopulmonary)

aortitis
    luetic a.

aortogram

aortography
    retrograde a.
    translumbar a.

AP
    anteroposterior
        AP view

apertura *pl.* aperturae
    a. externa aqueductus vestibuli
    a. externa canaliculi cochleae
    a. lateralis ventriculi quarti
    a. mediana ventriculi quarti
    a. pelvis inferior
    a. pelvis superior
    a. piriformis
    a. sinus frontalis
    a. sinus sphenoidalis
    aperturae superior et inferior fossae axillaris
    a. thoracis inferior
    a. thoracis superior
    a. tympanica canaliculi chordae tympani

aperturae (plural of apertura)

aperture
    inferior a. of pelvis
    inferior thoracic a.
    inferior a. of thorax
    superior thoracic a.
    superior a. of thorax

apex *pl.* apices
    a. auriculae
    a. auriculare
    a. capitis fibulae
    a. cartilaginis arytenoideae
    a. cordis
    a. cornus posterioris medullae spinalis
    a. dentis
    a. linguae
    a. lingualis

apex *(continued)*
    lung a.
    a. nasi
    a. ossis sacralis
    a. ossis sacri
    a. partis petrosae ossis
      temporalis
    a. patellae
    a. prostatae
    a. of prostate gland
    a. pulmonalis
    a. pulmonis
    a. vesicae
    a. vesicalis

apheresis

apical

apicalis

apices (plural of apex)

aplasia
    a. cutis congenita
    pure red cell a.

aplastic

apnea

apneic

apocrinitis

apoferritin

aponeuroses

aponeurosis *pl.* aponeuroses
    a. bicipitalis
    epicranial a.
    a. epicranialis
    a. glutealis
    a. linguae
    lingual a.
    a. musculi bicipitis brachii
    a. of occipitofrontal muscle
    a. palatina
    a. palmaris
    a. plantaris

apophysis
    a. of Ingrassia

apparatus
    Abbe-Zeiss a.
    Hilal embolization a.
    a. lacrimalis
    pilosebaceous a.

appearance
    bulbous a.
    cobblestone a.
    gracile a.
    ground-glass a.
    "honeycombed" a.
    mottled a.
    serrated a.
    "soap bubble" a.
    "stepladder" a.
    stippled a.
    streaky a.
    striated a.

appendage
    left atrial a.
    a's of the skin

appendical

appendiceal

appendices (plural of appendix)

appendicolith

appendicular

appendix *pl.* appendices
    a. epididymidis
    appendices epiploicae
    a. fibrosa hepatis
    appendices omentales
    perforated a.
    retrocecal a.
    a. testis
    vermiform a.
    a. vermiformis
    appendices vesiculosae
      epoophori

applicator
    Horwitz a.

apposition

approach
    femoral artery a.

approach *(continued)*
    jugular a.
    translumbar a.

approximal

apudoma

aquaeductus

aquagenic

aqueduct
    a. of Sylvius

aqueductus
    a. cerebri
    a. cochleae
    a. mesencephali
    a. vestibuli

ara-C (cytarabine)

arachnoid

arachnoidea mater
    a. m. cranialis
    a. m. encephali
    a. m. spinalis
    a. m. et pia mater

arachnoiditis
    adhesive a.

arbor *pl.* arbores
    a. bronchialis
    a. vitae cerebelli

arc
    bregmatolambdoid a.
    nasobregmatic a.
    naso-occipital a.

arcade

arcate

arch
    abdominothoracic a.
    diaphragmatic a., external
    diaphragmatic a., internal
    Haller's a's
    lumbocostal a. of diaphragm, external
    lumbocostal a. of diaphragm, internal

arch *(continued)*
    lumbocostal a. of Haller, lateral
    lumbocostal a. of Haller, medial
    neural a.
    orbital a. of frontal bone
    a. of pelvis
    Shenton's a.
    superciliary a.
    tendinous a.
    tendinous a. of diaphragm, external
    tendinous a. of diaphragm, internal
    tendinous a. of pelvic fascia
    a. of thoracic duct

archicerebellum

archicortex

architecture

arciform

Arctic anemia

arcual

arcuate

arcus
    a. anterior atlantis
    a. aortae
    a. cartilaginis cricoideae
    a. costalis
    a. costarum
    a. ductus thoracici
    a. inguinalis
    a. lumbocostalis lateralis
    a. lumbocostalis medialis
    a. palatoglossus
    a. palatopharyngeus
    a. palmaris profundus
    a. palmaris superficialis
    a. palpebralis inferior
    a. palpebralis superior
    a. pedis transversus distalis
    a. pedis transversus proximalis

arcus *(continued)*
- a. plantaris profundus
- a. posterior atlantis
- a. pubicus
- a. pubis
- a. superciliaris
- a. tendineus
- a. tendineus fasciae pelvis
- a. tendineus musculi levatoris ani
- a. tendineus musculi solei
- a. venae azygou
- a. venosus dorsalis pedis
- a. venosus jugularis
- a. venosus palmaris profundus
- a. venosus palmaris superficialis
- a. venosus plantaris
- a. vertebrae
- a. vertebralis
- a. zygomaticus

ARDS
- adult respiratory distress syndrome

area
- adnexal a's
- a. amygdaloidea anterior
- aortic a.
- Broca's a.
- a. cochleae
- a. cribrosa papillae renalis
- deltoid a.
- focal a.
- areae gastricae
- "hot" a.
- a. hypothalamica dorsalis
- a. hypothalamica intermedia
- a. hypothalamica lateralis
- a. hypothalamica posterior
- a. hypothalamica rostralis
- a. intercondylaris anterior tibiae
- a. intercondylaris posterior tibiae
- jugular a.
- Kiesselbach's a.

area *(continued)*
- a. nervi facialis
- a. nuda hepatis
- parieto-occipital a.
- parietotemporal a.
- perihilar a's
- perirenal a.
- periumbilical a.
- photopenic a.
- posterior parietal a.
- punched-out a's
- a. preoptica
- a. pretectalis
- a. retroolivaris
- sacrococcygeal a.
- skip a's
- a. subcallosa
- suprahilar a.
- temporoparietal a.
- a. vestibularis inferior meatus acustici interni
- a. vestibularis superior meatus acustici interni

areata

areatus

aregenerative

areola *pl.* areolae
- a. mammae
- a. of mammary gland
- a. of nipple
- a. papillaris
- umbilical a.

areolae (plural of areola)

areolar

argentaffinoma
- a. of bronchus

Arimidex

arm

armpit

Arneth
- A. count
- A. index
- A's classification
- A's formula

Arnold
    A's canal
    internal zygomatic foramen
        of A.
    A.-Chiari malformation
    A.-Chiari syndrome

arrector *pl.* arrectores
    a. pili

arrest
    cardiac a.
    maturation a.

arrhenoblastoma

arrhythmia

arsine

arteria *pl.* arteriae
    a. alveolaris inferior
    arteriae alveolares supe-
        riores anteriores
    a. alveolaris superior pos-
        terior
    a. angularis
    a. appendicularis
    a. arcuata pedis
    arteriae arcuatae renis
    a. auricularis posterior
    a. auricularis profunda
    a. axillaris
    arteriae azygoi vaginae
    a. basilaris
    a. brachialis
    a. brachialis superficialis
    a. buccalis
    a. bulbi penis
    a. bulbi vestibuli
    a. caecalis anterior
    a. caecalis posterior
    a. callosomarginalis
    a. canalis pterygoidei
    arteriae caroticotympani-
        cae
    a. carotis communis
    a. carotis externa
    a. carotis interna
    a. caudae pancreatis
    arteriae centrales anterola-
        terales

arteria *(continued)*
    arteriae centrales antero-
        mediales arteriae cerebri
        anterioris
    arteriae centrales antero-
        mediales arteriae com-
        municantis anterioris
    arteriae centrales postero-
        laterales
    arteriae centrales postero-
        mediales arteriae cerebri
        posterioris
    arteriae centrales postero-
        mediales arteriae com-
        municantis posterioris
    a. centralis retinae
    a. cerebri anterior
    a. cerebri media
    a. cerebri posterior
    a. cervicalis ascendens
    a. cervicalis profunda
    a. choroidea anterior
    arteriae ciliares anteriores
    arteriae ciliares posteriores
        breves
    arteriae ciliares posteriores
        longae
    a. circumflexa femoris lat-
        eralis
    a. circumflexa femoris me-
        dialis
    a. circumflexa humeri ante-
        rior
    a. circumflexa humeri pos-
        terior
    a. circumflexa ilium pro-
        funda
    a. circumflexa ilium superfi-
        cialis
    a. circumflexa scapulae
    a. colica dextra
    a. colica media
    a. colica sinistra
    a. collateralis media
    a. collateralis radialis
    a. collateralis ulnaris infe-
        rior
    a. collateralis ulnaris supe-
        rior

arteria *(continued)*
- a. comitans nervi ischiadici
- a. comitans nervi mediani
- a. communicans anterior
- a. communicans posterior
- arteriae conjunctivales anteriores
- arteriae conjunctivales posteriores
- a. coronaria dextra
- a. coronaria sinistra
- a. cremasterica
- a. cystica
- arteriae digitales dorsales manus
- arteriae digitales dorsales pedis
- arteriae digitales palmares communes
- arteriae digitales palmares propriae
- arteriae digitales plantares communes
- arteriae digitales plantares propriae
- a. dorsalis clitoridis
- a. dorsalis nasi
- a. dorsalis pedis
- a. dorsalis penis
- a. dorsalis scapulae
- a. ductus deferentis
- a. epigastrica inferior
- a. epigastrica superficialis
- a. epigastrica superior
- arteriae episclerales
- a. ethmoidalis anterior
- a. ethmoidalis posterior
- a. facialis
- a. femoralis
- a. fibularis
- a. frontobasalis lateralis
- a. frontobasalis medialis
- arteriae gastricae breves
- a. gastrica dextra
- a. gastrica posterior
- a. gastrica sinistra
- a. gastroduodenalis
- a. gastroomentalis dextra
- a. gastroomentalis sinistra

arteria *(continued)*
- a. descendens genus
- a. glutea inferior
- a. glutea superior
- arteriae helicinae penis
- a. hepatica communis
- a. hepatica propria
- a. hyaloidea
- a. hypophysialis inferior
- a. hypophysialis superior
- arteriae ileales
- a. ileocolica
- a. iliaca communis
- a. iliaca externa
- a. iliaca interna
- a. iliolumbalis
- a. inferior anterior cerebelli
- a. inferior lateralis genus
- a. inferior medialis genus
- a. inferior posterior cerebelli
- a. infraorbitalis
- arteriae insulares
- arteriae intercostales posteriores
- a. intercostalis posterior prima
- a. intercostalis posterior secunda
- a. intercostalis suprema
- arteriae interlobares renis
- arteriae interlobares renis
- arteriae interlobulares hepatis
- arteriae interlobulares renis
- arteriae interlobulares renis
- a. interossea anterior
- a. interossea communis
- a. interossea posterior
- a. interossea recurrens
- arteriae jejunales
- a. labialis inferior
- a. labialis superior
- a. labyrinthi
- a. labyrinthina
- a. lacrimalis
- a. laryngea inferior

arteria *(continued)*
- a. laryngea superior
- a. lienalis
- a. ligamenti teretis uteri
- a. lingualis
- a. lingularis
- a. lingularis inferior
- a. lingularis superior
- arteriae lobares inferiores pulmonis dextri
- arteriae lobares inferiores pulmonis sinistri
- a. lobaris media pulmonis dextri
- arteriae lobares superiores pulmonis dextri
- arteriae lobares superiores pulmonis sinistri
- a. lobi caudati
- arteriae lumbales
- arteriae lumbales imae
- a. malleolaris anterior lateralis
- a. malleolaris anterior medialis
- a. marginalis coli
- a. masseterica
- a. maxillaris
- a. media genus
- arteriae membri inferioris
- arteriae membri superioris
- a. meningea media
- a. meningea posterior
- arteriae mesencephalicae
- a. mesenterica inferior
- a. mesenterica superior
- arteriae metacarpales dorsales
- arteriae metacarpales palmares
- arteriae metatarsales dorsales
- arteriae metatarsales plantares
- arteriae musculares
- a. musculophrenica
- arteriae nasales posteriores laterales
- a. nutricia

arteria *(continued)*
- arteriae nutriciae femoris
- a. nutricia fibulae
- arteriae nutriciae humeri
- a. nutricia tibiae
- a. nutricia tibialis
- a. nutriens
- arteriae nutrientes femoris
- a. nutriens fibulae
- arteriae nutrientes humeri
- a. nutriens tibiae
- a. obturatoria
- a. obturatoria accessoria
- a. occipitalis
- a. occipitalis lateralis
- a. occipitalis medialis
- a. ophthalmica
- a. ovarica
- a. palatina ascendens
- a. palatina descendens
- a. palatina major
- arteriae palatinae minores
- arteriae palpebrales laterales
- arteriae palpebrales mediales
- a. pancreatica dorsalis
- a. pancreatica inferior
- a. pancreatica magna
- arteriae pancreaticoduodenales inferiores
- a. pancreaticoduodenalis superior anterior
- a. pancreaticoduodenalis superior posterior
- arteriae parietales anterior et posterior
- arteriae perforantes
- a. pericallosa
- a. pericardiacophrenica
- a. perinealis
- a. pharyngea ascendens
- a. phrenica inferior
- arteriae phrenicae superiores
- a. plantaris lateralis
- a. plantaris medialis
- a. plantaris profunda
- arteriae pontis

arteria *(continued)*
- a. poplitea
- a. prepancreatica
- a. princeps pollicis
- a. profunda brachii
- a. profunda clitoridis
- a. profunda femoris
- a. profunda linguae
- a. profunda penis
- a. pudenda externa profunda
- a. pudenda externa superficialis
- a. pudenda interna
- a. pulmonalis dextra
- a. pulmonalis sinistra
- a. radialis
- a. radialis indicis
- a. rectalis inferior
- a. rectalis media
- a. rectalis superior
- a. recurrens radialis
- a. recurrens tibialis anterior
- a. recurrens tibialis posterior
- a. recurrens ulnaris
- arteriae intrarenales
- a. renalis
- arteriae retroduodenales
- arteriae sacrales laterales
- a. sacralis mediana
- a. segmentalis anterior pulmonis dextri
- a. segmentalis anterior pulmonis sinistri
- a. segmentalis apicalis pulmonis dextri
- a. segmentalis apicalis pulmonis sinistri
- a. segmentalis basalis anterior pulmonis dextri
- a. segmentalis basalis anterior pulmonis sinistri
- a. segmentalis basalis lateralis pulmonis dextri
- a. segmentalis basalis lateralis pulmonis sinistri

arteria *(continued)*
- a. segmentalis basalis medialis pulmonis dextri
- a. segmentalis basalis medialis pulmonis sinistri
- a. segmentalis basalis posterior pulmonis dextri
- a. segmentalis basalis posterior pulmonis sinistri
- a. segmentalis lateralis pulmonis dextri
- a. segmentalis medialis pulmonis dextri
- a. segmentalis posterior pulmonis dextri
- a. segmentalis posterior pulmonis sinistri
- a. segmentalis superior pulmonis dextri
- a. segmentalis superior pulmonis sinistri
- a. segmenti anterioris hepatici
- a. segmenti anterioris inferioris renalis
- a. segmenti anterioris superioris renalis
- a. segmenti inferioris renalis
- a. segmenti lateralis hepatici
- a. segmenti medialis hepatici
- a. segmenti posterioris hepatici
- a. segmenti posterioris renalis
- a. segmenti superioris renalis
- arteriae sigmoideae
- a. sphenopalatina
- a. spinalis anterior
- a. splenica
- a. stylomastoidea
- a. subclavia
- a. subcostalis
- a. sublingualis
- a. submentalis
- a. subscapularis

arteria *(continued)*
- a. sulci centralis
- a. sulci postcentralis
- a. sulci precentralis
- a. superior cerebelli
- a. superior lateralis genus
- a. superior medialis genus
- a. supraduodenalis
- a. supraorbitalis
- a. suprarenalis inferior
- a. suprarenalis media
- arteriae suprarenales superiores
- a. suprascapularis
- a. supratrochlearis
- arteriae surales
- arteriae tarsales mediales
- a. tarsea lateralis
- arteriae tarseae mediales
- a. tarsalis lateralis
- a. temporalis anterior
- a. temporalis media
- a. temporalis profunda anterior
- a. temporalis profunda posterior
- a. temporalis superficialis
- a. testicularis
- a. thoracica interna
- a. thoracica lateralis
- a. thoracica superior
- a. thoracoacromialis
- a. thoracodorsalis
- a. thyroidea ima
- a. thyroidea inferior
- a. thyroidea superior
- a. tibialis anterior
- a. tibialis posterior
- a. transversa cervicis
- a. transversa colli
- a. transversa facialis
- a. transversa faciei
- a. tympanica anterior
- a. tympanica inferior
- a. tympanica posterior
- a. tympanica superior
- a. ulnaris
- a. umbilicalis
- a. urethralis

arteria *(continued)*
- a. uterina
- a. vaginalis
- a. vertebralis
- a. vesicalis inferior
- arteriae vesicales superiores
- a. zygomaticoorbitalis

arteriae (plural of arteria)

arterial

arteriogram

arteriograph

arteriography
- catheter a.
- coronary a.
- femoral run-off a.
- selective a.

arteriola *pl.* arteriolae
- a. glomerularis afferens
- a. glomerularis efferens
- a. macularis inferior
- a. macularis superior
- a. macularis media
- a. nasalis retinae inferior
- a. nasalis retinae superior
- arteriolae rectae renis
- arteriolae rectae spuriae
- a. temporalis retinae inferior
- a. temporalis retinae superior

arteriolae (plural of arteriola)

arteriorenal

arteriosclerosis

arteriosclerotic

arteritis *pl.* arteritides
- temporal a.

artery
- anterior cerebral a.
- anterior communicating a. (*sometimes dictated* "acom")

artery *(continued)*
>   anterior-inferior communi-
>   cating a.
>   a. of Drummond
>   basilar a.
>   basilic a.
>   brachial a.
>   carotid a.
>   cerebellar a.
>   circumflex a.
>   common carotid a.
>   common femoral a.
>   coronary a.
>   dorsalis pedis a.
>   femoral a.
>   inferior mesenteric a.
>   innominate a.
>   internal carotid a.
>   internal mammary a.
>   left anterior descending a.
>   main pulmonary a.
>   mammary a.
>   middle cerebral a.
>   nutrient a.
>   ophthalmic a.
>   pancreatoduodenal a.
>   pericallosal a.
>   peroneal a.
>   popliteal a.
>   posterior tibial a.
>   posterior-inferior cerebel-
>   lar a.
>   posterior-inferior communi-
>   cating a.
>   profunda femoral a.
>   pulmonary a.
>   radial a.
>   renal a.
>   subclavian a.
>   superficial femoral a. (SFA)
>   superficial mesenteric a.
>   (SMA)
>   temporal a's
>   thoracoacromial a.
>   tibial a.
>   umbilical a.
>   vertebral a's

arthritide

arthritis
>   degenerative a.
>   facet joint a.
>   facette joint a.
>   gouty a.
>   juvenile rheumatoid a.
>   (JRA)
>   psoriatic a.
>   pyogenic a.
>   rheumatoid a.
>   traumatic a.

arthrogram

arthrography
>   air a.

arthrologia

arthropathia
>   a. psoriatica

arthropathy
>   facet a.
>   facette a.
>   hemophilic a.
>   psoriatic a.

arthropneumography

arthropneumoradiography

arthrosis

articulare

articulating

articulatio *pl.* articulationes
>   a. acromioclavicularis
>   a. atlantoaxialis lateralis
>   a. atlantoaxialis mediana
>   a. atlantooccipitalis
>   a. calcaneocuboidea
>   a. capitis costae
>   articulationes carpi
>   articulationes carpometa-
>   carpales
>   a. carpometacarpalis polli-
>   cis
>   articulationes carpometa-
>   carpeae
>   a. carpometacarpea pollicis

articulatio *(continued)*
  articulationes columnae vertebralis
  a. complexa
  a. composita
  articulationes costochondrales
  a. costotransversaria
  articulationes costovertebrales
  a. cotylica
  a. coxae
  a. coxofemoralis
  articulationes cranii
  a. cricoarytenoidea
  a. cricothyroidea
  a. cubiti
  a. cuneonavicularis
  a. ellipsoidea
  a. genus
  a. glenohumeralis
  a. humeri
  a. humeroradialis
  a. humeroulnaris
  a. incudomallearis
  a. incudostapedialis
  articulationes intercarpales
  articulationes intercarpeae
  articulationes interchondrales
  articulationes intercuneiformes
  articulationes intermetacarpales
  articulationes intermetacarpeae
  articulationes intermetatarsales
  articulationes intermetatarseae
  articulationes interphalangeae manus
  articulationes interphalangeae pedis
  articulationes interphalangeales manus
  articulationes interphalangeales pedis
  articulationes intertarsales

articulatio *(continued)*
  a. lumbosacralis
  articulationes manus
  a. mediocarpalis
  a. mediocarpea
  articulationes membri inferioris liberi
  articulationes membri superioris liberi
  articulationes metacarpophalangeae
  articulationes metacarpophalangeales
  articulationes metatarsophalangeae
  articulationes metatarsophalangeales
  a. ossis pisiformis
  articulationes ossiculorum auditoriorum
  articulationes ossiculorum auditus
  articulationes pedis
  a. plana
  a. radiocarpalis
  a. radiocarpea
  a. radioulnaris distalis
  a. radioulnaris proximalis
  a. sacrococcygea
  a. sacroiliaca
  a. sellaris
  a. simplex
  a. spheroidea
  a. sternoclavicularis
  articulationes sternocostales
  a. subtalaris
  articulationes synoviales cranii
  a. talocalcanea
  a. talocalcaneonavicularis
  a. talocruralis
  a. tarsi transversa
  a. tarsi transversa [Choparti]
  articulationes tarsometatarsales
  articulationes tarsometatarseae

articulatio *(continued)*
    a. temporomandibularis
    articulationes thoracis
    a. trochoidea
    articulationes zygapophy-
      siales

articulation
    subtalar a.
    synovial a's of cranium

articulationes (plural of articu-
    latio)

artifact
    aliasing a.
    beam-hardening a.
    "magic angle" a.
    misregistration a.
    wraparound a.

artifactitious

artifactual

arylamine

arytenoid

asbestiform

asbestos
    amphibole a.
    blue a.
    brown a.
    chrysotile a.
    crocidolite a.
    serpentine a.
    white a.

asbestosis

A-scan

ascariasis

Ascaris lumbricoides

ascertain

Aschoff-Rokitansky sinuses

ascites

ascitic

ASD
    atrial septal defect

asepsis

aseptic

Askin's tumor

Ask-Upmark kidney

asparaginase

aspect
    anterior a. of cranium
    dorsal a.
    facial a. of cranium
    frontal a. of cranium
    inferior apical a. of the
      myocardium
    inferoapical a. of the left
      ventricle
    inferoapical a. of the myo-
      cardium
    inferior a. of cranium
    lateral a. of cranium
    occipital a. of cranium
    plantar a.
    sagittal a. of cranium
    superior a. of cranium
    temporal a. of cranium
    ventral a.
    vertical a. of cranium

aspergillosis

aspiration

aspirin

asplenia
    functional a.

asplenic

assay
    cancer antigen 125 (CA
      125) a.
    Clauss a.
    D-dimer a.
    fibrinogen a.
    renal vein renin a.
    stem cell a.

asteatodes

asteatosis

asterion

asternal

asthenia
    cutaneous a.

asthenic

asthma
    bronchial a.

asthmatic

astragalar

astragalus

astroblastoma

astrocytoma
    anaplastic a.
    cerebellar a.
    diffuse cerebellar a.
    a. fibrillare
    fibrillary a.
    gemistocytic a.
    Grade I a's
    Grade II a's
    Grade III a's
    Grade IV a's
    juvenile pilocytic a.
    malignant a.
    pilocytic a.
    piloid a.
    protoplasmic a.
    a. protoplasmaticum
    subependymal giant cell a.

asymmetric

asymmetry

asynclitism

ataxia
    Friedreich's a.

atelectasis
    discoid a.
    focal a. of the newborn
    platelike a.
    segmental a.

atelectatic

atherectomy

atheromatous
    a. calcification
    a. disease
    a. plaque formation

atherosclerosis

atherosclerotic
    a. disease
    a. plaque

athymia

athymism

atlantoaxial

atlantodental

atlas

atom
    recoil a.
    rest a.
    tagged a.

atonic

atony

atracurium besylate

atransferrinemia

atresia

atretic

atria (plural of atrium)

atrial

atrichosis

atrichous

atrium pl. atria
    a. dextrum
    a. meatus medii
    a. sinistrum

atrophedema

atrophia
    a. cutis
    a. cutis senilis
    a. maculosa

atrophie
    a. blanche

atrophie *(continued)*
    a. noire

atrophoderma
    a. biotripticum
    idiopathic a. of Pasini and
        Pierini
    a. maculatum
    a. neuriticum
    a. of Pasini and Pierini
    a. reticulatum symmetri-
        cum faciei
    a. senile
    a. vermicularis

atrophodermatosis

atrophodermia
    a. vermiculata

atrophy
    cerebral a.
    cortical a.
    disuse a.
    focal a.
    macular a.
    black a.
    Sudeck's a.

atropine

attack
    transient ischemic a. (TIA

attenuated

attenuation
    low a.

attitude
    fetal a.

atypia
    koilocytotic a.

Auberger blood group

Auer
    A. bodies
    A. rods

Aufranc-Turner prosthesis

Auger electron

aures (plural of auris)

auricula
    a. dextra
    a. sinistra

auricular

auricle

aurid

auris *pl.* aures
    a. externa
    a. interna
    a. media

aurochromoderma

auscultation

Austin Moore hip prosthesis

autoeczematization

autoerythrophagocytosis

autofluoroscope

autogram

autohemagglutination

autohemagglutinin

autohemolysin

autohemolysis

autohemolytic

autohemotherapy

autohemotransfusion

autohistoradiograph

Automeris

autoprothrombin
    a. II
    a. C

autoradiogram

autoradiograph

autoradiography

autosensitization
    erythrocyte a.

autosplenectomy

autotomographic

autotomography

autotransfusion
  intraoperative a.
  postoperative a.

AV, A-V
  arteriovenous
    Cimino AV shunt

avascularity

averaging
  volume a.

Avertin

axes (plural of axis)

axial
  a. and longitudinal images
  a. skeleton

axialis

axifugal

axilla *pl.* axillae

axillary
  a. segment of the right up-
    per lobe

axipetal

axis *pl.* axes
  a. bulbi externus

axis *(continued)*
  a. bulbi internus
  cephalocaudal a.
  dorsoventral a.
  a. lentis
  long a. of body
  a. opticus
  a. pelvis

Ayerza's disease

azacitidine

aziridine

azobenzene

azotemia
  prerenal a.

azotomycin

azurophil

azurophile

azurophilia

azurophilic

azygoesophageal

azygogram

azygography

azygomediastinal

azygos

azygous

baby
    collodion b.

baccate

bacciform

bacille Calmette-Guérin (BCG)

bacillus
    acid-fast b.
    b. Calmette-Guérin (BCG)

back

backflow
    pyelolymphatic b.
    pyelotubular b.
    pyelovenous b.

backscatter

BACOP
    bleomycin, Adriamycin
    (doxorubicin), cyclophos-
    phamide, Oncovin (vin-
    cristine), and prednisone

bacterid
    pustular b.

Baer's plane

Bäfverstedt's syndrome

bag
    colostomy b.
    Mosher b.

Baker's cyst

balanitis
    b. circumscripta plasmacel-
    lularis
    plasma cell b.
    b. plasmacellularis
    b. xerotica obliterans

balanoposthitis
    chronic circumscribed
    plasmocytic b.
    b. chronica circumscripta
    plasmocellularis

Ballance's sign

balloon
    ACX coronary artery b.
    Bardex b.
    Hunter b.
    Hunter-Sessions b.

ballooning of the disc spaces

"bamboo spine"

band
    Henle's b.
    omental b.

bandaletta

bandelette

bank
    blood b.

Bankart procedure for shoulder
    dislocation

Bannister's disease

Banti's disease

Baralyme

bar
    arch b's

barbotage

barbula
    b. hirci

Barclay's niche

Barcoo disease

Bardex balloon

barium
    b. bolus
    b. enema
    b. enema with air contrast
    study
    b.-filled
    b. mixture
    pocketing of b.
    retained b.
    b. sulfate
    b. suspension
    b. swallow

barium *(continued)*
    video b. swallow

barn

Barosperse

Barotrast

barrier
    blood-thymus b.
    protective b.
    protective b's, primary
    protective b's, secondary
    radiation b.

Bart's syndrome

Bartonella anemia

bartonelliasis

bartonellosis

basad

basal

basalis

basaloid

basaloma

base
    b. of cranium
    external b. of skull
    film b.
    lung b.
    b. of skull

basial

basialis

basicranial

basilad

basilar

basilaris
    b. cranii

basilateral

basilic

basinasial

basioccipital

basion

basis
    b. cartilaginis arytenoideae
    b. cochleae
    b. cordis
    b. cornus posterioris me-
        dullae spinalis
    b. cranii externa
    b. cranii interna
    b. modioli
    b. ossis metacarpalis
    b. ossis metacarpi
    b. ossis metatarsalis
    b. ossis metatarsi
    b. ossis sacri
    b. patellae
    b. pedunculi cerebri
    b. phalangis digitorum ma-
        nus
    b. phalangis digitorum
        pedis
    b. prostatae
    b. pulmonalis
    b. pulmonis
    b. stapedis

basophil

basophile

basophilia

basophilic

basophilism

basophilopenia

basophilous

bath
    alkaline b.
    colloid b.
    emollient b.
    oatmeal b.

BATO

battery pack

Baumann's angle

Bazex's syndrome

Bazin's disease

B-CAVe
  bleomycin, CCNU (lomustine), Adriamycin (doxorubicin), and vinblastine

B-cell
  B-c. lymphoma
  B-c. monocytoid lymphoma

BCG
  bacille Calmette-Guérin

beading

beam
  primary b.
  useful b.

Becker's nevus

becquerel

bed
  nail b.
  prostatic b.

bedsore

Behnken's unit

Beigel's disease

belemnoid

belly

belonoid

Benadryl

Bence Jones
  B. J. protein
  B. J. proteinemia
  B. J. proteinuria

benignancy, benignity

Bennett's fracture

Bentley button

benzanthracene

benzene

benzidine

benzocaine

benzo[a]pyrene

3,4-benzpyrene

benzquinamide hydrochloride

Bergman's sign

Bergonié-Tribondeau law

Berkow formula

Bernard-Soulier syndrome

Bertin
  columns of B.

Betadine

Beta HCG test

betatron

Bethesda unit

bezoar

Bg blood group

biasteric

bibasilar

bicalutamide

bicapsular

bicarbonate
  blood b.
  plasma b.

biciromab

bicisate

BiCNU

biconcave

biconvex

Bier
  B. block
  B.'s local anesthesia

Biett's collarette

bidermoma

bifid

bifidus

biforate

bifurcate

bifurcatio *pl.* bifurcationes
  b. aortae
  b. aortica
  b. carotidis
  b. tracheae
  b. trunci pulmonalis

bifurcation
  carotid b.
  tracheal b.

bifurcationes (plural of bifurcatio)

bilateral

bilateralism

bile

Billroth
  B. I gastrectomy
  B. I procedure
  B. II gastrectomy
  B. II gastrectomy proce-
    dure
  B.'s strands

bilobate

bilobular

bilobulate

bilocular

biloculate

Bilopaque

binomial

Binswanger's disease

biology
  radiation b.

biomarker

biomodulator

bionucleonics

biopsy
  brush b.
  CT-guided b.

biopsy *(continued)*
  excisional b.
  fine needle b.
  percutaneous b.
  percutaneous needle b.
  punch b.
  shave b.
  stereotactic b.
  transbronchial lung b.

biopsy-proven

biparietal

bipartite

bipedal

biperforate

biphenamine hydrochloride

biphenyl
  polychlorinated b.

p-biphenylamine

BIRADS
  Breast Imaging Reporting
    and Data System

biramous

Birbeck granules

birthmark

bisaxillary

bis(chloromethyl)ether

biseptate

bismuthia

2,3-bisphosphoglycerate

bisphosphonate

bispinous

bistephanic

bistratal

bitemporal

bituberous

bivalved

biventer

biventral

BKA
    below-knee amputation

Blackfan
    B.-Diamond anemia
    B.-Diamond syndrome

blackhead

bladder
    chyle b.
    cord b.
    fluid-filled urinary b.
    neurogenic b.
    urinary b.

Blalock-Taussig operation

Blancophor

blankophore

blast

blastoma
    pulmonary b.

blastomatoid

blastomatous

blastomogenic

blastomogenous

blastomycosis
    European b.

bleb
    emphysematous b.

bleeder

bleeding
    gastrointestinal b.
    variceal b.

bleomycin
    b. sulfate

blepharoadenoma

blepharoatheroma

blepharoncus

blister
    blood b.
    water b.

block
    ankle b.
    Bier b.
    brachial plexus b.
    caudal b.
    cervical plexus b.
    cryogenic b.
    elbow b.
    epidural b.
    femoral b.
    field b.
    intercostal b.
    intercostal nerve b.
    intranasal b.
    intraspinal b.
    intravenous (IV) b.
    lumbar plexus b.
    nerve b.
    paracervical b.
    paraneural b.
    parasacral b.
    paravertebral b.
    perineural b.
    presacral b.
    pudendal b.
    sacral b.
    saddle b.
    sciatic b.
    spinal b.
    splanchnic b.
    stellate b.
    stellate ganglion b.
    subarachnoid b.
    sympathetic b.
    transsacral b.
    uterosacral b.
    vagal b.
    vagus nerve b.
    wrist b.

blockade
    combined androgen b.

blocking

blood
    arterial b.

blood *(continued)*
    citrated b.
    cord b.
    defibrinated b.
    intraventricular b.
    laky b.
    peripheral b.
    sludged b.
    venous b.
    whole b.

blood group
    ABO b. g.
    Auberger b. g.
    Bg b. g.
    Cartwright b. g.
    Chido-Rodgers b. g.
    Colton b. g.
    Cromer b. g.
    Diego b. g.
    Dombrock b. g.
    Duffy b. g.
    Gerbich b. g.
    Hh b. g.
    high frequency b. g.
    I b. g.
    Kell b. g.
    Kidd b. g.
    Knops b. g.
    Lan b. g.
    Lewis b. g.
    low frequency b. g.
    Lutheran b. g.
    MNSs b. g.
    P b. g.
    Rh b. g.
    Scianna b. g.
    Sid b. g.
    Vel b. g.
    Wright b. g.
    Xg b. g.
    Yt b. g.

bloodstream

blue
    Evans b.

Blue Max balloon catheter

Blumenbach
    B's clivus

Blumenbach *(continued)*
    B's plane

Blumensaat's line

blush
    tumor b.

B-mode ultrasound examination

Bochdalek
    foramen of B.
    foramen of B. hernia
    B. hernia

Bockhart's impetigo

body
    anococcygeal b.
    Auer b's
    bull's eye b.
    cancer b's
    Deetjen's b.
    dense b.
    elementary b.
    embryoid b's
    fat b. of ischioanal fossa
    foreign b.
    b. habitus
    Hassall's b's
    HX b's
    intraocular foreign b.
    lamellar b.
    loose b.
    malpighian b's
    malpighian b's of spleen
    metallic foreign b.
    Mott b's
    b. of nail
    no-threshold b's
    Odland b.
    opaque foreign b.
    pacchionian b's
    b. of the pancreas
    pearly b's
    pineal b.
    pituitary b.
    platelet dense b.
    Plimmer's b's
    psammoma b.
    radiopaque foreign b.
    b. of the stomach

body *(continued)*
 Symington's b.
 thoracic vertebral b's
 threshold b's
 uterine b.
 b. of the uterus
 Verocay b's
 vertebral b.
 Weibel-Palade b's

Boeck's sarcoid (or sarcoidosis)

Boerhaave's syndrome

Böhler
 B's angle
 B's splint

Bohr effect

boil
 blind b.

Bolton-nasion plane

bolus
 barium b.
 food b.
 b. injection

bomb

bombard

Bombay phenotype

bombesin

bone
 b. age
 b.-on-b. contact
 b's of cranium
 b's of skull
 bregmatic b.
 cancellous b.
 carpal navicular b.
 cranial b's
 cuboid b.
 cuneiform b.
 dermal b.
 b. dowel graft
 epactal b.
 epactal b., proper

bone *(continued)*
 ethmoid b.
 exoccipital b.
 facial b's
 fetal cranial b's
 b. flap
 flat b.
 frontal b.
 b. graft
 greater multangular b.
 hamate b.
 hook of the hamate b.
 hyoid b.
 incarial b.
 b. infarct
 innominate b.
 interparietal b.
 irregular b.
 b. island
 b. length studies
 lesser multangular b.
 long b's
 lunate b.
 malar b.
 membrane b.
 mesethmoid b.
 metacarpal b.
 metatarsal b.
 multangular b.
 navicular b.
 nonlamellated b.
 occipital b.
 parietal b.
 pelvic b's
 periosteal b.
 petrous b.
 b. plug
 pneumatic b.
 preinterparietal b.
 Riolan's b's
 rudimentary b.
 scaphoid b.
 sesamoid b.
 short b.
 solid b.
 sphenoid b.
 b. spicule
 squamous b.

bone *(continued)*
    b. strut
    supernumerary b.
    suprainterparietal b.
    sutural b.
    tarsal navicular b.
    temporal b.
    temporal b's
    wormian b.
    wormian b's

bonelet

bony
    b. nonunion *(frequently dictated* "non-bony union")

boot
    Unna's b.
    Unna's paste b.

border
    diaphragmatic b.
    frontal b. of parietal bone
    parietal b. of squamous part of temporal bone
    posterior b. of petrous part of temporal bone
    posterior b. of petrous portion of temporal bone
    sagittal b. of parietal bone
    squamous b. of parietal bone
    superior b. of petrous part of temporal bone
    superior b. of petrous portion of temporal bone

borderline

Borrmann's classification

Bosniak type B renal cyst

boss
    parietal b's

bosselated

bosselation

Boston exanthem

bouquet

Bowen
    B's disease
    B's precancerous dermatosis

bowenoid

box
    anatomical snuff-b.
    brain b.

bowing

Braasch bulb technique

brace

bracelet

brachia

brachiocephalic

brachiocrural

brachiocubital

brachiofaciolingual

brachium
    b. colliculi inferioris
    b. colliculi superioris

brachycheilia

brachychily

brachytherapy

bradycardia

Bragg curve

brain stem

branch
    collateral b's
    geniculate b's
    intracranial b's

branchioma

Braune's muscle

breast
    b. implants
    b. parenchyma
    pendulous b's
    stromal pattern of the b's

breech

bregma

bremsstrahlung

Brenner
    B. nodules
    B. tumor

Breschet's canals

Brescia-Cimino AV fistula

BrIDA

bridge
    nasal b.

bridging
    bony b.

bridle

Brill-Symmers disease

brim
    pelvic b.
    b. of the pelvis

Brinton's disease

broad-based

Broadbent
    B. registration point
    B.-Bolton plane

Brockenbrough transseptal
  catheter

Broden view

Broders
    B's classification
    B's index

Brodie's abscess

bromhidrosis

bromidrosis

bromochlorotrifluoroethane

bromoderma

bronchi (plural of bronchus)

bronchial

bronchiectasis

bronchioles

bronchiolitis

bronchiolus *pl.* broncholi

bronchitis
    asthmatic b.

bronchogram
    air b.

bronchographic

bronchography

bronchopneumonia

bronchoradiography

bronchoscopy

bronchospasm

bronchus *pl.* bronchi
    bronchi lobares
    main stem b.
    bronchi principales dexter/
      sinister
    bronchi segmentales

Brooke's tumor

brow

Brown-Séquard syndrome

Bruch's glands

bruit

Brunner's glands

Brunsting's syndrome

Bryant's triangle

B-scan

bubble
    b. of air
    gastric air b.

bubonulus

bucca

buckling of the cortex

Bucky film

Budd-Chiari syndrome

buffer
  bicarbonate b.

buffering
  secondary b.

bulb
  carotid b.
  duodenal b.
  b. of hair

bulbar

bulbi (plural of bulbus)

bulbiform

bulboid

bulbus *pl.* bulbi
  b. aortae
  b. cornus posterioris ven-
    triculi lateralis
  b. encephali
  b. inferior venae jugularis
  b. oculi
  b. olfactorius
  b. penis
  b. pili
  b. superior venae jugularis
  b. vestibuli vaginae

bulging
  disk b.

bulla *pl.* bullae
  b. ethmoidalis cavi nasi
  b. ethmoidalis ossis eth-
    moidalis

bullosis
  diabetic b.

bullous

bundle of His

bupivacaine hydrochloride

buprenorphine hydrochloride

Burkitt
  B's lymphoma

Burkitt *(continued)*
  B's tumor

burn
  brush b.
  chemical b.
  contact b.
  electric b.
  electrical b.
  flash b.
  friction b.
  radiation b.
  sun b.
  thermal b.
  x-ray b.

Burns
  B's ligament
  B's space

bursa *pl.* bursae
  anserine b.
  bicipitoradial b.
  b. anserina
  b. bicipitoradialis
  b. cubitalis interossea
  cubitoradial b.
  deltoid b.
  b. iliopectinea
  iliopectineal b.
  infrahyoid b.
  b. infrahyoidea
  b. infrapatellaris profunda
  bursae intermusculares
    musculorum gluteorum
  b. intratendinea olecrani
  b. ischiadica musculi glutei
    maximi
  b. ischiadica musculi obtu-
    ratorii interni
  b. musculi bicipitis femoris
    superior
  b. musculi coracobrachialis
  b. musculi piriformis
  b. musculi semimembra-
    nosi
  b. musculi tensoris veli pal-
    atini
  olecranon b.
  omental b.
  b. omentalis

bursa *(continued)*
  prepatellar b.
  b. pharyngea
  pharyngeal b.
  b. pharyngealis
  retrohyoid b.
  b. retrohyoidea
  b. sciatica musculi glutei
    maximi
  b. sciatica musculi obtura-
    torii interni
  subacromial b.
  b. subacromialis
  b. subcutanea
  b. subcutanea acromialis
  b. subcutanea calcanea
  b. subcutanea infrapatel-
    laris
  b. subcutanea malleoli lat-
    eralis
  b. subcutanea malleoli me-
    dialis
  b. subcutanea olecrani
  b. subcutanea prepatellaris
  b. subcutanea prominen-
    tiae laryngeae
  b. subcutanea prominen-
    tiae laryngealis
  b. subcutanea tuberositatis
    tibiae
  subcutaneous b.
  subdeltoid b.
  b. subdeltoidea
  b. subfascialis
  b. subfascialis prepatellaris
  b. submuscularis
  b. subtendinea
  b. subtendinea iliaca
  b. subtendinea musculi bi-
    cipitis femoris inferior
  b. subtendinea musculi
    gastrocnemii lateralis
  b. subtendinea musculi
    gastrocnemii medialis
  b. subtendinea musculi in-
    fraspinati
  b. subtendinea musculi la-
    tissimi dorsi

bursa *(continued)*
  b. subtendinea musculi ob-
    turatorii interni
  bursae subtendineae mus-
    culi sartorii
  b. subtendinea musculi
    subscapularis
  b. subtendinea musculi ter-
    etis majoris
  b. subtendinea musculi ti-
    bialis anterioris
  b. subtendinea musculi ti-
    bialis posterioris
  b. subtendinea musculi tra-
    pezii
  b. subtendinea musculi tri-
    cipitis brachii
  b. subtendinea olecrani
  b. subtendinea prepatel-
    laris
  suprapatellar b.
  b. suprapatellaris
  trochanteric b.
  b. trochanterica musculi
    glutei maximi
  bursae trochantericae mus-
    culi glutei medii
  b. trochanterica musculi
    glutei minimi
  b. trochanterica subcuta-
    nea

bursae (plural of bursa)

bursal

bursitis
  olecranon b.
  pes anserinus b.

burst
  spider b.

Buruli ulcer

Buschke
  B.-Löwenstein tumor
  B.-Ollendorff syndrome

busulfan

butamben
  b. picrate

Butesin

butterfly

buttocks

button
Bentley b.

butyl
b. aminobenzoate

bypass
gastrojejunal b.

CABG (*sometimes dictated*
    "cabbage")
    coronary artery bypass
        graft

cachexia
    cancerous c.

cadaver

cadaveric

cadaverous

caecum
    c. cupulare ductus coch-
        learis
    c. vestibulare ductus coch-
        learis

caecus

Caffey
    C's disease
    C's syndrome

cage
    metallic c.
    thoracic c.
    titanium c.

calamus

calcaneal

calcaneus *pl.* calcanei

calcar
    c. avis

calcareous

calcarine

calcification
    adrenal c.
    amorphous c.
    anterior spinal ligament c.
    arteriovascular c.
    bursal c.
    cartilaginous c.
    curvilinear c.
    "eggshell" c.
    falx c.
    heavy vascular c.

calcification *(continued)*
    hilar c.
    intimal c.
    intracranial c.
    intraductal c's
    ligamentous c.
    mitral annulus c.
    neoplastic c.
    nodular c.
    pancreatic c.
    pathological intracranial
        c's
    pearl-like c.
    peritendinous c.
    peritendinous or bursal c.
    phlebolith-like c's
    pleural c's
    popcorn type c.
    psammomatous c.
    punctate c.
    splenic c.
    sutural c's
    teacup c's
    tendinous c.
    urinary tract c.
    vascular c.

calcified

calcinosis
    c. circumscripta
    c. cutis

calcium
    c. 45
    c. 47
    c. cyclamate
    c. ipodate

Caldwell
    C. view
    C.'s position
    C.'s projection
    C.-Luc procedure

calculus *pl.* calculi
    biliary c.
    obstructive c.
    renal c.
    staghorn c.
    ureteral c.

caliceal

calices (plural of calix)

calicine

caliculi (plural of caliculus)

caliculus
    c. gustatorius

caliectasis

calix *pl.* calices
    calices renales
    calices renales majores
    calices renales minores

Callison's fluid

callositas

callosity

callous

callus

calotte

calvaria *pl.* calvariae

calvarial

calvities

calx

calyectasis (variant of caliectasis)

calyceal (variant of caliceal)

calyx (variant of calix) *pl.* calyces

camera
    Anger c.
    c. anterior bulbi
    gamma c.
    c. posterior bulbi
    scintillation c.
    c. vitrea bulbi

Cameron's lines

campylobacter

Canada-Cronkhite syndrome

canal
    acoustic c.
    adductor c.
    Alcock's c.
    anal c.
    Arnold's c.
    auditory c.
    Breschet's c's
    condylar c.
    condyloid c.
    condyloid c., anterior
    diploic c's
    Dorello's c.
    hair c.
    hypoglossal c.
    inguinal c.
    internal auditory c.
    lymphatic c.
    medullary c.
    neural c.
    obturator c.
    perivascular c.
    pyloric c.
    c's of Recklinghausen
    semicircular c.
    serous c.
    spinal c.
    supraorbital c.
    Van Hoorne's c.

canales (plural of canalis)

canalicular (*not* canicular, as sometimes dictated)

canaliculus *pl.* canaliculi
    canaliculi caroticotympanici
    c. chordae tympani
    c. cochleae
    cochlear c.
    innominate c.
    c. innominatus
    c. lacrimalis
    c. mastoideus
    c. petrosus
    petrous c.
    c. tympanicus

canalis *pl.* canales
    c. adductorius

canalis *(continued)*
    canales alveolares maxillae
    c. analis
    c. caroticus
    c. carpi
    c. centralis medullae spinalis
    c. cervicis uteri
    c. condylaris
    canales diploici
    c. facialis [Fallopii]
    c. femoralis
    c. gastricus
    c. hyaloideus
    c. hypoglossalis
    canales incisivi
    c. infraorbitalis
    c. inguinalis
    canales longitudinales modioli
    c. musculotubarius
    c. nasolacrimalis
    c. nervi facialis
    c. nervi hypoglossi
    c. nutricius
    c. nutriens
    c. obturatorius
    c. opticus
    c. palatinus major
    canales palatini minores
    c. palatovaginalis
    canales paraurethrales urethrae masculinae
    c. pterygoideus
    c. pudendalis
    c. pyloricus
    c. sacralis
    c. semicircularis anterior
    c. semicircularis lateralis
    canales semicirculares ossei
    c. semicircularis posterior
    c. spiralis cochleae
    c. spiralis modioli
    c. vertebralis
    c. vomerorostralis
    c. vomerovaginalis
cancellated

cancellus *pl.* cancelli

cancellous

cancer
    c. à deux
    aniline c.
    betel c.
    buyo cheek c.
    cerebriform c.
    chimney-sweeps' c.
    clay pipe c.
    colloid c.
    contact c.
    cystic c.
    dendritic c.
    duct c.
    dye workers' c.
    encephaloid c.
    c. en cuirasse
    endometrial c.
    endothelial c.
    epithelial c.
    glandular c.
    c. in situ
    kang c.
    kangri c.
    latent c.
    medullary c.
    melanotic c.
    mule-spinners' c.
    non–small cell lung c.
    occult c.
    paraffin c.
    pitch workers' c.
    scar c.
    schistosomal bladder c.
    scirrhous c.
    small-cell lung c.
    soft c.
    soot c.
    spindle cell c.
    tar c.
    tubular c.

canceremia

cancericidal

cancerigenic

cancerocidal

cancerogenic

cancerous

cancerphobia

cancriform

cancroid

Candida granuloma

candidiasis
    cutaneous c.

candidid

canities

Cannon
    C's point
    C's ring

cannula

cannulated

cannulation

cannulization

canthus
    outer c.

Cantor tube

cap
    duodenal c.
    phrygian c.
    skull c.
    c. of Zinn

capacity
    iron-binding c.
    total iron-binding c.

capillary
    lymph c.
    lymphatic c.

capillus *pl.* capilli

capita

capitate

capitellar

capitellum

capitopedal

capitular

capitulum
    c. humeri
    c. of humerus

capnogram

capnograph

capnography

capnohepatography

capsula *pl.* capsulae
    c. adiposa
    c. adiposa renis
    c. articularis
    c. articularis costotransver-
        saria
    c. articularis cricoaryteno-
        idea
    c. articularis cricothyro-
        idea
    c. externa
    c. extrema
    c. fibrosa
    c. fibrosa glandulae thyro-
        ideae
    c. fibrosa perivascularis
    c. fibrosa renis
    c. ganglii
    c. interna
    c. lentis
    c. nodi lymphatici
    c. nodi lymphoidei
    c. prostatica
    c. serosa lienis
    c. splenis
    c. tonsillaris

capsulae (plural of capsula)

capsular

capsule
    adherent c.
    adipose c.
    fibrous c.
    fibrous c. of spleen

capsule *(continued)*
 joint c.
 c. of lymph node
 serous c. of spleen
 c. of spleen
 tonsillar c.

capsulitis
 adhesive c.

Captopril renal scan

capture
 electron c.

caput *pl.* capita
 c. breve musculi bicipitis brachii
 c. breve musculi bicipitis femoris
 c. cornus posterioris medullae spinalis
 c. costae
 c. epididymidis
 c. femoris
 c. fibulae
 c. fibulare
 c. humerale musculi flexoris carpi ulnaris
 c. humeroulnare musculi flexoris digitorum superficialis
 c. humeri
 c. laterale musculi gastrocnemii
 c. laterale musculi tricipitis brachii
 c. lienis
 c. longum musculi bicipitis brachii
 c. longum musculi bicipitis femoris
 c. longum musculi tricipitis brachii
 c. mallei
 c. mediale musculi gastrocnemii
 c. mediale musculi tricipitis brachii
 c. musculi
 c. nuclei caudati

caput *(continued)*
 c. obliquum musculi adductoris hallucis
 c. obliquum musculi adductoris pollicis
 c. ossis metacarpi
 c. ossis metatarsi
 c. pancreatis
 c. pancreatis
 c. phalangis manus
 c. phalangis pedis
 c. radii
 c. rectum musculi recti femoris
 c. reflexum musculi recti femoris
 c. stapedis
 c. talare
 c. tali
 c. transversum musculi adductoris hallucis
 c. transversum musculi adductoris pollicis
 c. ulnae
 c. ulnare musculi flexoris carpi ulnaris
 c. ulnare musculi pronatoris teretis

capita (plural of caput)

carbaminohemoglobin

carbhemoglobin

carbohemoglobin

carbon
 c. 11
 c. 14
 c. monoxide C 11

carboplatin

carboxyhemoglobinemia

carbuncle

carbuncular

carbunculoid

carbunculosis

carcass

carcinemia

carcinocythemia

carcinoembryonic

carcinogen
    epigenetic c.
    genotoxic c.

carcinogenesis

carcinogenic

carcinogenicity

carcinoid
    c. of the appendix
    bronchial c.
    c. of bronchus

carcinolysis

carcinolytic

carcinoma *pl.* carcinomata
    acinar c.
    acinic cell c.
    acinous c.
    adenocystic c.
    adenoid cystic c.
    adenoid squamous cell c.
    c. adenomatosum
    adenosquamous c.
    adnexal c.
    c. of adrenal cortex
    adrenocortical c.
    aldosterone-producing c.
    aldosterone-secreting c.
    alveolar c.
    alveolar cell c.
    ameloblastic c.
    ampullary c.
    anaplastic c. of thyroid
      gland
    apocrine c.
    apple-core c. of the colon
    basal cell c.
    basal cell c., alveolar
    basal cell c., comedo

carcinoma *(continued)*
    basal cell c., cystic
    basal cell c., morphea-like
    basal cell c., multicentric
    basal cell c., nodulo-ulcera-
      tive
    basal cell c., pigmented
    basal cell c., sclerosing
    basal cell c., superficial
    basaloid c.
    basosquamous cell c.
    bile duct c.
    bile duct c., extrahepatic
    bile duct c., intrahepatic
    bilharzial c.
    bronchioalveolar c.
    bronchiolar c.
    bronchioloalveolar c.
    bronchoalveolar c.
    bronchoalveolar cell c.
    bronchogenic c.
    cecal c.
    cerebriform c.
    cholangiocellular c.
    chorionic c.
    choroid plexus c.
    clear cell c.
    cloacogenic anal c.
    colloid c.
    comedo c.
    corpus c.
    c. of corpus uteri
    cortisol-producing c.
    cribriform c.
    cribriform c.
    cylindrical c.
    cylindrical cell c.
    duct c.
    ductal c.
    ductal c. in situ
    ductal c. of the prostate
    eccrine c.
    embryonal c.
    c. en cuirasse
    endometrial c.
    c. of endometrium
    endometrioid c.
    epidermoid c.

carcinoma *(continued)*
  esophageal c.
  c. ex mixed tumor
  c. ex pleomorphic ade-
    noma
  exophytic c.
  fibrolamellar c.
  c. fibrosum
  follicular c. of thyroid
    gland
  gastric c.
  gelatiniform c.
  gelatinous c.
  giant cell c.
  giant cell c. of thyroid
    gland
  c. gigantocellulare
  glandular c.
  granulosa cell c.
  hepatocellular c.
  Hürthle cell c.
  hypernephroid c.
  infantile embryonal c.
  infiltrating ductal cell c.
  inflammatory c. of the
    breast
  c. in situ
  intraductal c.
  intraepidermal c.
  intraepithelial c.
  juvenile embryonal c.
  Kulchitzky-cell c.
  large cell c.
  leptomeningeal c.
  lobular c.
  lobular c.
  lobular c., infiltrating
  lobular c., invasive
  lobular c. in situ
  lymphoepithelial c.
  c. medullare
  medullary c.
  medullary c. of thyroid
    gland
  medullary thyroid c.
  melanotic c.
  meningeal c.
  Merkel cell c.
  metatypical cell c.

carcinoma *(continued)*
  micropapillary c.
  c. molle
  mucinous c.
  c. muciparum
  c. mucocellulare
  mucoepidermoid c.
  c. mucosum
  mucous c.
  napkin-ring c.
  nasopharyngeal c.
  neuroendocrine c. of the
    skin
  noninfiltrating c.
  non–small cell c.
  non–small cell lung c.
  oat cell c.
  c. ossificans
  osteoid c.
  ovarian c.
  Paget's c.
  papillary c.
  papillary c. of thyroid
    gland
  periampullary c.
  preinvasive c.
  prickle cell c.
  prickle cell c.
  primary intraosseous c.
  prostatic c.
  renal cell c.
  scar c.
  schistosomal bladder c.
  schneiderian c.
  scirrhous c.
  sebaceous c.
  signet-ring cell c.
  c. simplex
  small cell c.
  small cell lung c.
  spindle cell c.
  c. spongiosum
  squamous c.
  squamous cell c.
  terminal duct c.
  thyroid c., anaplastic
  thyroid c., follicular
  thyroid c., medullary
  thyroid c., papillary

carcinoma *(continued)*
    trabecular c. of the skin
    transitional cell c.
    tubular c.
    undifferentiated c. of thyroid gland
    uterine corpus c.
    verrucous c.
    villous c.
    c. villosum
    yolk sac c.

carcinomata (plural of carcinoma)

carcinomatoid

carcinomatosis
    leptomeningeal c.
    meningeal c.

carcinomatous

carcinosarcoma
    embryonal c.

carcinostatic

cardia
    c. of the stomach

cardiac
    c. arrest
    c. catheterization
    c. decompensation
    c. dilatation
    c. enlargement
    c. failure
    c. output
    c. series

Cardiografin

cardioangiography

cardiocairograph

cardiography
    ultrasonic c.

cardiohepatic

cardiokymographic

cardiokymography

Cardiolite

cardiomediastinum

cardiomediastinal
    c. shadow

cardiomegaly

cardiomyopathy

cardionephric

cardioneural

cardioprotectant

cardioprotective

cardiopulmonary

cardiorenal

cardiorespiratory

cardiospasm

CardioTec

cardiothymic shadow

cardiotoxicity

cardiovascular

cardiovascular-renal

cardioversion

cardioverter
    implantable c.-defibrillator

caries
    dental c.

carina *pl.* carinae
    c. tracheae
    c. tracheae
    c. urethralis vaginae

carinae (plural of carina)

carinal

carinate

carination

Carman
    C's sign
    C.-Kirklin meniscus sign

Carman *(continued)*
    C.-Kirklin sign

C-arm fluoroscopic unit

carmustine

Carney
    C's complex
    C's syndrome
    C's triad

carotenosis

Carpule

carpus

carrier

carrier-free

Carrión's disease

Carter-Rowe view

cartilage
    articular c.
    auricular c.
    costal c.
    hyaline c.
    triticeal c.

cartilago *pl.* cartilagines
    c. alaris major
    cartilagines alares minores
    cartilagines et articulationes laryngeales
    cartilagines et articulationes laryngis
    c. arytenoidea
    c. auriculae
    c. auricularis
    c. corniculata
    c. costalis
    c. cricoidea
    c. cuneiformis
    c. epiglottica
    c. epiphysialis
    c. meatus acustici
    cartilagines nasales
    cartilagines nasales accessoriae
    cartilagines nasi

cartilago *(continued)*
    cartilagines nasi accessoriae
    c. septi nasi
    c. sesamoidea ligamenti vocalis
    c. thyroidea
    cartilagines tracheales
    c. triticea
    c. tubae auditivae
    c. vomeronasalis
    c. tubae auditoriae

Cartwright blood group

carubicin hydrochloride

caruncle

caruncula
    carunculae hymenales
    c. lacrimalis

carunculae

Casal
    C's collar
    C's necklace

cascade
    coagulation c.

Casodex

Casper plate

cassette

cast
    hair c.
    plaster c.

Castillo catheter

Castleman's disease

CAT
    computerized axial tomograph
    CAT scan (also CT scan)

catagen

catapophysis

category
    ACR (American College of

Radiology) c. (followed
by a numeral, usually 1, 2,
3 or 4)

cathemoglobin

catheter
acorn-tipped c.
Amplatz coronary c.
angiographic c.
atherectomy c.
balloon c.
Bardex c.
Blue Max balloon c.
Brockenbrough transsep-
tal c.
cardiac c.
Castillo c.
c. tip
central venous pressure
(CVP) c.
cobra c.
Councill c.
Cournand c.
CVP (central venous pres-
sure) c.
double lumen c.
drainage c.
end-hole c.
Foley c.
French c. (preceded by a
number, such as 5)
French pigtail c. (preceded
by a number)
Gensini c.
Gensini coronary c.
Grollman c.
Groshong c.
Gruentzig balloon c.
Gruentzig dilatation c.
headhunter c.
H1H c.
Hickman c.
indwelling c.
indwelling Foley c.
Infusaport c.
intrathoracic c.
Judkins coronary c.

catheter *(continued)*
Judkins pigtail left ventriculography c.
jugular c.
left coronary c.
Lunderquist c.
Mallinckrodt c.
Mani cerebral c.
Medi Omni II c.
multipurpose c.
multisidehole c.
mushroom c.
NIH c.
PICC (peripherally inserted
central catheter)
pigtail c.
right coronary c.
Ring biliary drainage c.
self-retaining c.
sidewinder c.
Simmons c.
Sones coronary c.
SOS c.
Swan-Ganz c.
Tenckhoff peritoneal c.
Torcon blue c.
triple-lumen c.
umbilical c.
whistle-tip c.
yellow bend c.

catheterization
cardiac c.
selective c.
transseptal c.

cauda *pl.* caudae
c. epididymidis
c. equina
c. helicis
c. nuclei caudati
c. pancreatis

caudad

caudae (plural of cauda)

caudal

caudalis

caudally

caudalward

caudate

caudocephalad

cava

cave
Meckel's c.

cavern

caverna
cavernae corporum caver-
nosorum penis
cavernae corporis spon-
giosi

cavernosal

cavernosography
dynamic infusion c.

cavernosometry
dynamic infusion c.

cavernous

cavitas *pl.* cavitates
c. abdominis
c. abdominis et pelvis
c. abdominalis
c. articularis
c. conchae
c. conchalis
c. cranii
c. glenoidalis
c. infraglottica
c. laryngis
c. medullaris
c. nasi
c. oris
c. pelvica
c. pelvina
c. pelvis
c. pericardiaca
c. pericardialis
c. peritonealis
c. pharyngis
c. pleuralis
c. thoracica
c. thoracis

cavitas *(continued)*
c. tympanica
c. tympani
c. uteri

cavitates (plural of cavitas)

cavity
abdominal c.
abdominopelvic c.
body c.
cranial c.
endometrial c.
glenoid c.
ischioanal c.
ischiorectal c.
lymph c's
mediastinal c., anterior
mediastinal c., middle
mediastinal c., posterior
mediastinal c., superior
nasal c.
oral c.
pectoral c.
pelvic c.
peritoneal c.
pleural c.
rectoischiadic c.
serous c.
splanchnic c.
thin-walled c.
thoracic c.
uterine c.
visceral c.

cavography

cavum
c. conchae
c. rectoischiadicum
c. septi pellucidi
c. veli interpositum
c. vergae

CCNU (lomustine)

2-CdA (cladribine)

CDDP (cisplatin)

CEA
carcinoembryonic antigen

cecal

cecum *pl.* ceca
  c. mobile
  mobile c.

Celestin's tube

celioma

cell
  air c's, posterior ethmoidal
  band c.
  basal c.
  berry c.
  blast c.
  blood c.
  bowenoid c's
  counting c.
  dendritic c's
  dendritic c's, follicular
  diploic c's
  Dorothy Reed c's
  emigrated c.
  epidermic c's
  erythroid c's
  Ferrata's c.
  foot c's
  gametoid c's
  granular c.
  grape c.
  hairy c.
  heckle c.
  Hodgkin's c's
  juvenile c.
  lacunar c.
  Langerhans' c's
  M c's
  malpighian c.
  marrow c.
  mastoid air c's
  matrix c's
  Merkel-Ranvier c's
  morular c.
  Mott c.
  mulberry c.
  myeloid c.
  myeloma c.
  nevus c.
  oat c's

cell *(continued)*
  oat-shaped c's
  packed red blood c's
  Paget's c.
  pagetoid c.
  physaliferous c's
  physaliphorous c's
  polychromatic c's
  polychromatophil c's
  popcorn c.
  prickle c.
  progenitor c.
  progenitor c., hematopoi-
    etic
  progenitor c's, peripheral
    blood
  pulpar c's
  red c.
  red blood c.
  red blood c's
  Reed c's
  Reed-Sternberg c's
  rhagiocrine c.
  Rieder's c.
  RS c's
  segmented c.
  Sézary c.
  signet-ring c.
  smudge c.
  spider c.
  stab c.
  staff c.
  star c's
  stem c.
  stem c., hematopoietic
  stem c's, peripheral blood
  Sternberg's giant c's
  Sternberg-Reed c's
  Thoma-Zeiss counting c.
  white c.
  white blood c.

cellula *pl.* cellulae
  cellulae ethmoidales
  cellulae ethmoidales ante-
    riores
  cellulae ethmoidales me-
    diae
  cellulae ethmoidales pos-
    teriores

cellula *(continued)*
 cellulae mastoideae
 cellulae pneumaticae tubae
  auditivae
 cellulae pneumaticae tubae
  auditoriae
 cellulae tympanicae

cellulae (plural of cellula)

cellular

cellularity

cellule

cellulitis
 anaerobic c.
 clostridial anaerobic c.
 dissecting c. of scalp
 eosinophilic c.
 facial c.
 finger c.
 gangrenous c.
 indurated c.
 necrotizing c.
 nonclostridial anaerobic c.
 phlegmonous c.

cementoblastoma

cementoma
 true c.

center
 accessory ossification c.
 ossification c.
 phrenic c.

centigray

centra

centrad

centralis

centraxonial

centriciput

centrifugal

centrilobular

centripetal

centrolobular

centrum
 c. ossificationis
 c. perinei
 c. tendineum diaphragma-
  tis

cephalad

cephalgia

cephalhematocele
 Stromeyer's c.

cephalhematoma

cephalic

cephalocaudad

cephalocaudal

cephalography

cephalohematocele

cephalohematoma

cephalometer

cephalorhachidian

cephalostat

cephalothoracic

cerebella (plural of cerebellum)

cerebellar

cerebellum *pl.* cerebella

cerebra (plural of cerebrum)

cerebral

cerebrocardiac

cerebromalacia

cerebro-ocular

cerebrotendinous

cerebrum *pl.* cerebra

Cerenkov radiation

Ceretec

ceroplasty

Cerubidine

cervical

cervicalis

cervicoaxillary

cervicobrachial

cervicodorsal

cervico-occipital

cervicoscapular

cervicothoracic

cervix *pl.* cervices
    c. cornus posterioris me-
        dullae spinalis
    c. uteri
    uterine c.
    c. vesicae

cesium (Cs)

chafe

chain
    α c.
    globin c.
    β c.
    δ c.
    ε c.
    γ c.
    ζ c.

chalazodermia

chamber
    Abbe-Zeiss counting c.
    air-equivalent ionization c.
    counting c.
    free-air ionization c.
    ionization c.
    thimble c.
    Thoma-Zeiss counting c.
    tissue-equivalent ioniza-
        tion c.
    Zappert's c.

Chamberlain-Towne view

Chance fracture

change
    atelectatic c's

change *(continued)*
    cystic c's
    discoid atelectatic c's
    emphysematous c's
    geriatric c's
    hypertrophic c's
    osteoarthritic c's
    osteoporotic c's
    pagetoid c's
    postpneumonectomy radia-
        tion c's
    postthoracotomy c's
    prediverticular c's
    senescent c's
    senile c's
    sensorineural c's

channel
    lymph c's
    perineural c.

Chaoul tube

chapped

Charcot joint

Charnley-Mueller prosthesis

chart
    Greulich-Pyle c. for bone
        age

cheilitis
    Miescher's granuloma-
        tous c.
    granulomatous c.

cheilocarcinoma

cheiropompholyx

cheloid

cheloma

chemabrasion

chemexfoliation

chemodectoma

chemoembolization

chemonucleolysis

chemoprotectant

chemoradiotherapy

chemosurgery
    Mohs' c.

chemotherapy
    adjuvant c.
    combination c.
    induction c.
    Mohs c.
    neoadjuvant c.
    preoperative c.
    presurgical c.
    primary c.
    regional c.

chest
    flail c.
    c. for ribs

cheyletiellosis

CHF
    congestive heart failure

chiasm
    optic c.

chiasma
    c. tendinum digitorum ma-
        nus
    c. opticum

chiasmal

chiasmata

chiasmatic

chiasmic

Chiba needle

Chido-Rodgers blood group

Chilaiditi
    C's sign
    C's syndrome

chilblain, chilblains

CHILD syndrome

Chlamydia

chloasma

chloracne

chlorambucil

chloride
    thallous c. Tl 201

chlormerodrin

2-chlorodeoxyadenosine

chloroethylene

chloroleukemia

chloroma

chloronaphthalene

chloroprene

chloroprocaine hydrochloride

chloropropylene oxide

choana

choanae

choanoid

cholangioadenoma

cholangiocarcinoma
    hilar c.
    peripheral c.

cholangiodrainage

cholangiogram
    T-tube c.
    intraoperative c.
    intravenous c. (IVC)
    operative c.

cholangiography
    fine needle transhepatic c.
    operative c.
    percutaneous c.
    transhepatic c.
    transjugular c.

cholangiohepatoma

cholangioma

cholangiopancreatography
    endoscopic retrograde c.
    (ERCP

cholanthrene

Cholebrine

cholecystitis
    acalculous c.
    emphysematous c.

cholecystocholangiogram

cholecystogram
    oral c. (OCG

cholecystography

cholecystolithiasis

cholecystosis
    percutaneous c.

choledochoduodenostomy

choledochogram

choledochography

cholelithiasis

cholera
    pancreatic c.

cholescintigram

cholescintigraphy

cholesteatoma *pl.* cholesteato-
    mas, cholesteatomata
    congenital c.
    intracranial c.

cholesteatomatous

cholesterolosis
    hyperplastic c.

cholesterosis
    extracellular c.

Choletec

Cholex

Cholografin

chondritis

chondroangioma

chondroblastoma
    benign c.

chondrocalcinosis

chondrocranium

chondrodermatitis
    c. nodularis chronica heli-
    cis

chondrodysplasia
    hereditary deforming c.

chondroendothelioma

chondrofibroma

chondroglossus

chondrolipoma

chondroma
    juxtacortical c.
    periosteal c.
    true c.

chondromalacia

chondromatosis
    synovial c.

chondromyoma

chondromyxoma

chondromyxosarcoma

chondrosarcoma
    central c.
    clear cell c.
    dedifferentiated c.
    juxtacortical c.
    mesenchymal c.
    myxoid c.
    periosteal c.
    peripheral c.

chondrosarcomatosis

chondrosarcomatous

chondrosteoma

CHOP
    cyclophosphamide, hy-
    droxydaunomycin (doxo-
    rubicin), Oncovin (vin-
    cristine), and prednisone

CHOP-BLEO
    bleomycin, cyclophospha-

mide, hydroxydaunomy-
cin (doxorubicin), On-
covin (vincristine), and
prednisone

chorangioma

chorda *pl.* chordae
c. obliqua membranae in-
terosseae antebrachii
chordae tendineae cordis
c. tympani

chordae (plural of chorda)

chordoblastoma

chordocarcinoma

chordoepithelioma

chordoma

chordosarcoma

choreoacanthocytosis

chorioadenoma
c. destruens

chorioangiofibroma

chorioangioma

chorioblastoma

choriocarcinoma

chorioepithelioma
c. malignum

chorioma

chorionepithelioma

choristoblastoma

choristoma

choroidea

Christian-Weber disease

Christensen temporomandibular joint prosthesis

Christmas
C. disease
C. factor

chromaffinoma
medullary c.

chromatoblast

chromhidrosis

chromidrosis

chromium
c. 51

chromoblastomycosis

chromomere

chromomycosis

chromophage

chromophototherapy

chromosome
Ph^1 c.
Philadelphia c.

chromotherapy

chromotoxic

chromotrichia

chromotrichial

chronicity

chronic laxative use

chrotoplast

chrysene

chrysiasis

chrysoderma

chrysotile

chylangioma

chylectasia

chylocyst

chylorrhea

Chymodiactin

cicatrix *pl.* cicatrices

cicatricial

cilium *pl.* cilia

Cimino
    C. AV shunt
    C. dialysis shunt

cineangiocardiography

cineangiograph

cineangiography

cinedensigraphy

cinefluorography

cinematography

cinematoradiography

cinephlebography
    ascending functional c.

cineradiofluorography

cineradiography

cineurography

cingula (plural of cingulum)

cingulate

cingule

cingulum *pl.* cingula
    c. membri inferioris
    c. membri superioris
    c. pectorale
    c. pelvicum

circle of Willis

circulation
    collateral c.
    fourth c.
    intracranial c.
    lymph c.
    posterior fossa c.

circulus *pl.* circuli
    c. arteriosus
    c. arteriosus cerebri
    c. arteriosus iridis major
    c. arteriosus iridis minor
    c. vasculosus
    c. vasculosus nervi optici

circumaxillary

circumduction

circumferentia
    c. articularis capitis radii
    c. articularis capitis ulnae

circumnuclear

circumvallate

cirrhosis
    Laënnec's c.

cirsoid

cisatracurium besylate

cisplatin

cistern
    ambient c.
    basal c's
    interpeduncular c.
    c. of Pecquet
    perimesencephalic c.
    pontine c.
    prepontine c.
    quadrigeminal c.
    subarachnoid c's
    sylvian c.
    trigeminal c.

cisternal

cisterna *pl.* cisternae
    c. ambiens
    c. cerebellomedullaris posterior
    c. chiasmatica
    c. chyli
    c. fossae lateralis cerebri
    c. interpeduncularis
    c. magna
    cisternae subarachnoideae

cisternae (plural of cisterna)

cisternographic

cisternography
    air c.
    metrizamide c.
    radionuclide c.

Citanest

Clado's ligament

cladosporiosis
    c. epidermica

cladribine (2-CdA)

clamp
    Crutchfield c's

clasmatocyte

classification
    Arneth's c.
    Borrmann's c.
    Broders' c.
    Dukes' c.
    FIGO c.
    French-American-British
        (FAB) c.
    Kiel c.
    Lennert's c.
    Lukes-Collins C.
    Lund-Browder c.
    McNeer c.
    Rappaport C.
    Rye C. (of Hodgkin's dis-
        ease)
    REAL C. (of lymphomas)
    Revised European Ameri-
        can Lymphoma C.
    Wolfe's c. of breast carci-
        noma

clastic

clastothrix

claudication
    intermittent c.

Clauss
    C. assay
    C. method

claustrum *pl.* claustra

clavacin

clavicle

clavicula

clavicular

claviformin

clavus
    c. durus
    c. mollis
    c. syphiliticus

clearance
    plasma iron c.

cleft
    anal c.
    clunial c.
    gluteal c.
    Hahn's c's
    intergluteal c.
    Larrey's c.
    natal c.

cleidocranial

Cleopatra view

clinoid

clip
    metallic surgical c's
    skin c's
    surgical c's

clition

clival

clivography

clivus
    basilar c.
    c. basilaris
    Blumenbach's c.
    c. blumenbachii
    c. ossis occipitalis
    c. ossis sphenoidalis

C-loop

Cloquet
    C.'s gland
    C.'s node

clot
    blood c.

clotting

clubbing of the calices

cluneal

clunes

CMF
    cyclophosphamide, metho-
    trexate, and 5-fluorouracil

C-MOPP
    cyclophosphamide, On-
    covin (vincristine), pro-
    carbazine, and predni-
    sone

CNS
    central nervous system

coadaptation

coagulability

coagulable

coagulant

coagulate

coagulation
    blood c.
    diffuse intravascular c.
    disseminated intravascu-
        lar c.

coagulative

coagulogram

coagulopathy
    consumption c.

coagulum

coalescence

coalescent

coaptation

coarctation of the aorta

coat
    adventitial c.
    adventitious c.
    albugineous c.
    buffy c.
    external c. of viscera
    fibrous c.

coat (continued)
    mucous c.
    muscular c.
    proper c.
    proper c. of corium
    proper c. of dermis
    serous c.
    submucous c.
    subserous c.
    vascular c. of viscera
    white c.

coating of the mucosa

cobalt
    c. 57
    c. 58
    c. 60
    c. 60

Cobb angle

cobblestoning of the mucosa

cocaine
    c. hydrochloride

cocainization

cocainize

cocarcinogen

cocarcinogenesis

coccidioidomycosis

coccyx

cochlea

codeine
    c. phosphate
    c. sulfate

Codman
    C's triangle
    C's tumor

coefficient
    absorption c.
    apparent diffuse c. (ADC)
    homogeneity c.
    linear absorption c.
    linear attenuation c.
    mass absorption c.

coefficient *(continued)*
    mass attenuation c.

coeur
    c. en sabot

cofactor
    heparin c. II
    platelet c. I
    platelet c. II

Cohnheim's theory

coil
    Gianturco c's

coin lesion of the lung

colaspase

COLD
    chronic obstructive lung
      disease

cold

coldsore

Cole's sign

colectomy

colitis
    amebic c.
    Crohn's c.
    granulomatous c.
    mucous c.
    seronegative arthritis spastic c.
    supraspinatus tendinitis
    ulcerative c.

colla (plural of collum)

collapse

collar
    Casal's c.
    c. of pearls
    venereal c.
    c. of Venus

collarette
    Biett's c.

collateral

collection
    cholecystic fluid c.
    extra-axial c's
    pericholecystic fluid c.

Colles
    C's fracture
    C's space

colliculus *pl.* colliculi
    c. cartilaginis arytenoideae
    c. facialis
    c. inferior
    c. seminalis
    c. superior

collimation

collimator

colloid
    stannous sulfur c.

collum *pl.* colla
    c. anatomicum humeri
    c. chirurgicum humeri
    c. costae
    c. folliculi pili
    c. glandis penis
    c. mallei
    c. femoris
    c. radii
    c. scapulae
    c. tali
    c. vesicae biliaris
    c. vesicae felleae

colon
    c. ascendens
    ascending c.
    c. descendens
    descending c.
    familial polyposis of the c.
    fecal-filled c.
    hepatic flexure of the c.
    irritable c.
    lead-pipe c.
    sigmoid c.
    c. sigmoideum
    splenic flexure of the c.
    transverse c.
    c. transversum

colonization

colonoscopy

colophony

colostomy
    permanent c.

Colton blood group

columella *pl.* columellae

column
    c's of abdominal ring
    c's of Bertin
    dye c.
    spinal c.
    tracheal air c.
    vertebral c.

columna *pl.* columnae
    columnae anales
    columni ani
    c. anterior medullae spinalis
    c. autonomica medullae spinalis
    c. fornicis
    columnae griseae medullae spinalis
    c. intermedia medullae spinalis
    c. posterior medullae spinalis
    columnae renales
    c. rugarum anterior vaginae
    c. rugarum posterior vaginae
    columnae rugarum vaginae

columnae (plural of columna)

columnization of contrast material

comedo
    closed c.
    open c.

comedocarcinoma

comedogenic

commissura *pl.* commissurae
    c. alba anterior medullae spinalis
    c. alba posterior medullae spinalis
    c. anterior
    c. colliculi inferioris
    c. colliculi superioris
    c. epithalamica
    c. fornicis
    c. grisea anterior medullae spinalis
    c. grisea posterior medullae spinalis
    c. habenularum
    c. labiorum anterior
    c. labiorum oris
    c. labiorum posterior
    c. lateralis palpebrarum
    c. medialis palpebrarum
    c. posterior
    c. supraoptica dorsalis
    c. supraoptica ventralis

commissurae (plural of commissura)

commissural

commissure

commissurotomy

communicans

communis

compartimentum
    c. superficiale perinei

compartment
    extra-axial c's
    c. of the knee
    medial c. of the knee
    superficial perineal c.

complex
    Carney's c.
    Eisenmenger c.
    Ghon c.
    renal sinus c.

complexion

complexus
   c. olivaris inferior
   c. stimulans cordis

component
   plasma thromboplastin c.

compression
   vertebral c.

Compton effect

c-*onc*

concatenation of shadows

concavity

concentration
   mean corpuscular hemo-
      globin c.
   minimal alveolar c.

concha *pl.* conchae
   c. auriculae
   c. auricularis
   c. bullosa
   c. of cranium
   c. nasalis inferior
   c. nasalis media
   c. nasalis superior
   c. nasalis suprema
   c. nasi inferior
   c. nasi media
   c. nasi superior
   c. nasi suprema
   c. sphenoidalis

conchae (plural of concha)

concomitant

conduit
   ileal conduit

condylar

condyle
   mandibular c.

condyli (plural of condylus)

condyloid

condyloma *pl.* condylomata
   c. acuminatum

condyloma *(continued)*
   flat c.
   giant c.
   c. latum
   pointed c.

condylomata (plural of condyloma)

condylomatoid

condylomatosis

condylomatous

condylus *pl.* condyli
   c. humeri
   c. lateralis femoris
   c. lateralis tibiae
   c. medialis femoris
   c. medialis tibiae
   c. occipitalis

cone-shaped

conexus

confertus

configuration
   geriatric c.
   global c.
   globular c.
   hourglass c.
   trefoil c.

confluence

confluens
   c. sinuum

confluent

congelation

congenital

congestion
   passive c. of the lungs
   pulmonary vascular c.
   pulmonary venous c.

conglobate

conglobation

conglutination

coni (plural of conus)

conjugata
   c. anatomica pelvis
   c. diagonalis pelvis
   c. externa pelvis
   c. mediana pelvis
   c. recta pelvis
   c. vera pelvis

conjugation

connexus
   c. intertendinei

Conray

consolidation

constant
   decay c.
   disintegration c.
   radioactive c.

constitution
   lymphatic c.

constrictor

contamination

content
   disc water c.
   disk water c.
   gastric c's
   overlying bowel c.

contiguous

contraction
   tertiary c's

contracture
   Dupuytren's c.
   flexion c.

contralateral

contrast
   film c.
   high c.
   long-scale c.
   low c.
   short-scale c.
   subject c.

contrast material
   columnization of c. m.

contrast material *(continued)*
   c. m.
   flow of c. m.
   iodinated c. m.
   ionic c. m.
   layering of c. m.
   nonionic c. m.
   water-soluble c. m.

contusion

conus *pl.* coni
   c. arteriosus
   c. elasticus
   coni epididymidis
   c. medullaris

conversion
   internal c.

convertin

convexity
   parietal c.

convoluted

convolution

convolutional

convolutionary

Cook enforcer

Cooley
   C's anemia
   C's disease

Coolidge tube

Cooper
   inguinal ligament of C.
   C's ligament

COP
   cyclophosphamide, On-
      covin (vincristine), and
      prednisone

COP-BLAM
   cyclophosphamide, On-
      covin (vincristine), pred-
      nisone, bleomycin, Adria-
      mycin (doxorubicin), and
      Matulane (procarbazine)

COPD
   chronic obstructive pulmonary disease

COPP
   cyclophosphamide, Oncovin (vincristine), procarbazine, and prednisone

copper
   c. 64
   c. 67
   c. 67

Copper-7 intrauterine device

coprolith

copula

cor
   c. pulmonale

cord
   Billroth's c's
   cervical c.
   lymph c's
   medullary c's
   red pulp c's
   spinal c.
   splenic c's
   vocal c's

cordate

cordiform

core

corium

corn
   hard c.
   soft c.

cornea

corneocyte

corneous

corneum

corniculate

cornification

cornified

cornoid

cornu *pl.* cornua
   c. anterius medullae spinalis
   c. anterius ventriculi lateralis
   c. coccygeum
   c. coccyx
   c. cutaneum
   c. frontale ventriculi lateralis
   c. inferius cartilaginis thyroideae
   c. inferius marginis falciformis
   c. inferius ventriculi lateralis
   c. laterale medullae spinalis
   c. majus ossis hyoidei
   c. minus ossis hyoidei
   c. occipitale ventriculi lateralis
   c. posterius medullae spinalis
   c. posterius ventriculi lateralis
   sacral c.
   c. sacrale
   c. superius cartilaginis thyroideae
   c. superius marginis falciformis
   c. temporale ventriculi lateralis
   c. uteri
   c. uterinum

cornua (plural of cornu)

cornual

cornuate

corona *pl.* coronae
   c. ciliaris
   c. glandis penis
   c. radiata

coronad

coronae (plural of corona)

coronal

coronale

coronalis

coronary

coronoid

corpectomy (vertebrectomy)

corpora (plural of corpus)

corpulence

corpulent

corpus *pl.* corpora
  c. adiposum fossae is-
    chioanalis
  c. adiposum fossae ischio-
    rectalis
  c. adiposum infrapatellare
  c. adiposum orbitae
  c. adiposum pararenale
  c. adiposum preepiglotti-
    cum
  c. albicans
  c. amygdaloideum
  c. anococcygeum
  c. callosum
  c. cavernosum clitoridis
  c. cavernosum penis
  c. cerebelli
  c. ciliare
  c. claviculae
  c. claviculare
  c. clitoridis
  c. costae
  c. epididymidis
  c. fibulae
  c. fornicis
  c. gastricum
  c. geniculatum laterale
  c. geniculatum mediale
  c. glandulae sudoriferae
  c. humeri
  c. incudis
  c. linguae

corpus *(continued)*
  c. luteum
  c. mammillare
  c. mammae
  c. maxillae
  c. medullare cerebelli
  c. nuclei caudati
  c. ossis hyoidei
  c. ossis ilii
  c. ossis ilium
  c. ossis ischii
  c. ossis metacarpi
  c. ossis metatarsi
  c. ossis pubis
  c. ossis sphenoidalis
  c. pancreatis
  corpora paraaortica
  c. penis
  c. perineale
  c. phalangis manus
  c. phalangis pedis
  c. pineale
  c. pineale
  c. radii
  c. spongiosum penis
  c. sterni
  c. striatum
  c. tali
  c. tibiae
  c. tibiale
  c. trapezoideum
  c. ulnae
  c. unguis
  c. uteri
  c. vertebrae
  c. vertebrale
  c. vesicae biliaris
  c. vesicae felleae
  c. vesicae urinariae
  c. vitreum

corpuscle
  blood c.
  blood c., red
  blood c., white
  bridge c.
  chyle c.
  concentric c's
  dust c's

corpuscle *(continued)*
    Gierke's c's
    Hassall's c's
    Leber's c's
    lymph c's
    lymphoid c's
    malpighian c's of spleen
    red c.
    reticulated c.
    splenic c's
    thymus c's
    white c.

corpuscular

corpusculum *pl.* corpuscula

correlation
    clinical c.

Correra's line

corrugator

cortex *pl.* cortices
    cerebellar c.
    c. cerebelli
    c. cerebri
    c. glandulae suprarenalis
    c. lentis
    motor c.
    c. nodi lymphatici
    c. nodi lymphoidei
    c. ovarii
    c. renalis
    c. thymi
    c. of thymus

cortical

corticate

cortices (plural of cortex)

corticotropinoma

cortisone

corymbiform

corymbose

Corynebacterium
    C. acnes

Cosmegen

cosmesis

cosmetic

costa *pl.* costae
    c. cervicalis
    costae fluctuantes
    costae fluitantes
    c. prima
    c. secunda
    costae spuriae
    costae verae

costae (plural of costa)

costophrenic

costopleural

cothromboplastin

Cotting's operation

cotyloid

Coulter counter

Coumadin

Councill catheter

count
    Arneth c.
    blood c.
    blood c., complete
    blood c., differential
    blood cell c.
    differential c's
    erythrocyte c.
    filament-nonfilament c.
    leukocyte c.
    leukocyte c., differential
    leukocyte c., total
    neutrophil lobe c.
    platelet c.
    red blood cell c.
    red cell c.
    reticulocyte c.
    white blood cell c.
    white cell c.

counter
    Coulter c.
    Geiger c.
    Geiger-Müller c.

counter *(continued)*
    proportional c.
    scintillation c.

countertransport
    sodium-lithium c.

counting
    liquid scintillation c.

coup
    c. de sabre
    en c. de sabre

Cournand catheter

Courvoisier-Terrier syndrome

Coutard
    C's law
    C's method

cowage

Cowper's glands

CPA
    cerebellopontine angle

CPD
    cephalopelvic dispropor-
    tion

cpm
    counts per minute

craniad

cranial

cranialis

cranioacromial

craniocervical

craniopharyngioma

craniostenosis

craniosynostosis

cranium
    cerebral c.
    c. cerebrale

crassamentum

crater

cream
    leukocytic c.

crease
    flexion c.
    palmar c.

crena
    c. analis
    c. ani
    c. clunium
    c. interglutealis

crenate

crenated

crenocytosis

crepitance

crepitation

crepitus

crest
    basilar c. of occipital bone
    cerebral c's of cranial bone
    frontal c.
    frontal c., external
    frontal c., internal
    c. of the ilium
    c's of the ilia
    iliac c.
    c. of matrix of nail
    occipital c., external
    occipital c., internal
    temporal c. of frontal bone

CREST syndrome (calcinosis,
    Raynaud's phenomenon,
    esophageal dysmotility, scler-
    odactyly, and telangiectasia)

cribrate

cribration

cribriform

crines

crinis

crisantaspase

crisis
- aplastic c.
- blast c.
- carcinoid c.
- deglobulinization c.
- hemolytic c.
- megaloblastic c.
- sickle cell c.
- vaso-occlusive c.

crista *pl.* cristae
- c. ampullaris
- c. arcuata cartilaginis arytenoideae
- c. basilaris ductus cochlearis
- c. capitis costae
- c. capituli costae
- c. colli costae
- c. conchalis corporis maxillae
- c. conchalis ossis palatini
- cristae cutis
- c. ethmoidalis maxillae
- c. ethmoidalis ossis palatini
- c. fenestrae cochleae
- c. frontalis
- c. galli
- c. iliaca
- c. infratemporalis
- c. intertrochanterica
- c. lacrimalis anterior
- c. lacrimalis posterior
- c. matricis unguis
- c. medialis fibulae
- c. musculi supinatoris
- c. nasalis maxillae
- c. nasalis ossis palatini
- c. obturatoria
- c. occipitalis externa
- c. occipitalis interna
- c. pubica
- c. sacralis intermedia
- c. sacralis lateralis
- c. sacralis mediana
- c. sacralis medialis
- c. sphenoidalis

crista *(continued)*
- c. spiralis ductus cochlearis
- c. supracondylaris lateralis humeri
- c. supracondylaris medialis humeri
- c. supraepicondylaris lateralis humeri
- c. supraepicondylaris medialis humeri
- c. supramastoidea
- c. supraventricularis
- c. temporalis
- c. terminalis atrii dextri
- c. transversa meati acustici interni
- c. tuberculi majoris
- c. tuberculi minoris
- c. urethralis
- c. vestibuli

cristae (plural of crista)

cristal

criterion
- radiographic criteria

crocidolite

Crohn
- C's disease
- C's gastritis

Cromer blood group

Cronkhite-Canada syndrome

Crookes' space

cross-filling

crossmatch

crossmatching

cross-resistance

crossway

croup

Crouzon's disease

Crow-Fukase syndrome

Crowe's sign

crown

CRST syndrome

cruciate

cruciform

cruor

crura (plural of crus)

crural

crus *pl.* crura
    c. anterius capsulae inter-
       nae
    c. anterius stapedis
    crura anthelicis
    c. breve incudis
    c. cerebri
    c. clitoridis
    c. dextrum diaphragmatis
    c. dextrum fasciculi atrio-
       ventricularis
    crura of diaphragm
    c. of diaphragm, left
    c. of diaphragm, right
    crura diaphragmatis
    c. fornicis
    c. helicis
    c. inferius marginis falcifor-
       mis
    c. laterale anuli inguinalis
       superficialis
    c. laterale cartilaginis alaris
       majoris
    c. longum incudis
    c. mediale anuli inguinalis
       superficialis
    c. mediale cartilaginis
       alaris majoris
    crura membranacea ampul-
       laria ductus semicircu-
       laris
    c. membranaceum com-
       mune ductus semicircu-
       laris
    c. membranaceum simplex
       ductus semicircularis

crus *(continued)*
    crura ossea
    crura ossea ampullaria
    c. osseum commune
    c. osseum simplex
    c. penis
    c. posterius capsulae inter-
       nae
    c. posterius stapedis
    c. primum lobuli ansiformis
    c. secundum lobuli ansifor-
       mis
    c. sinistrum diaphragmatis
    c. sinistrum fasciculi atrio-
       ventricularis
    c. superius marginis falci-
       formis

crustosus

Crutchfield
    C. clamps
    C. tongs

crux
    cruces pilorum

cryoanesthesia

cryocrit

cryofibrinogenemia

cryoglobulinemia
    essential mixed c.

cryoprecipitability

cryoprecipitate

cryoprecipitation

cryoprotective

cryoprotein

crypt

crypta *pl.* cryptae
    cryptae mucosae
    cryptae tonsillares tonsillae
       palatinae
    cryptae tonsillares tonsillae
       pharyngeae
    cryptae tonsillae

crypta *(continued)*
    cryptae tonsillares tonsillae
      lingualis
    cryptae tonsillares tonsillae
      tubariae
    cryptae tonsillae tonsillae
      palatinae
    cryptae tonsillae tonsillae
      pharyngeae
    cryptae tonsillares tonsillae
      pharyngealis

cryptae (plural of crypta)

cryptitis

cryptococcosis
    cutaneous c.

cryptoscope
    Satvioni's c.

cryptoscopy

crystal
    scintillation c.
    Teichmann's c's

Cs
    cesium

C-section

CSF
    cerebrospinal fluid
      CSF-density

CT
    computed tomography
      CT scan
      CT gantry
      CT-guided biopsy
      spiral CT scan

CTR
    cardiothoracic ratio

CTS
    carpal tunnel syndrome

cubital

cubitalis

cubitus

cuff

cuffing
    peribronchial c.

cul-de-sac

culling

culmen
    c. cerebelli
    c. of cerebellum

culmina

culture
    blood c.

cumulus *pl.* cumuli

cuneate

cunei (plural of cuneus)

cuneiform

cuneus *pl.* cunei

cuniculus *pl.* cuniculi

cup
    Diogenes' c.

cupola (variant of cupula)

cupping of the calices

cupula *pl.* cupulae
    c. ampullaris
    c. cochleae
    c. cristae ampullaris
    c. pleurae
    c. pleuralis

cupulae (plural of cupula)

curet, curette

curie

curie-hour

curietherapy

curioscopy

Curling's ulcer

current
    fulguration c.
    saturation c.

curvatura
    c. major gastris
    c. minor gastris

curvature
    greater c. of the stomach
    lesser c. of the stomach
    lumbar c.
    reversal of the normal lor-
        dotic c.

curve
    Bragg c.
    dose-effect c.
    dose-frequency c.
    dose-intensity c.
    dose-response c.
    isodose c's
    oxygen dissociation c.
    oxygen-hemoglobin disso-
        ciation c.
    oxyhemoglobin dissocia-
        tion c.
    Price-Jones c.

Cushing's disease

cushion

cusp
    c. of the hemidiaphragm

cuspis pl. cuspides
    c. anterior valvae atrioven-
        tricularis dextrae
    c. anterior valvae atrioven-
        tricularis sinistrae
    cuspides commisurales
    c. posterior valvae atrio-
        ventricularis dextrae
    c. posterior valvae atrio-
        ventricularis sinistrae
    c. septalis valvae atrioven-
        tricularis dextrae

cut
    tomographic c's

cutaneous

cuticle
    c. of root sheath

cuticula pl. cuticulae

cutis
    c. anserina
    c. laxa
    c. marmorata
    c. rhomboidalis nuchae
    c. verticis gyrata

CVA
    cerebrovascular accident

CVB
    CCNU (lomustine), vinblas-
        tine, and bleomycin

CVP
    central venous pressure
        CVP catheter
        CVP line
    cyclophosphamide, vincris-
        tine, and prednisone

cyanhemoglobin

cyanmethemoglobin

cyanmetmyoglobin

cyanosed

cyanosis
    false c.
    hereditary methemoglobi-
        nemic c.
    c. lienis

cyanotic

cycad

Cycas

cycasin

cyclamate

cyclamic acid

cycle
    hair c.
    isohydric c.

cyclophosphamide

cyclopropane

cyclotron

cylindroma

cylindromatous

cymba
    c. conchae auriculae

cymbiform

cyst
    aneurysmal bone c.
    atheromatous c.
    Baker's c.
    blue dome c.
    Bosniak type B renal c.
    branchial cleft c.
    coelomic c.
    craniobuccal c's
    craniopharyngeal c's
    dentigerous c.
    dermoid c.
    echinococcal c.
    epidermal c.
    epidermal inclusion c.
    epidermoid c.
    epithelial c.
    follicular c.
    ganglion c.
    implantation c.
    inclusion c.
    intrapituitary c's
    keratinizing c.
    keratinous c.
    meibomian c.
    meniscal c.
    multiloculated c.
    myxoid c.
    nabothian c.
    pancreatic c.
    parapelvic c.
    pericardial c.
    peripancreatic c.
    peripelvic c.

cyst *(continued)*
    pilar c.
    piliferous c.
    pilonidal c.
    popliteal c.
    c. or polyp (*not* "sister
      polyp")
    porencephalic c.
    pseudomucinous c.
    trichilemmal c., proliferat-
      ing

cystadenocarcinoma
    mucinous c.
    papillary c.
    pseudomembranous c.
    serous c.

cystadenoma
    apocrine c.
    bile duct c.
    mucinous c.
    papillary c.
    papillary c. lymphomato-
      sum
    papillary c. of thyroid
    pseudomucinous c.
    serous c.

cystectomy
    radical c.

cystic

cystides

cystiform

cystis

cystoadenoma

cystogram

cystography
    delayed c.
    voiding c.

Cystokon

Cystografin

cystoma

cystomatous

cystomorphous

cystoprostatectomy
   radical c.

cystopyelography

cyst or polyp (*not* "sister
   polyp")

cystoradiography

cystosarcoma
   c. phyllodes

cystoscope

cystoscopy

cystoureterogram

cystourethrogram
   voiding c.

cystourethrography
   chain c.
   voiding c.

cytapheresis

cytarabine

cytoanalyzer

cytological

cytology

cytolysate
   blood c.

Cytomel

cytopenia

cytoreduction

Cytoxan

Cytosar-U

dacarbazine

Dacron graft

dacryon

dacryoscintigraphy

dactinomycin

dakryon

dance
hilar d.
hilus d.

dandruff

Dandy-Walker syndrome

D antigen

Darier
D's disease
D's sign
D.-White disease

Daubenton
D's line
D's plane

daughter

daunomycin

daunorubicin
d. hydrochloride

DaunoXome

o,p-DDD (mitotane)

DDP (cisplatin)

deactivation

debilitated

debility

débouchement

débridement

debris
metallic d.

Decadron

decamethonium

Decapeptyl

decay
alpha d.
beta d.
free induction d.
positron d.
radioactive d.

decholesterolization

deciduoma
d. malignum

decitabine

declive

decoagulant

decompensation
cardiac d.

decompression

decortication of the lung

decubital

decubitus
lateral d.

decurrent

decussate

decussatio *pl.* decussationes
d. fibrarum nervorum trochlearium
d. lemnisci medialis
d. pedunculorum cerebellarium superiorum
d. pyramidum
decussationes tegmentales
d. tegmentalis anterior
d. tegmentalis posterior

decussation

decussationes (plural of decussatio)

dedifferentiation

deep
d.-seated

deep to the nipple

Deetjen's body

defecography

defect
  atrial septal d. (ASD)
  craniotomy d.
  extradural d.
  fibrous cortical d.
  filling d.
  fixed perfusion d.
  interatrial septal d.
  intraluminal filling d.
  intravascular filling d.
  intrinsic or extrinsic fill-
    ing d.
  lucent d.
  matching d's
  metaphyseal fibrous d.
  mismatched perfusion d.
  perfusion d.
  punched-out bony d's
  saucer-shaped d.
  subsegmental perfusion d.
  transverse bar d.
  trephine d's

deferens

deferent

defibrinated

defibrination

defibrinogenation

deficiency
  plasma thromboplastin an-
    tecedent d.
  PTA d.

deflorescence

defluvium
  d. unguium

defluxion

deformability

deformation

deformity
  Åkerlund d.
  boutonniere d.
  cloverleaf d.
  clubfoot d.
  contracture d.
  coxa valga hip d.
  coxa vara hip d.
  dextroscoliotic d.
  equinovarus d.
  flexion d.
  fracture d.
  funnel chest d.
  gibbous d.
  hammertoe d.
  pectus carinatum d.
  pectus excavatum d.
  pectus recurvatum d.
    (*same as* pectus excava-
    tum)
  phrygian cap d.
  pigeon-breast d.
  rotoscoliotic d.
  "round back" d.
  silver fork d.
  Sprengel's d.
  valgus d.
  varus d.

degeneration
  cerebellar d., paraneoplas-
    tic
  cerebellar d., paraneoplas-
    tic subacute
  olivopontocerebellar d.

deglutition

deglycerolize

Degos
  D. acanthoma
  D's disease
  D's syndrome

dehiscence

delivery from below

dell

delle

delling

deltoid

demarcation

Demerol

demineralization of bones

demipenniform

demise
    fetal d.

demonstrator

De Morgan's spots

demyelinization

dendriform

dendritic

dendroid

Dennie's sign

Dennis tube

dens
    dentes acustici
    d. axis
    d. view of the cervical
      spine

densitometer

densitometry

density
    background d.
    heterogeneous d.
    inherent d.
    ionization d.
    low d.
    magnetic flux d.
    near-water d.
    streaky d.

dentate

dentiform

dentinoma

dentinosteoid

dentoid

dentoma

deoxyhemoglobin

dependent

depigmentation

depilate

depilation

depilatory

deposition of tracer

depression
    pacchionian d's
    precordial d.

de Quervain's disease

derangement

Dercum's disease

derivative
    hematoporphyrin d.

derma

dermabrader

dermabrasion

dermad

dermal

dermamyiasis

dermatitis *pl.* dermatitides
    actinic d.
    allergic d.
    allergic contact d.
    ammonia d.
    d. artefacta
    ashy d.
    atopic d.
    berlock d.
    berloque d.
    brown-tail moth d.
    d. bullosa striata pratensis
    d. calorica
    caterpillar d.

dermatitis *(continued)*
    cercarial d.
    contact d.
    contagious pustular d.
    cosmetic d.
    dhobie mark d.
    diaper d.
    eczematous d.
    d. exfoliativa
    d. exfoliativa neonatorum
    exfoliative d.
    exudative discoid and lich-
      enoid d.
    factitial d.
    d. gangrenosa infantum
    d. herpetiformis
    d. hiemalis
    industrial d.
    infectious eczematous d.
    insect d.
    irritant d.
    Jacquet's d.
    livedoid d.
    marine d.
    meadow d.
    meadow-grass d.
    d. medicamentosa
    moth d.
    napkin d.
    nickel d.
    nummular eczematous d.
    occupational d.
    onion mite d.
    d. papillaris capillitii
    Pelodera d.
    perfume d.
    periocular d.
    perioral d.
    photoallergic contact d.
    photocontact d.
    phototoxic d.
    phytophototoxic d.
    pigmented purpuric lichen-
      oid d.
    poison ivy d.
    poison oak d.
    poison sumac d.
    precancerous d.
    primary irritant d.

dermatitis *(continued)*
    radiation d.
    rat-mite d.
    d. repens
    rhabditic d.
    rhus d.
    roentgen-ray d.
    sabra d.
    schistosome d.
    seborrheic d.
    d. seborrheica
    stasis d.
    d. striata pratensis bullosa
    swimmers' d.
    uncinarial d.
    d. vegetans
    d. venenata
    verrucose d.
    verrucous d.
    vesicular d.
    x-ray d.

dermatoarthritis
    lipid d.
    lipoid d.

dermatochalasis, dermatochala-
zia

dermatodysplasia

dermatofibroma
    d. protuberans

dermatofibrosarcoma
    d. protuberans

dermatofibrosis
    d. lenticularis disseminata

dermatoglyphics

dermatographic

dermatographism
    black d.
    white d.

dermatologic, dermatological

dermatologist

dermatology

dermatolysis

dermatomegaly

dermatomycosis
  d. furfuracea

dermatomyiasis

dermatomyoma

dermatomyositis

dermatopathic

dermatopathy

dermatophiliasis

dermatophilosis

dermatophyte

dermatophytid

dermatophytosis

dermatorrhagia

dermatorrhexis

dermatosclerosis

dermatosis
  acute febrile neutrophil-
    ic d.
  ashy d. of Ramirez
  Bowen's precancerous d.
  chronic bullous d. of child-
    hood
  d. cenicienta
  dermatolytic bullous d.
  industrial d.
  lichenoid d.
  linear IgA d. of adulthood
  linear IgA d. of childhood
  d. papulosa nigra
  precancerous d.
  progressive pigmentary d.
  Schamberg's d.
  Schamberg's progressive
    pigmented purpuric d.
  subcorneal pustular d.
  transient acantholytic d.

dermatotherapy

dermatotropic

dermatozoiasis

dermatozoonosis

dermic

dermis

dermographism

dermoid

dermopathic

dermopathy
  diabetic d.

dermosynovitis

dermotropic

dermovascular

descendens

descending

desflurane

deshydremia

desiccated

desiccation

Desjardins' point

desmocranium

desmocytoma

desmoid
  periosteal d.

desmoma

desmosome
  half d.

desquamation
  furfuraceous d.
  lamellar d. of the newborn

desquamative

desquamatory

destruction
  mucosal d.

detail
  fetal d.

detail *(continued)*
    fine d.
    intraluminal d.

detection
    coincidence d.

detector
    radiation d.

detrusor

deuterion

deuterium
    d. oxide

deuteron

deuton

deviation
    d. to the left
    d. to the right
    standard d.

device
    contraceptive d.
    Copper-7 intrauterine d.
    halo traction d.
    immobilization d.
    intrauterine d. (IUD)
    intrauterine contraceptive
      d. (IUCD)
    load-sharing internal fixa-
      tion d.
    prosthetic d.

dexrazoxane

DEXA
    dual energy x-ray absorp-
      tion
        DEXA scan

dexter

dextrad

dextral

dextroposition

dextroscoliosis

dextrosinistral

dextroversion

diabetes mellitus

diabetic

diabetid

diagnosis
    differential d.

dialysis
    lymph d.
    peritoneal d.

diameter
    anteroposterior d.
    anterotransverse d.
    bicristal d.
    biparietal d.
    bisacromial d.
    bitemporal d.
    cranial d's
    craniometric d.
    frontomental d.
    fronto-occipital d.
    longitudinal d., inferior
    mento-occipital d.
    mentoparietal d.
    d. obliqua pelvis
    occipitofrontal d.
    occipitomental d.
    parietal d.
    posterotransverse d.
    sagittal d.
    suboccipitobregmatic d.
    temporal d.
    d. transversa pelvis
    transverse d.
    vertebromammary d.
    vertical d.

p-diaminodiphenyl

cis-diamminedichloroplatinum

Diamond
    D.-Blackfan anemia
    D.-Blackfan syndrome

diapedesis

diapedetic

diaphoresis

diaphoretic

diaphragm
  pelvic d.
  d. of pelvis
  polyarcuate d.
  Potter-Bucky d.
  respiratory d.
  thoracic d.

diaphragma *pl.* diaphragmata
  d. pelvis
  d. sellae
  d. thoraco-abdominale

diaphragmatic

diaphysis *pl.* diaphyses

diapiresis

diarrhea

diarrheal

diarthrosis

diascope

diascopy

diastasis recti

diastematomyelia

diastole

diathesis
  hemorrhagic d.

diatrizoate
  d. meglumine
  d. sodium

diatrizoic acid

diaziquone

diazoma

dibenzanthracene

dibromochloropropane

dibromodulcitol

1,2-dibromoethane

dibucaine
  d. hydrochloride

3,3-dichlorobenzidine

1,2-dichloroethane

dictyoma

didermoma

Didiée's projection

Diego blood group

diencephalon

diener

1,4-diethylene dioxide

diethylenetriamine pentaacetic
  acid

diethylstilbestrol

digastric

digit

supernumerary digit

digitalis

digitatio *pl.* digitationes
  digitationes hippocampi

digitiform

digitus *pl.* digiti
  d. anularis
  digiti manus
  d. medius
  d. minimus manus
  d. minimus pedis
  digiti pedis
  d. primus (I) manus
  d. primus (I) pedis
  d. quartus (IV) manus
  d. quartus (IV) pedis
  d. quintus (V) manus
  d. quintus (V) pedis
  d. secundus (II) manus
  d. secundus (II) pedis

digitus *(continued)*
    d. tertius (III) manus
    d. tertius (III) pedis

Di Guglielmo's syndrome

diktyoma

dikwakwadi

dilatation
    aneurysmal d.
    biliary d.
    cardiac d.
    ductal d.
    ex vacuo d.
    fusiform d.
    gaseous d.
    junctional d.
    poststenotic d.
    sulcal d.

dilation

dilatator

dilator
    Amplatz d.

dimer
    D d.

dimethisoquin hydrochloride

p-dimethylaminoazobenzene

7,12-dimethyl-
    benz[a]anthracene

dimethylnitrosamine

dimethylphenanthrene

dimethyl phthalate

dimethyl sulfate

diminution

dimple

dimpling
    d. of the skin

dinitrogen
    d. monoxide

Diodrast

Diogenes' cup

Dionosil

dioxane

dioxin

DIP
    distal interphalangeal
        DIP joint

diperodon

diphenyldiimide

diphenylnitrosamine

2,3-diphosphoglycerate

diphosphonate
    methylene d.

diphtheria
    cutaneous d.

diploë

diploetic

diploic

diplon

diplopia

Diprivan

diprotrizoate

"dirty fat"

disc *(also* disk)

discharge
    nipple d.

disci (plural of discus)

disciform

discocyte

discogram

discography

disc space–thecal sac interface

discrepancy

discriminator

discus *pl.* disci
    d. articularis

discus *(continued)*
    d. articularis articulationis
        acromioclavicularis
    d. articularis articulationis
        radioulnaris distalis
    d. articularis articulationis
        sternoclavicularis
    d. interpubicus
    disci intervertebrales
    d. nervi optici
disease
    Addison's d.
    alpha chain d.
    Alzheimer's d.
    Amiodarone lung d.
    Anders' d.
    aortic valvular d.
    Ayerza's d.
    Bannister's d.
    Banti's d.
    Barcoo d.
    Bazin's d.
    Beigel's d.
    Binswanger's d.
    Bowen's d.
    Brill-Symmers d.
    Brinton's d.
    Caffey's d.
    calcium pyrophosphate
        deposition d. (CPPD)
        (pseudogout)
    calcium pyrophosphate di-
        hydrate deposition d.
        (CPPD) (pseudogout)
    Carrión's d.
    Castleman's d.
    Christian-Weber d.
    Christmas d.
    chronic granulomatous d.
    chronic granulomatous d.
        of childhood
    chronic obstructive lung d.
        (COLD)
    chronic obstructive pulmo-
        nary d. (COPD)
    collagen vascular d.
    Cooley's d.
    creeping d.

disease *(continued)*
    Crohn's d.
    Crouzon's d.
    Cushing's d.
    Darier's d.
    Darier-White d.
    de Quervain's d.
    degenerative joint d. (DJD)
    degenerative disk (or
        disk) d.
    Degos' d.
    demyelinating d.
    Dercum's d.
    disk (or disc) d.
    discogenic d.
    diskogenic d.
    diverticular d.
    Duhring's d.
    embolic d.
    end-stage renal d.
    Engelmann's d.
    fibrocystic d.
    Flegel's d.
    Fordyce's d.
    Forestier's d.
    Fox-Fordyce d.
    Gaisböck's d.
    gamma chain d.
    gamma chain d.
    Gamna's d.
    Gandy-Nanta d.
    gastroesophageal reflux d.
        (GERD)
    Gaucher's d.
    gestational trophoblastic d.
    Gilbert's d. (zhēl-bārz')
    Glanzmann's d.
    glycogen storage d.
    grass d.
    granulomatous d.
    Graves' d.
    Habermann's d.
    Hailey-Hailey d.
    hand-foot-and-mouth d.
    Hand-Schüller-Christian d.
    Hansen's d.
    d. of the Hapsburgs Hashi-
        moto's d.
    heavy chain d's

disease *(continued)*

Hebra's d.
Heckathorn's d.
hemoglobin C d.
hemoglobin C–thalasse-
    mia d.
hemoglobin D d.
hemoglobin d.
hemoglobin E d.
hemoglobin E–thalasse-
    mia d.
hemoglobin H d.
hemoglobin SC d.
hemoglobin SD d.
hemolytic d. of the new-
    born
hemorrhagic d. of the new-
    born
hepatocellular d.
Herlitz's d.
Hippel's d.
Hippel-Lindau d.
Hirschsprung's d.
Hodgkin's d.
Hodgkin's d., lymphocyte
    depletion type
Hodgkin's d., lymphocyte
    predominance type
Hodgkin's d., mixed cellu-
    larity type
Hodgkin's d., nodular scle-
    rosis type
Hutchinson's d.
hyaline membrane d.
hypertensive cardiovascu-
    lar d.
immunoproliferative small
    intestine d.
ischemic d.
inflammatory bowel d.
Johnson-Stevens d.
Kikuchi's d.
Kikuchi-Fujimoto d.
Kimura's d.
knight's d.
Kyrle's d.
Larsen's d.
Leriche's d.

disease *(continued)*

Letterer-Siwe d.
Lewandowsky-Lutz d.
Lindau's d.
Lindau-von Hippel d.
Lutembacher's d.
Lyell's d.
lymphoproliferative d's
lymphoreticular d's
Madelung's d.
Majocchi's d.
Malibu d.
margarine d.
Mediterranean d.
Meleda d.
Ménétrier's d.
metabolic bone d.
metastatic d.
metastatic bone d.
microdrepanocytic d.
mitral valvular d.
Milton's d.
Morquio's d.
Moschcowitz's d.
mu chain d.
Mucha's d.
Mucha-Habermann d.
mule-spinners' d.
myeloproliferative d's
neoplastic d.
obstructive airway d.
obstructive lung d.
obstructive pulmonary d.
oid-oid d.
Ollier's d.
Osgood-Schlatter d.
Osler's d.
Osler-Vaquez d.
Owren's d.
ox-warble d.
Paget's d.
Paget's d. of the bone
Paget's d. of the breast
Paget's d., extramammary
Paget's d., vulvar
Parkinson's d.
Pellegrini-Stieda d.

disease *(continued)*
    pelvic inflammatory d.
      (PID)
    peptic ulcer d. (PUD)
    Peyronie's d.
    polycystic kidney d.
    polycystic liver d.
    polycystic d. of the ovary
    Pringle's d.
    pulmonary embolic d.
    pulmonary parenchymal d.
    pulmonary thromboembol-
      ic d.
    Quincke's d.
    Reed-Hodgkin d.
    Rh hemolytic d.
    Ritter's d.
    Rosai-Dorfman d.
    sandworm d.
    Schamberg's d.
    Scheuermann's d.
    Schönlein's d.
    sickle cell d.
    sickle cell–hemoglobin C d.
    sickle cell–hemoglobin D d.
    sickle cell–thalassemia d.
    silo-filler's d.
    Simmond's d.
    sinus d.
    Sneddon-Wilkinson d.
    Sternberg's d.
    storage pool d.
    Symmers's d.
    Tay-Sachs d.
    thalassemia–sickle cell d.
    transient respiratory d. of
      the newborn (TRND)
    trophoblastic d.
    Unna-Thost d.
    vagabonds' d.
    vagrants' d.
    Vaquez' d.
    Vaquez-Osler d.
    vascular occlusive d.
    von Hippel's d.
    von Hippel-Lindau d.
    von Recklinghausen's d.
    von Willebrand's d.

disease *(continued)*
    Weber-Christian d.
    Werlhof's d.
    Werner Schultz d.
    Whipple d.
    white spot d.
    Winkler's d.
    Woringer-Kolopp d.

disgerminoma

DISH
    diffuse idiopathic skeletal
      hyperostosis

DISIDA
    disofenin
        DISIDA scan

disintegration
    radioactive d.

disk *(also* disc*)*
    blood d.
    Molnar d.

diskectomy *(also* discectomy*)*

diskogenic *(also* discogenic*)*

diskogram *(also* discogram*)*

diskography *(also* discography*)*

disk space–thecal sac interface

dislocation

disofenin

disorder
    plasma cell d's
    myeloproliferative d's
    lymphoreticular d's
    lymphoproliferative d's
    metabolic bone d.

displacement
    palmar d.
    shaft's width d.
    volar d.

disproportion
    cephalopelvic d. (CPD

disseminated

dissect

dissection
> d. of the aorta
> axillary d.
> axillary lymph node d.
> radical neck d.

dissector

dissepiment

distad

distal

distalis

distally

distance
> interdomal d.
> interpediculate d.
> source-skin d.
> target-skin d.

distantia
> d. intercristalis
> d. interspinosa
> d. intertrochanterica

distended

distention
> gaseous d.
> gastric d.
> jugular venous d.

distortion
> barrel d.
> pincushion d.

distraction

distribution (of an artery, a nerve, etc.)
> dose d.
> loop d.
> d. of a nerve
> skew d.

districhiasis

distrix

diuresis

diuretic

diverticular

diverticulitis

diverticulogram

diverticulosis

diverticulum *pl.* diverticula
> diverticula ampullae ductus deferentis
> bladder d.
> cricopharyngeal d.
> duodenal d.
> epiphrenic d.
> functional d.
> gastric d.
> Hutch d.
> Meckel's d.
> pulsion d.
> traction d.
> Zenker's d.

division
> lingular d. of the left lung

D5 $\frac{1}{2}$ normal saline

DMFO (eflornithene)

Dobbhoff
> mercury tip of the D. tube
> tip of the D. tube
> D. tube

dobutamine

docetaxel

dolabrate

dolabriform

dolichocephalic

dolichocephaly

dolichoderus

dolichofacial

dolichohieric

dolichokerkic

dolichoknemic

dolichomorphic

dolichoprosopic

domain
    kringle d.

Dombrock blood group

dome
    d's of the hemidiaphragms
    d. of the liver

donor
    universal d.

Doppler
    color D. echocardiography
    color flow D. imaging
    continuous wave D. echo-
        cardiography
    echocardiography
    pulsed wave D. echocardi-
        ography
    D. studies

Dorello's canal

Dorothy Reed cells

dorsa (plural of dorsum)

dorsad

dorsal

dorsalis

dorsiduct

dorsiflexion

dorsimesal

dorsocephalad

dorsointercostal

dorsolateral

dorsolumbar

dorsomedian

dorsomesial

dorsonuchal

dorsoradial

dorsoventrad

dorsoventral

dorsum *pl.* dorsa
    d. linguae
    d. manus
    d. nasi
    d. pedis
    d. penis
    d. of penis
    d. sellae

dose
    absorbed d.
    air d.
    cumulative d.
    cumulative radiation d.
    depth d.
    doubling d.
    epilating d.
    erythema d.
    exit d.
    exposure d.
    fatal d.
    integral d.
    integral absorbed d.
    lethal d.
    lethal d., median
    maximum d.
    maximum permissible d.
    maximum tolerated d.
    organ tolerance d.
    permissible d.
    radiation absorbed d.
    skin d.
    threshold d.
    threshold erythema d.
    tissue d.
    tolerance d.
    volume d.

dosimeter

dosimetric

dosimetrist

dosimetry
    biological d.

dosimetry *(continued)*
    physical d.

Douglas
    line of D.
    semicircular line of D.

Down syndrome

down

Doxil

doxorubicin
    d. hydrochloride

Drabkin's solution

drain
    Penrose d.
    radiopaque d.
    rubber d.

drainage
    gravity d.
    lymphatic d.
    percutaneous d.
    percutaneous biliary d.

drepanocytosis

Dresbach's syndrome

dressing
    occlusive d.

drip
    Reno M d.

dromostanolone propionate

dropacism

drostanolone propionate

drug-induced

Drummond

artery of Drummond

drumstick

drusen

DSA
    digital subtraction angiography

DTIC, Dtic (dacarbazine)

DTIC-Dome

dualism

duazomycin

Dubreuilh
    circumscribed precancerous melanosis of D.

ductal

duct
    aberrant d.
    alimentary d.
    biliary d's
    chyliferous d.
    common bile d.
    common hepatic d.
    cystic d.
    efferent d.
    excretory d.
    extrahepatic d's
    hepatic d.
    intercalated d.
    interlobular d's
    intrahepatic d's
    lymphatic d's
    lymphatic d., left
    lymphatic d., right
    major intrahepatic d's
    nasolacrimal d.
    d. of Pecquet
    salivary d.
    secretory d.
    Stensen's d.
    sudoriferous d.
    sweat d.
    thoracic d.
    thoracic d., right
    Wharton's d.

ductule
    aberrant d's

ductulus *pl.* ductuli
    ductuli aberrantes
    d. aberrans inferior
    d. aberrans superior

ductulus *(continued)*
  ductuli efferentes testis
  ductuli excretorii glandulae
    lacrimalis
  ductuli prostatici
  ductuli transversi epoö-
    phori
ductus
  d. arteriosus
  d. biliaris
  d. choledochus
  d. cochlearis
  d. cysticus
  d. deferens
  d. deferens vestigialis
  d. ejaculatorius
  d. endolymphaticus
  d. epididymidis
  d. excretorius glandulae
    seminalis
  d. excretorius glandulae
    vesiculosae
  d. excretorius vesiculae
    seminalis
  d. glandulae bulboureth-
    ralis
  d. hepaticus communis
  d. hepaticus dexter
  d. hepaticus sinister
  d. incisivus
  d. lactiferi
  d. lobi caudati dexter
  d. lobi caudati sinister
  d. longitudinalis epoöphori
  d. lymphatici
  d. lymphaticus dexter
  d. nasolacrimalis
  d. pancreaticus
  d. pancreaticus accesso-
    rius
  d. paraurethrales urethrae
    femininae
  d. paraurethrales urethrae
    masculinae
  patent d. arteriosus (PDA)
  d. reuniens
  d. semicirculares
  d. semicircularis anterior

ductus *(continued)*
  d. semicircularis lateralis
  d. semicircularis posterior
  d. sudoriferus
  d. thoracicus
  d. thoracicus dexter
  d. thyroglossalis
  d. utriculosaccularis
  d. venosus

Duffy blood group

Duke
  D's method
  D's test

Dukes' classification

duodenitis
  Crohn's d.

duodenogram

duodenum

Dupuytren's contracture

dura mater
  d. m. of brain
  d. m. cranialis
  d. m. encephali
  d. m. of spinal cord
  d. m. spinalis

Duranest

dust
  blood d.
  chromatin d.

DVT
  deep venous thrombosis

dwarf
  achondroplastic d.

DWI
  diffusion weighted images

DXA
  dual energy x-ray absorp-
    tion
      DXA scan

Dyclone

dyclonine hydrochloride

dyschondroplasia

dyschromia

dyscrasia
    blood d.
    plasma cell d's

dysembryoma

dysentery
    amebic d.

dyserythropoiesis

dysfibrinogenemia

dysfunction
    neuromuscular d.

dysgerminoma

dyshematopoiesis

dyshematopoietic

dyshemopoiesis

dyshemopoietic

dyshesion

dyshidrosis

dyshydrosis

dysidrosis

dyskeratoma
    warty d.

dyskeratosis
    d. congenita
    congenital d.
    isolated d. follicularis

dyskeratotic

dysmotility
    esophageal d.

dysmyelopoiesis

dysostosis
    cleidocranial d.

dysphagia

dysphasia

dyspigmentation

dysplasia
    cervical d.
    d. of cervix
    fibromuscular d.
    fibrous d.
    mammary d.

dysplastic

dyspnea
    paroxysmal nocturnal d.
        (PND

dyspneic

dyspoiesis

dysproteinemia

dysrhythmia

dysrhythmic

dyssebacea

dyssebacia

dystrophia
    d. mediana canaliformis
    d. unguis mediana canali-
        formis
    d. unguium

dystocia

dystrophic

dystrophy
    muscular dystrophy

dysuria

E antigen

Eaton-Lambert syndrome

Ebstein's pearl

eburnation

ecchondroma

ecchondrosis
  e. physaliphora

ecchymosis *pl.* ecchymoses

eccrine

eccrisis

echinosis

echo
  homogeneous liver echoes
  spin e.

echocardiography
  contrast e.
  Doppler e.
  Doppler e., color
  Doppler e., continuous
    wave
  Doppler e., pulsed wave
  M-mode e.
  two-dimensional e.

echogenic

echogenicity

echogram

echography

echolucent

echo-ranging

echotexture

écorché

ectad

ectal

ectasia

ectatic

ecthyma
  contagious e.
  e. gangrenosum

ecthymiform

ectodermosis
  e. erosiva pluriorificialis

ectoentad

ectopia
  cross-fused e.

ectopic

ectopy
  cross-fused e.

eczema
  allergic e.
  asteatotic e.
  atopic e.
  e. craquelé
  dyshidrotic e.
  flexural e.
  e. herpeticum
  infantile e.
  e. intertrigo
  e. marginatum
  nummular e.
  seborrheic e.
  e. vaccinatum
  xerotic e.

eczematization

eczematogenic

eczematoid

eczematous

ED50

edema
  alveolar e.
  angioneurotic e.
  circumscribed e.
  frank pulmonary e.
  giant e.
  hereditary angioneurotic e.
  interstitial e.
  lymphatic e.

edema *(continued)*
    Milton's e.
    pedal e.
    periodic e.
    periorbital e.
    periosteal e.
    peripheral e.
    pretibial e.
    pulmonary e.
    Quincke's e.

edematous

edentulous

edge
    heaped-up e's
    shelving e.

effect
    Bohr e.
    Compton e.
    Fahraeus-Lindqvist e.
    Haldane e.
    heel e.
    isomorphic e.
    Mach e.
    mass e.
    tramlike e. in the liver

effectiveness
    relative biological e.

efferential

efflorescence

effluvium
    anagen e.
    telogen e.

effort
    shallow inspiratory e.

effusion
    layering-out of pleural e.
    pericardial e.
    pleural e.

eflornithine hydrochloride

Efudex

Eisenmenger complex

eisodic

EKG
    electrocardiogram
        EKG leads

Eklund view

Elant's triangle

elastica

elastofibroma

elastoidosis
    nodular e.

elastolysis
    generalized e.
    perifollicular e.
    postinflammatory e.

elastoma
    juvenile e.

elastosis
    actinic e.
    nodular e. of Favre and Ra-
        couchot
    e. perforans serpiginosa
    perforating e.
    senile e.
    solar e.

electroanesthesia

electrodermal

electrode
    e's over the chest wall
    monitoring e's

electrokymogram

electrokymograph

electrokymography

electrolysis

electrolytic

electrolyzable

electrometer

electromyogram (EMG)

electron
    Auger e.

electron *(continued)*
    emission e.
    free e.
    valence e.

electroscope

eleidin

element
    fibroglandular e's
    formed e's of the blood
    glandular e's
    posterior e's
    stromal e's
    tracer e.

elephantiasis
    e. neuromatosa

elevated (right or left) hemidia-
    phragm

elevation
    diaphragmatic e.
    e. of the floor of the uri-
      nary bladder
    periosteal e.
    tactile e's

elinin

Elliot's sign

elliptical

elliptocytosis
    hereditary e.
    spherocytic e.

elliptocytotic

elongation

Elspar

eman

emanation
    actinium e.
    thorium e.

emanating

embolism
    lymph e.
    lymphogenous e.

embolism *(continued)*
    pulmonary e.
    tumor e.

embolization

embolus *pl.* emboli
    cancer e.
    pulmonary e.
    tumor e.

embryoma
    e. of kidney

embryomorphous

emergence

emesis

Emete-con

EMG
    electromyogram

EMI scanner

emigration

eminence
    articular e. of temporal
      bone
    cruciate e.
    cruciform e. of occipital
      bone
    frontal e.
    jugular e.
    hypothenar e.
    malar e.
    olivary e. of sphenoid bone
    parietal e.
    thenar e.

eminentia *pl.* eminentiae
    e. arcuata
    e. articularis ossis tempo-
      ralis
    e. collateralis ventriculi lat-
      eralis
    e. conchae
    e. cruciata
    e. cruciformis
    e. fossae triangularis auric-
      ulae
    e. frontalis

eminentia *(continued)*
 e. hypothenaris
 e. iliopubica
 e. intercondylaris
 e. jugularis
 e. maxillae
 e. medialis fossae rhomboi-
  deae
 e. parietalis
 e. pyramidalis
 e. scaphae
 e. thenaris

emission
 positron e.

emphysema
 bullous e.
 compensatory e.
 cutaneous e.
 mediastinal e.
 pulmonary e.
 subcutaneous e.

empyema

emulsion
 photographic e.

emunctory

enameloblastoma

enarthrosis

en bloc

encasement

encephalitis

encephalocele

encephalography

encephaloid

encephaloma

encephalon

encephalopathy

enchondroma
 multiple congenital e's

enchondromatosis
 multiple e.

enchondromatosis *(continued)*
 skeletal e.

enchondromatous

enchondrosarcoma

enchondrosis

encroachment

endarterectomy

endocardial

endocarditis

endocardium

endoceliac

endocorpuscular

endoepidermal

endoglobar

endoglobular

endolympha

endometria

endometrioid

endometrium

endometrioma

endometriosis

endometry

end-on

endoneurium

endopelvic

endophytic

endoradiography

endosalpingoma

endoscanning

endoscopic

endoscopy

endosonography

endosteoma

endosteum

endostoma

endothelia (plural of endothelium)

endothelioblastoma

endothelioma
    e. angiomatosum
    e. angiomatosum
    dural e.
    perithelial e.

endotheliomatosis

endotheliosarcoma

endothelium *pl.* endothelia

endothoracic

endotracheal (ET)
    e. junction

end-point of stress

enema
    barium e.
    contrast e.
    double-contrast e.
    Fleet e. (*not* Fleet's)
    single contrast barium e.
    small bowel e.

energy
    atomic e.
    nuclear e.

enflurane

enforcer
    Cook e.

Engelmann's disease

engorged

engorgement

enhancement
    contrast e.
    edge e.
    gyral e.

enlargement
    biventricular e.

enlargement *(continued)*
    cardiac e.
    chamber e.
    hilar e.
    marked e.

enolase
    neuron-specific e.

en plaque

ensiform

entad

ental

enteritis
    regional e.

enteroclysis

enterocolitis
    necrotizing e. (NEC)

enterorenal

Entero Vu

enthesis

enthesitis

enthesopathy

entity

entoectad

entomion

eosinocyte

eosinopenia

eosinophil

eosinophile

eosinophilia

eosinophilic

eosinophilopoietin

eosinophilosis

eosinophilous

eosinotactic

epactal

epaxial

ependyma

ependymoblastoma

ependymocytoma

ependymoma

ephelides

ephelis

epicarcinogen

epichlorohydrin

epicondylar

epicondyle

epicondylus *pl.* epicondylitis
    e. lateralis femoris
    e. lateralis humeri
    e. medialis femoris
    e. medialis humeri

epicranium

epicranius

epiderm

epidermal

epidermatitis

epidermic

epidermicula

epidermidalization

epidermis *pl.* epidermides

epidermitis

epidermodysplasia
    e. verruciformis

epidermoid

epidermoidoma

epidermolysis
    e. bullosa
    e. bullosa, acquired
    e. bullosa acquisita
    e. bullosa dystrophica

epidermolysis *(continued)*
    e. bullosa dystrophica, albopapuloid
    e. bullosa dystrophica, dominant
    e. bullosa dystrophica, dysplastic
    e. bullosa dystrophica, hyperplastic
    e. bullosa dystrophica, polydysplastic
    e. bullosa dystrophica, recessive
    e. bullosa hereditaria
    e. bullosa, junctional
    e. bullosa letalis
    e. bullosa simplex
    e. bullosa simplex, generalized
    e. bullosa simplex, localized
    toxic bullous e.

epidermolytic

epidermomycosis

epidermophytid

epidermophytosis

epididymis *pl.* epididymides

epidurography

epiduroscopy

epifascial

epigastric

epigastrium

epiglottis

epiglottitis

epilate

epilation

epimysium

epinephrine

epineurium

epiphyseal

epiphysis *pl.* epiphyses
    femoral e.
    fetal e's
    e's at the knees

epiphysitis
    juvenile e.

epipleural

epipodophyllotoxin

epirubicin

episode
    syncopal e.

epispinal

episplenitis

epithalamus

epithelia (plural of epithelium)

epithelialization

epitheliogenesis
    e. imperfecta

epithelioma
    e. adenoides cysticum
    basal cell e.
    benign calcifying e.
    calcified e.
    calcifying e.
    calcifying e. of Malherbe
    chorionic e.
    diffuse e.
    Ferguson Smith e.
    Malherbe's calcifying e.
    malignant e.
    multiple self-healing squa-
        mous e.
    sebaceous e.
    self-healing squamous e.

epitheliomatosis

epitheliomatous

epithelite

epithelium *pl.* epithelia
    e. anterius corneae
    e. lentis

epithelium *(continued)*
    e. mucosae
    e. pigmentosum iridis
    e. posterius corneae

epitrochlear

epitympanum

Epogen

eponychium

epoophoron

epulis *pl.* epulides
    congenital e.
    giant cell e.
    e. gigantocellularis
    e. granulomatosa
    e. of newborn

epulofibroma

epuloid

equator
    e. bulbi oculi
    e. lentis

equatorial

equiaxial

equilibrium
    radioactive e.

equivalent
    aluminum e.
    concrete e.
    dose e.
    lead e.

equivocal finding

Erb's paralysis

ERCP
    endoscopic retrograde
        cholangiopancreatogra-
        phy

erectile

erector

Ergamisol

ergometer

erose

erosio
    e. interdigitalis blastomyce-
        tica

erosion
    bony e.

erosive

ERPF
    effective renal plasma flow

eruption
    creeping e.
    drug e.
    fixed e.
    fixed drug e.
    Kaposi's varicelliform e.
    polymorphous light e.
    seabather's e.
    serum e.

eruptive

erysipelas
    gangrenous e.
    necrotizing e.

erysipelatous

erysipeloid

erysipelotoxin

erythema
    e. annulare
    e. annulare centrifugum
    e. annulare rheumaticum
    e. caloricum
    e. chromicum figuratum
        melanodermicum
    e. circinatum
    e. circinatum rheumaticum
    cold e.
    diaper e.
    e. dyschromicum perstans
    e. elevatum diutinum
    figurate e.
    e. figuratum
    e. figuratum perstans
    e. fugax
    gyrate e.

erythema *(continued)*
    e. gyratum
    e. gyratum perstans
    e. gyratum repens
    e. ab igne
    e. induratum
    e. iris
    Jacquet's e.
    e. marginatum
    e. marginatum rheumati-
        cum
    e. migrans
    e. multiforme
    e. multiforme majus
    e. multiforme minus
    necrolytic migratory e.
    e. necroticans
    e. nodosum
    e. nodosum leprosum
    e. nodosum migrans
    palmar e., e palmare
    e. pernio
    e. streptogenes
    toxic e.
    e. toxicum
    e. toxicum neonatorum

erythematoedematous

erythematous

erythemogenic

erythrasma

erythremia

erythrism

erythristic

erythroblast
    acidophilic e.
    basophilic e.
    early e.
    eosinophilic e.
    intermediate e.
    definitive e's
    late e.
    polychromatic e.
    polychromatophilic e.
    primitive e's
    orthochromatic e.

erythroblast *(continued)*
    oxyphilic e.
    primordial e's

erythroblastemia

erythroblastic

erythroblastoma

erythroblastopenia
    transient e. of childhood

erythroblastosis
    e. fetalis
    e. neonatorum

erythroblastotic

erythrocatalysis

erythroclasis

erythroclastic

erythrocyanosis

erythrocytapheresis

erythrocyte
    immature e.
    normochromic e.
    nucleated e.
    polychromatic e.
    polychromatophilic e.

erythrocythemia

erythrocytic

erythrocytoblast

erythrocytolysin

erythrocytolysis

erythrocytometer

erythrocytometry

erythrocytopenia

erythrocytophagous

erythrocytophagy

erythrocytopoiesis

erythrocytorrhexis

erythrocytoschisis

erythrocytosis
    benign e.
    stress e.

erythrodegenerative

erythroderma
    e. desquamativum
    e. psoriaticum
    Sézary e.

erythrodermia

erythrogenesis
    e. imperfecta

erythrogenic

erythroid

erythrokatalysis

erythrokeratodermia

erythrokinetics

erythroleukemia
    acute e.

erythroleukothrombocythemia

erythrolysin

erythrolysis

erythrometer

erythrometry

erythron

erythroneocytosis

erythropenia

erythrophage

erythrophagia

erythrophagocytic

erythrophagocytosis

erythrophagous

erythrophore

erythroplakia
    speckled e.

erythroplasia
    e. of Queyrat

erythroplasia *(continued)*
    Zoon's e.

erythroplastid

erythropoiesis

erythropoietic

erythropoietin

erythrorrhexis

érythrose
    é. péribuccale pigmentaire
        of Brocq

erythrosis

erythrostasis

eschar

escutcheon

eseptate

esophageal

esophagitis
    reflux e.

esophagogastroscopy

esophagogastric (EG)

esophagogram
    barium-water e.

esophagography

esophagotracheal

esophagram

esophagus

esthesioneuroblastoma

estramustine phosphate

estrophilin

ET
    endotracheal
        ET junction
        ET tube

ether
    anesthetic e.
    diethyl e.

etherization

etherize

Ethiodol

ethmoiditis

ethopropazine hydrochloride

Ethrane

ethyl
    e. aminobenzoate
    e. chloride
    e. ether

ethylene
    e. dibromide
    e. dichloride
    e. oxide

ethyleneimine

ethylenimine

Ethyol

etidocaine hydrochloride

etidronate

etiolation

etiology

etoposide

eukeratin

Euproctis

eusplenia

euthymism

evacuation

evagination

Evans
    E. blue
    E's syndrome

eventration of the (left or right)
    hemidiaphragm

eversion
    nipple e.

evert

evertor

evidence
  presumptive e.
  scintigraphic e.

Ewald's node

Ewing
  E's sarcoma
  E's tumor

exacerbation

exametazime

examination
  B-mode ultrasound e.
  cystoscopic e.
  double-contrast e.
  gastroscopic e.
  mammographic e.
  proctoscopic e.
  sigmoidoscopic e.
  small bowel follow-
    through e.

exanthem
  Boston e.

exanthema *pl.* exanthemata

exanthematous

excavatio *pl.* excavationes
  e. disci
  e. rectouterina
  e. rectovesicalis
  e. vesicouterina

excavation
  ischiorectal e.
  rectoischiadic e.

excavationes (plural of excavatio)

exchange
  plasma e.

excision
  disc e.

excision *(continued)*
  disk e.
  intracapsular e.
  marginal e.
  radical e.
  wide e.

excitation

exclave

excoriation
  neurotic e.

excrescence

excretion

excursion

exemia

exercise
  flexion and extension exer-
    cises

exfoliation
  lamellar e. of newborn

exitus
  e. pelvis

exophytic

exoserosis

exostosis *pl.* exostoses
  e. bursata
  e. cartilaginea
  hereditary multiple e's
  ivory e.
  multiple e's
  multiple cartilaginous e's
  multiple osteocartilaginous
    e's
  osteocartilaginous e.
  subungual e.

exostotic

expander
  plasma volume e.

expansion of the lungs

experiment
  Müller's e.

expiration

exposure
    acute e.
    air e.
    chronic e.

exsanguinotransfusion

exstrophy

extender
    artificial plasma e.

extension

extensor

externus

extima

extirpation of the bladder

extra-abdominal

extra-arachnoid

extrabulbar

extracapsular

extracorpuscular

extraluminal

extralymphatic

extramural

extraperineal

extraperitoneal

extrarenal

extraserous

extrathoracic

extratubal

extrauterine

extravasation

extremital

extremitas *pl.* extremitates
    e. acromialis claviculae
    e. anterior lienis
    e. anterior splenis
    e. inferior
    e. inferior lienis
    e. inferior renis
    e. inferior testis
    e. posterior lienis
    e. posterior splenis
    e. sternalis claviculae
    e. superior
    e. superior lienis
    e. superior renis
    e. superior testis
    e. tubalis ovarii
    e. tubaria ovarii
    e. uterina ovarii

extremitates (plural of extremitas)

extremity
    lower e.
    upper e.

extrinsic

extrusion
    disc e.
    disk e.

exudate
    pleural e.

exudative

fabella

Faber's syndrome

fabism

face
  moon f.

face-lift

facet
  articular f's
  f. for malleus
  odd f.

facette (variant of facette)

facial

facies
  f. anterior corneae
  f. anterior glandulae supra-
    renalis
  f. anterior iridis
  f. anterior lateralis humeri
  f. anterior lentis
  f. anterior corporis maxil-
    lae
  f. anterior medialis humeri
  f. anterior palpebrae
  f. anterior partis petrosae
    ossis temporalis
  f. anterior patellae
  f. anterior prostatae
  f. anterior pyramidis ossis
    temporalis
  f. anterior radii
  f. anterior renis
  f. anterior scapulae
  f. anterior ulnae
  f. anteroinferior corporis
    pancreatis
  f. anterolateralis cartila-
    ginis arytenoideae
  f. anterolateralis humeri
  f. anteromedialis humeri
  f. anterosuperior corporis
    pancreatis
  f. articularis acromialis
    claviculae

facies *(continued)*
  f. articularis anterior dentis
  f. articularis arytenoidea
    cartilaginis cricoideae
  f. articularis calcanea ante-
    rior tali
  f. articularis calcanea me-
    dia tali
  f. articularis calcanea pos-
    terior tali
  f. articularis capitis costae
  f. articularis capitis fibulae
  f. articularis carpalis radii
  f. articularis cartilaginis ar-
    ytenoidea
  f. articularis cuboidea cal-
    canei
  f. articularis fibularis tibiae
  f. articularis fossae mandi-
    bularis
  f. articularis inferior atlan-
    tis
  f. articularis inferior tibiae
  f. articularis navicularis tali
  f. articularis ossium
  f. articularis patellae
  f. articularis posterior den-
    tis
  f. articularis sternalis clavi-
    culae
  f. articularis superior atlan-
    tis
  f. articularis superior tibiae
  f. articularis superior verte-
    brae
  f. articularis talaris anterior
    calcanei
  f. articularis talaris media
    calcanei
  f. articularis talaris poste-
    rior calcanei
  f. articularis thyroidea car-
    tilaginis cricoideae
  f. articularis tuberculi cos-
    tae
  f. auricularis ossis ilii
  f. auricularis ossis ilium

facies *(continued)*
- f. auricularis ossis sacri
- f. cerebralis alae majoris
- f. cerebralis ossis frontalis
- f. cerebralis ossis parietalis
- f. cerebralis partis squamosae ossis temporalis
- f. colica lienis
- f. colica splenis
- f. costalis pulmonis
- f. costalis scapulae
- cushingoid f.
- f. diaphragmatica cordis
- f. diaphragmatica hepatis
- f. diaphragmatica lienis
- f. diaphragmatica pulmonis
- f. diaphragmatica splenis
- f. dorsales digitorum manus
- f. dorsales digitorum pedis
- f. dorsalis ossis sacri
- f. externa ossis frontalis
- f. externa ossis parietalis
- f. frontalis ossis frontalis
- f. gastrica lienis
- f. gastrica splenis
- f. glutealis ossis ilii
- f. glutea ossis ilii
- f. inferior linguae
- f. inferior pancreatis
- f. inferior partis petrosae
  ossis temporalis
- f. inferior pyramidis ossis
  temporalis
- f. inferolateralis prostatae
- f. infratemporalis corporis
  maxillae
- f. interlobaris pulmonis
- f. interna ossis frontalis
- f. interna ossis parietalis
- f. intervertebralis
- f. intestinalis uteri
- f. lateralis fibulae
- f. lateralis ossis zygomatici
- f. lateralis ovarii
- f. lateralis radii
- f. lateralis testis
- f. lateralis tibiae

facies *(continued)*
- leonine f.
- f. leontina
- f. lunata acetabuli
- f. malleolaris lateralis tali
- f. malleolaris medialis tali
- f. maxillaris alae majoris
- f. maxillaris laminae perpendicularis ossis palatini
- f. medialis cartilaginis arytenoideae
- f. medialis fibulae
- f. medialis et inferior hemispherii cerebri
- f. medialis ovarii
- f. medialis testis
- f. medialis tibiae
- f. medialis ulnae
- f. mediastinalis pulmonis
- f. nasalis laminae horizontalis ossis palatini
- f. nasalis laminae perpendicularis ossis palatini
- f. nasalis corporis maxillae
- f. orbitalis alae magnae
- f. orbitalis alae majoris
- f. orbitalis corporis maxillae
- f. orbitalis ossis frontalis
- f. orbitalis ossis zygomatici
- f. palatina laminae horizontalis ossis palatini
- f. palmares digitorum manus
- f. parietalis ossis parietalis
- f. pelvica ossis sacri
- f. pelvina ossis sacri
- f. plantares digitorum pedis
- f. poplitea femoris
- f. posterior cartilaginis arytenoideae
- f. posterior corneae
- f. posterior fibulae
- f. posterior glandulae suprarenalis
- f. posterior humeri
- f. posterior iridis
- f. posterior lentis

facies *(continued)*
- f. posterior corporis pancreatis
- f. posterior corporis pancreatis
- f. posterior palpebrae
- f. posterior partis petrosae ossis temporalis
- f. posterior prostatae
- f. posterior pyramidis ossis temporalis
- f. posterior radii
- f. posterior renis
- f. posterior scapulae
- f. posterior tibiae
- f. posterior ulnae
- f. pulmonalis cordis
- f. pulmonalis dextra/sinistra cordis
- f. renalis glandulae suprarenalis
- f. renalis lienis
- f. renalis splenis
- f. sacropelvica ossis ilii
- f. sternocostalis cordis
- f. superior trochleae tali
- f. superolateralis cerebri
- f. superolateralis hemispherii cerebri
- f. symphyseos ossis pubis
- f. symphysialis ossis pubis
- f. temporalis alae majoris
- f. temporalis ossis frontalis
- f. temporalis ossis zygomatici
- f. temporalis partis squamosae ossis temporalis
- f. urethralis penis
- f. vesicalis uteri
- f. visceralis hepatis
- f. visceralis lienis
- f. visceralis splenis

faciobrachial

facioscapulohumeral

factor
- f. I
- f. II
- f. III

factor *(continued)*
- f. IV
- f. V
- f. VI
- f. VII
- f. VIII
- f. IX
- f. X
- f. XI
- f. XII
- f. XIII
- accelerator f.
- activation f.
- adherence f.
- antihemophilic f.
- antihemophilic f. A
- antihemophilic f. B
- antihemophilic f. C
- autocrine growth f.
- Christmas f.
- coagulation f's
- colony-stimulating f's
- contact f.
- epidermal growth f.
- epidermal growth f., human
- epithelial growth f.
- erythropoietic stimulating f.
- fibrin-stabilizing f.
- Fitzgerald f.
- Fletcher f.
- glass f.
- granulocyte colony-stimulating f.
- granulocyte-macrophage colony-stimulating f.
- Hageman f.
- hematopoietic growth f's
- labile f.
- Laki-Lorand f.
- macrophage colony-stimulating f.
- macrophage-derived growth f.
- platelet f's
- platelet f. 1
- platelet f. 2
- platelet f. 3
- platelet f. 4

factor *(continued)*
    platelet-derived growth f.
    Prower f.
    Rh f.
    Rhesus f.
    stable f.
    Stuart f.
    Stuart-Prower f.
    tissue f.
    transforming growth f.
    tumor-angiogenesis f.
    von Willebrand's f.

faex *pl.* feces

fagopyrism

Fahraeus
    F. method
    F.-Lindqvist effect

failure
    bone marrow f.
    cardiac f.
    congestive heart f. (CHF)
    frank congestive heart f.
    heart f.
    kidney f.
    passive congestive heart f.
    renal f.

falcate

falces (plural of falx)

falcial

falciform

falcular

falx *pl.* falces
    f. cerebelli
    f. cerebri
    f. inguinalis
    f. of cerebrum

Fallot
    tetralogy of F.

Fanconi
    F.'s anemia
    F.'s syndrome

Farre's tubercles

fascia *pl.* fasciae
    antebrachial f.
    f. antebrachii
    aponeurotic f.
    f. axillaris
    axillary f.
    f. brachii
    buccinator f.
    f. buccopharyngea
    buccopharyngeal f.
    f. buccopharyngealis
    f. cervicalis
    clavipectoral f.
    f. clavipectoralis
    f. clitoridis
    f. of clitoris
    cremasteric f.
    f. cremasterica
    f. cribrosa
    f. cruris
    deep f.
    deltoid f.
    f. deltoidea
    dorsal f. of hand
    f. dorsalis manus
    f. dorsalis pedis
    endopelvic f.
    f. endopelvina
    endothoracic f.
    f. endothoracica
    external intercostal f.
    extraperitoneal f.
    f. extraperitonealis
    fibroareolar f.
    Gerota's f.
    hypogastric f.
    f. iliaca
    f. inferior diaphragmatis
      pelvis
    f. lata
    masseteric f.
    f. masseterica
    muscular fasciae of eye
    fasciae musculares bulbi
    fasciae musculares occuli
    f. nuchae
    nuchal f.
    f. nuchalis

fascia *(continued)*
   obturator f.
   f. obturatoria
   orbital fasciae
   fasciae orbitales
   f. parietalis thoracis
   parietal f. of thorax
   parotid f.
   f. parotidea
   pectoral f.
   f. pectoralis
   pelvic f.
   pelvic f., parietal
   f. pelvica parietalis
   f. pelvica
   f. pelvis
   f. pelvis parietalis
   f. pelvis visceralis
   f. penis profunda
   f. penis superficialis
   f. perinei superficialis
   peritoneoperineal f.
   f. peritoneoperinealis
   f. pharyngobasilaris
   phrenicopleural f.
   f. phrenicopleuralis
   f. profunda
   f. prostatae
   f. of prostate
   rectoabdominal f.
   renal f.
   f. renalis
   Richet's f.
   Scarpa's f.
   f. spermatica externa
   f. spermatica interna
   superficial f.
   f. superficialis
   f. superior diaphragmatis
      pelvis
   temporal f.
   f. temporalis
   thoracic f.
   f. thoracica
   f. thoracolumbalis
   thoracolumbar f.
   f. transversalis
   transverse f.
   triangular f. of Macalister

fascia *(continued)*
   Treitz's f.

fasciae (plural of fasciae)

fascial

fascicle

fascicular

fasciculated

fasciculation

fasciculus *pl.* fasciculi
   f. atrioventricularis
   f. cuneatus medullae oblon-
      gatae
   f. cuneatus medullae spina-
      lis
   f. gracilis medullae oblon-
      gatae
   f. gracilis medullae spinalis
   f. interfascicularis
   f. lateralis plexus brachialis
   f. longitudinalis dorsalis
   f. longitudinalis inferior
      cerebri
   fasciculi longitudinales liga-
      menti cruciformis atlantis
   f. longitudinalis medialis
   f. longitudinalis posterior
   f. longitudinalis superior
      cerebri
   f. mammillotegmentalis
   f. mammillothalamicus
   f. medialis plexus brachi-
      alis
   f. medialis telencephali
   f. occipitofrontalis inferior
   f. occipitofrontalis superior
   f. posterior plexus brachi-
      alis
   f. proprius anterior medul-
      lae spinalis
   f. proprius lateralis medul-
      lae spinalis
   f. proprius posterior me-
      dullae spinalis
   f. semilunaris
   septomarginal f.
   f. septomarginalis

fasciculus *(continued)*
    f. subcallosus
    f. subthalamicus
    f. sulcomarginalis
    f. thalamicus
    fasciculi transversi aponeu-
        rosis plantaris
    unciform f.
    uncinate f.
    f. uncinatus

fasciitis
    intravascular f.
    necrotizing f.
    nodular f.
    plantar f.
    proliferative f.
    pseudosarcomatous f.

fasciola *pl.* fasciolae

fasciolar

fast spin echo (FSE)

fat
    mesenteric f.

fat saturated images (*may be dictated* "fat sat")

fauces

faveolar

faveolate

faveolus

favid

favism

Favre-Racouchot syndrome

febrile

fecal

feces
    inspissated f.
    semiliquid f.

fecalith

felon

Felty's syndrome

femora

femtocurie

femur

fenestra *pl.* fenestrae
    f. vestibuli

fenestrae (plural of fenestra)

fenestrated

fenestration

fentanyl citrate

Ferguson Smith epithelioma

ferpentetate

Ferrata's cell

ferriheme

ferritin

ferroheme

ferrokinetic

ferrokinetics

ferrum

fetal

fetography

fetometry
    roentgen f.

α-fetoprotein

fetus

Feuerstein-Mims syndrome

fever
    eruptive f.
    exanthematous f.
    Oroya f.
    rheumatic f.

fiber
    decussating f's
    hair f.

fiber *(continued)*
    Herxheimer's f's
    U f's

fibra *pl.* fibrae
    fibrae arcuatae cerebri
    fibrae arcuatae externae
      anteriores
    fibrae arcuatae externae
      posteriores
    fibrae arcuatae internae
    f. associationis
    fibrae associationis breves
    fibrae associationis longae
    fibrae associationis telence-
      phali
    fibrae circulares musculi
      ciliaris
    f. commissuralis
    fibrae commissurales telen-
      cephali
    fibrae corticopontinae
    fibrae corticoreticulares
    fibrae corticorubrales
    fibrae corticospinales
    fibrae corticothalamicae
    fibrae frontopontinae
    fibrae intercrurales
    fibrae intrathalamicae
    fibrae lentis
    fibrae meridionales musculi
      ciliaris
    fibrae obliquae gastricae
    fibrae obliquae ventriculi
    fibrae paraventriculohypo-
      physiales
    fibrae parietopontinae
    fibrae periventriculares
    fibrae pontis longitudinales
    fibrae pontis transversae
    fibrae pontocerebellares
    f. projectionis
    fibrae striae terminalis
    fibrae supraopticohypo-
      physiales
    fibrae temporopontinae
    fibrae thalamoparietales
    fibrae zonulares

fibrae (plural of fibra)

fibril
    anchoring f.

fibrillation
    paroxysmal atrial f.

fibrin
    stroma f.

fibrinase

fibrinocellular

fibrinogen

fibrinogenase

fibrinogenemia

fibrinogenesis

fibrinogenic

fibrinogenolysis

fibrinogenolytic

fibrinogenopenia

fibrinogenopenic

fibrinogenous

fibrinolysin

fibrinolysis

fibrinolytic

fibrinopeptide

fibrinoplatelet

fibrinous

fibroadenoma
    giant f. of the breast
    intracanalicular f.
    pericanalicular f.

fibroangioma
    nasopharyngeal f.

fibroblastoma
    perineural f.

fibrocalcareous

fibrocarcinoma

fibrocartilage
    basal f.
    basilar f.

fibrocartilago *pl.* fibrocarti-
lagines
    f. basilaris
    f. basalis

fibrocaseous

fibrochondroma

fibroenchondroma

fibroepithelioma
    premalignant f.

fibrofolliculoma

fibroid
    uterine f's

fibrolipoma

fibrolipomatous

fibroma
    ameloblastic f.
    cementifying f.
    cemento-ossifying f.
    chondromyxoid f.
    cutaneous f.
    cystic f.
    desmoplastic f.
    f. durum
    hard f.
    intracanalicular f.
    juvenile nasopharyngeal f.
    f. molle
    f. molluscum
    f. myxomatodes
    nonodontogenic f.
    nonossifying f.
    nonosteogenic f.
    odontogenic f.
    odontogenic f., peripheral
    ossifying f.
    ossifying f. of bone
    ossifying f., peripheral
    parasitic f.
    f. pendulum

fibroma *(continued)*
    perifollicular f.
    periungual f.
    soft f.
    telangiectatic f.
    f. thecocellulare xanthoma-
      todes
    f. xanthoma

fibromatogenic

fibromatoid

fibromatosis
    aggressive f.
    palmar f.
    plantar f.
    subcutaneous pseudosar-
      comatous f.
    f. ventriculi

fibromatous

fibromyoma
    f. uteri

fibromyxoma

fibromyxosarcoma

fibroneuroma

fibronodular

fibro-odontoma
    ameloblastic f.-o.

fibro-osteoma

fibropapilloma

fibrosarcoma
    ameloblastic f.
    odontogenic f.

fibrosis
    cystic f.
    nodular subepidermal f.
    ossifying retroperitoneal f.
    radiation f.
    retroperitoneal f.

fibrotic

fibrous

fibroxanthoma
  atypical f.

fibroxanthosarcoma

fibula *pl.* fibulae, fibulas

fibular

fibularis

field
  extended f.
  gamma f.
  inverted Y f.
  involved f.
  lung f.
  mantle f.
  para-aortic f.
  penumbra f.

FIGO classification

figuratum

figure
  flame f.

fila (plural of filum)

filament
  lymphatic anchoring f's

filgrastim

filling
  subintimal f.

filling-in

film
  drain-out f.
  f. badge
  Bucky f.
  f. diameter
  flat f. of the abdomen
  in-department f's
  intraoperative f's
  mobility f's
  motion on the f's
  occlusal f's
  overhead f's
  pelvic f's for IUD localization

film *(continued)*
  plain f.
  Polaroid f's
  portable f's
  portable chest f.
  postexercise f's
  postreduction f's
  postvoiding f's
  preliminary f.
  run-off f's
  semierect portable chest f.
  spot f.
  subtraction f's
  weight-bearing f's
  x-ray f.

filter
  Wood's f.

filtration

filum *pl.* fila
  fila olfactoria
  fila radicularia nervi spinalis
  f. terminale

fimbria *pl.* fimbriae
  f. hippocampi
  f. ovarica
  fimbriae tubae uterinae

fimbriated

fimbriation

fimbriatum

finding
  angiographic f's
  atypical f's
  incidental f.

finger
  blubber f.
  fifth f.
  fourth f.
  index f. (forefinger)
  little f.
  middle f.
  ring f.
  seal f.
  tulip f's

fingernail

fingerprint

fire
St. Anthony's f.

first carpal row

fissile

fission
nuclear f.

fissionable

fissula

fissura *pl.* fissurae
f. antitragohelicina
fissurae cerebelli
f. choroidea ventriculi lateralis
f. horizontalis cerebelli
f. horizontalis pulmonis dextri
f. intercruralis cerebelli
f. ligamenti teretis
f. ligamenti venosi
f. longitudinalis cerebralis
f. longitudinalis cerebri
f. mediana anterior medullae oblongatae
f. mediana anterior medullae spinalis
f. obliqua pulmonis
f. orbitalis inferior
f. orbitalis superior
f. petrooccipitalis
f. petrosquamosa
f. petrotympanica
f. postpyramidalis
f. posterolateralis cerebelli
f. preclivalis
f. prima cerebelli
f. pterygomaxillaris
f. secunda cerebelli
f. sphenopetrosa
f. transversa cerebri
f. tympanomastoidea
f. tympanosquamosa

fissurae (plural of fissura)

fissural

fissure
calcarine f.
choroidal f.
craniofacial f.
interhemispheric f.
interlobar f.
longitudinal f.
palpebral f.
parietosphenoid f.
petrosquamosal f.
petrosquamous f.
pontine f.
sylvian f.

fistula
Brescia-Cimino AV f.
choledochoduodenal f.
enterocolic f.
lymphatic f.
f. lymphatica
pilonidal f.
rectovaginal f.
tracheoesophageal (TE) f.
vesicovaginal f.

fistulogram

Fitzgerald factor

fixation
open reduction and internal f. (ORIF)
f. plate and screws

flaccid

FLAIR
fluid-attenuated inversion recovery
FLAIR images

flange
shaft f.

flank

flap
intimal f.

flare

flattening

Fleckinger view (*same as* swimmer's view)

Fleet enema (*not* Fleet's)

Flegel's disease

flesh
  goose f.

Fletcher factor

fleurette

flexion
  f. contracture
  f. deformity
  f. and extension exercises
  f. and extension views
  plantar f.

Flexner-Wintersteiner rosette

flexor

flexuose

flexura *pl.* flexurae
  f. anorectalis recti
  f. coli dextra
  f. coli hepatica
  f. coli sinistra
  f. coli splenica
  f. duodeni inferior
  f. duodeni superior
  f. duodenojejunalis
  f. perinealis recti
  f. sacralis recti

flexurae (plural of flexura)

flexural

flexure
  hepatic f. of the colon
  sigmoid f.
  splenic f. of the colon

flocculation

flocculent

flocculus

floor
  f. of the orbit

floor *(continued)*
  orbital f.
  f. of the urinary bladder

florid

floxuridine

flow
  f. of barium
  collateral f.
  f. of contrast material
  effective renal plasma f.
    (ERPF)
  hepatofugal f.
  hepatopetal f.
  hold-up in f.
  f. pattern
  pulmonary blood f.
  f. study

Fludara

fludarabine phosphate

fludeoxyglucose F 18

fluid
  amnionic f.
  amniotic f.
  ascitic f.
  Callison's f.
  cerebrospinal f. (CSF)
  cerebrospinal f. pathways
  encapsulated f.
  free f.
  f. level
  f.-filled urinary bladder
  f.-f. level
  f. overload
  pericardial f.
  Piazza's f.
  pleural f.
  serous f.
  straw-colored f.
  Toison's f.
  Wickersheimer's f.

fluid-filled

flumen
  flumina pilorum

flunitrazepam

fluorine
  f. 18

fluorocyte

fluorodeoxyglucose

fluorodopa F 18

fluorography

fluorometer

fluororadiography

fluoroscope
  biplane f.

fluoroscopic

fluoroscopically

fluoroscopy

fluorouracil

Fluosol-DC

Fluothane

flush
  carcinoid f.

flutamide

flux
  magnetic f.

focal

focus *pl.* foci

fogo
  f. selvagem

fold
  aryepiglottic f's
  axillary f., anterior
  axillary f., posterior
  epigastric f.
  falciform f. of fascia lata
  gastric f's
  gluteal f.
  interdigital f.
  intergluteal f.
  Kerckring's f's
  lacrimal f's
  mucosal f.

fold *(continued)*
  mucous f.
  nail f.
  nasolabial f.
  serosal f.
  serous f.
  skin f's
  thickened f's
  umbilical f., lateral
  umbilical f., medial
  umbilical f., median
  umbilical f., middle
  Vater's f.

folded upon itself

Folex

Foley
  F. catheter
  indwelling F. catheter

folium *pl.* folia
  folia cerebelli
  f. vermis

follicle
  aggregated f's
  aggregated lymphatic f's
  gastric f's
  graafian f.
  hair f.
  lenticular f's
  lingual f's
  lymph f.
  lymph f's of stomach
  lymphatic f's, solitary
  lymphatic f's of small intes-
    tine, aggregated
  lymphatic f's of small intes-
    tine, solitary
  lymphatic f's, laryngeal
  lymphatic f's of large intes-
    tine, solitary
  lymphatic f's of tongue
  lymphatic f's of vermiform
    appendix, aggregated
  lymphoid f.
  lymphoid f's, solitary
  lymphoid f's of large intes-
    tine, solitary

follicle *(continued)*
  lymphoid f's of small intestine, aggregated
  lymphoid f's of small intestine, solitary
  lymphoid f's of vermiform appendix, aggregated
  sebaceous f.
  f's of tongue
  lymphatic f.

folliclis

follicular

folliculi (plural of folliculus)

folliculitis
  f. abscedens et suffodiens
  agminate f.
  f. barbae
  f. decalvans
  eosinophilic pustular f.
  gram-negative f.
  keloidal f.
  f. keloidalis
  f. ulerythematosa reticulata
  f. varioliformis

folliculoma
  f. lipidique

folliculosis

folliculus *pl.* folliculi
  folliculi linguales
  f. lymphaticus
  folliculi lymphatici aggregati
  folliculi lymphatici aggregati appendicis vermiformis
  folliculi lymphatici gastrici
  folliculi lymphatici laryngei
  folliculi lymphatici lienales
  folliculi lymphatici recti
  folliculi lymphatici solitarii intestini crassi
  folliculi lymphatici solitarii intestini tenuis
  folliculi lymphatici splenici
  folliculi ovarici vesiculosi
  f. pili

folliculus *(continued)*
  folliculi lymphatici solitarii

Fonio's solution

fontanelle (*also* fontanel)

fonticulus
  f. gutturis

food particles

foot
  athlete's f.
  Hong Kong f.
  immersion f.
  immersion f., tropical
  Morton's f.
  mossy f.
  trench f.

foramen *pl.* foramina
  aortic f.
  f. of Bochdalek
  f. of Bochdalek hernia
  f. caecum linguae
  f. caecum medullae oblongatae
  f. caecum ossis frontalis
  caval f.
  f. cecum of frontal bone
  cecal f.
  f. cecum of tongue
  condyloid f., anterior
  condyloid f., posterior
  conjugate f.
  f. costotransversarium
  costotransverse f.
  cribroethmoid f.
  foramina cribrosa ossis ethmoidalis
  emissary f.
  emissary f., sphenoidal
  f. epiploicum
  esophageal f.
  foramina ethmoidalia
  f. ethmoidale anterius
  f. ethmoidale posterius
  frontal f.
  f. frontale
  frontoethmoidal f.
  foramina incisiva

foramen *(continued)*
- infraorbital f.
- f. infraorbitale
- f. interventriculare
- intervertebral f.
- f. intervertebrale
- foramina intervertebralia ossis sacri
- f. ischiadicum majus
- f. ischiadicum minus
- jugular f.
- f. jugulare
- f. lacerum
- left f., inferior
- left f., superior
- f. magnum
- f. of Luschka
- f. of Magendie
- f. of Morgagni hernia
- morgagnian f.
- mastoid f.
- f. mastoideum
- nasal foramina
- foramina nasalia
- foramina nervosa
- f. nutricium
- f. nutriens
- nutrient f.
- obturator f.
- f. obturatum
- f. obturatorium
- occipital f., great
- occipital f., inferior
- f. occipitale magnum
- olfactory foramina
- omental f.
- f. omentale
- optic f.
- orbitomalar f.
- f. ovale
- f. ovale cordis
- f. ovale ossis sphenoidalis
- f. palatinum majus
- foramina palatina minora
- foramina papillaria renis
- papillary foramina of kidney
- parietal f.
- f. parietale

foramen *(continued)*
- f. petrosum
- quadrate f.
- right f.
- Rosenmüller's fossa
- f. rotundum ossis sphenoidalis
- foramina sacralia anteriora
- foramina sacralia pelvica
- foramina sacralia posteriora
- f. sciaticum majus
- f. sciaticum minus
- f. singulare
- f. sphenopalatinum
- f. spinosum
- stylomastoid f.
- f. stylomastoideum
- supraorbital f.
- f. supraorbitale
- f. thyroideum
- f. transversarium
- f. venae cavae
- foramina venarum minimarum atrii dextri
- f. venosum
- venous f.
- f. vertebrale
- f. Vesalii
- f. of Vesalius
- zygomatic f. of Arnold, internal
- zygomatic f. of Meckel, internal
- zygomaticofacial f.
- f. zygomaticofaciale
- zygomatico-orbital f.
- f. zygomaticoorbitale
- zygomaticotemporal f.
- f. zygomaticotemporale

foramina (plural of foramen)

foraminiferous

foraminulum

Forane

forceps
- epilating f.
- f. frontalis

forceps *(continued)*
    f. major
    f. minor
    f. occipitalis

forcipate

Fordyce
    angiokeratoma of F.
    F.'s disease
    F.'s granules
    F.'s spots

forearm

forefinger

forefoot

forehead

form
    band f.
    juvenile f.
    young f.

formaldehyde

formatio *pl.* formationes
    f. reticularis
    f. reticularis spinalis
    f. reticularis tegmenti pontis
    f. reticularis tegmenti mesencephali

formation
    bleb f.
    callous f.
    rouleau f.
    f. of rouleaux
    periosteal new bone f.
    plaque f.
    subchondral cyst f.

formationes (plural of formatio)

formula
    Arneth's f.
    Berkow f.

formulation
    Working F.
    Working F. of National Cancer Institute

formulation *(continued)*
    Working F. of Non-Hodgkin's Lymphomas for Clinical Usage

fornicate

fornix
    f. conjunctivae inferior
    f. conjunctivae superior
    f. gastricus
    f. pharyngis
    f. sacci lacrimalis
    f. of stomach
    f. vaginae
    f. ventricularis
    f. ventriculi

Forsius
    F.-Eriksson syndrome
    F.-Eriksson type ocular albinism

Forssell's sinus

fossa *pl.* fossae
    acetabular f.
    f. acetabuli
    antecubital f.
    f. antihelica
    f. axillaris
    Biesiadecki's f.
    f. carotica
    f. cerebellaris
    f. cerebralis
    condylar f.
    f. condylaris
    condyloid f., posterior
    f. condyloidea
    f. coronoidea humeri
    f. cranii anterior
    f. cranii media
    f. cranii posterior
    f. cubitalis
    digital f., superior
    epigastric f.
    f. epigastrica
    floccular f.
    f. glandulae lacrimalis
    glenoid f.
    greater f. of Scarpa

fossa *(continued)*
- f. hyaloidea
- hypogastric f.
- f. hypophysialis
- f. iliaca
- f. iliacosubfascialis
- f. iliopectinea
- incudal f.
- f. incudis
- f. infraclavicularis
- f. infraspinata
- f. infratemporalis
- inguinal f., external
- inguinal f., internal
- inguinal f., lateral
- inguinal f., medial
- inguinal f., middle
- f. inguinalis lateralis
- f. inguinalis medialis
- f. intercondylaris femoris
- f. interpeduncularis
- f. ischioanalis
- ischiorectal f.
- f. ischiorectalis
- jugular f.
- f. jugularis
- f. jugularis ossis temporalis
- f. jugularis ossis temporalis
- f. lateralis cerebralis
- f. lateralis cerebri
- lesser f. of Scarpa
- f. malleoli lateralis
- mandibular f.
- f. mandibularis
- mastoid f. of temporal bone
- middle cranial f.
- Mohrenheim's f.
- f. navicularis urethrae
- f. navicularis urethrae [Morgagnii]
- f. olecrani
- f. ovalis cordis
- f. ovarica
- f. paravesicalis
- parietal f.
- perineal f.
- pituitary f.
- f. poplitea

fossa *(continued)*
- popliteal f.
- postcondyloid f.
- posterior f.
- pterygoid f.
- f. pterygoidea ossis sphenoidalis
- f. pterygopalatina
- pterygopalatine f.
- pyriform f.
- f. radialis humeri
- rhomboid f.
- f. rhomboidea
- f. sacci lacrimalis
- f. scaphoidea ossis sphenoidalis
- f. scarpae major
- sigmoid f.
- sigmoid f. of temporal bone
- f. subarcuata ossis temporalis
- f. subscapularis
- f. supraclavicularis major
- f. supraclavicularis minor
- f. supraspinata
- f. supratonsillaris
- f. supravesicalis
- temporal f.
- f. temporalis
- f. tonsillaris
- f. triangularis auriculae
- f. trochanterica
- umbilical f., medial
- urachal f.
- vermian f.
- f. vesicae biliaris
- f. vesicae felleae
- vestibular f.
- f. vestibuli vaginae
- zygomatic f.

fossae (plural of fossa)

fossette

fossula *pl.* fossulae
- f. fenestrae cochleae
- f. fenestrae vestibuli
- f. petrosa
- fossulae tonsillares tonsillae palatinae

fossula *(continued)*
  fossulae tonsillares tonsillae pharyngeae
  f. of petrous ganglion
  fossulae tonsillae tonsillae palatinae
  fossulae tonsillae tonsillae pharyngeae
  fossulae tonsillae tonsillae pharyngealis
  fossulae tonsillares tonsillae pharyngealis

fossulae (plural of fossula)

fossulate

fovea *pl.* foveae
  f. articularis capitis radii
  f. capitis femoris
  f. cardiaca
  f. centralis retinae
  f. costalis inferior
  f. costalis processus transversi
  f. costalis superior
  dental f. of atlas
  f. dentis atlantis
  glandular foveae of Luschka
  f. inferior
  inguinal f., external
  inguinal f., internal
  inguinal f., lateral
  inguinal f., medial
  inguinal f., middle
  f. inguinalis lateralis
  f. inguinalis medialis
  interligamentous f. of peritoneum
  f. oblonga cartilaginis arytenoideae
  f. superior
  f. supravesicalis peritonaei
  f. triangularis cartilaginis arytenoideae
  f. trochlearis

foveae (plural of fovea)

foveate

foveation

foveola *pl.* foveolae
  f. coccygea
  foveolae gastricae
  foveolae granulares
  foveolae granulares [Pachioni]
  f. retinae
  f. suprameatalis
  f. suprameatica

foveolae (plural of foveola)

foveolar

foveolate

Fowler's position

Fox-Fordyce disease

fraction
  ejection f.
  left ventricular ejection f.
  plasma f's

fractional

fractionate

fractionation
  dose f.
  plasma f.

fracture
  avulsion f.
  capillary f.
  Bennett's f.
  bimalleolar f.
  blow-out f.
  buckle f.
  burst type f.
  capillary f.
  Chance f.
  chip f.
  Colles' f.
  comminuted f.
  compound f.
  compound, comminuted f.
  compound, complex f.
  contrecoup f.
  depressed skull f.
  f.-dislocation

fracture *(continued)*
  epiphyseal f.
  fishmouth f.
  f. fragments
  greenstick f.
  hangman's f.
  healing f.
  hip f.
  impacted f.
  incomplete f.
  intertrochanteric f.
  Jefferson f.
  Jones f.
  linear f.
  Lisfranc f.
  march f.
  metaphyseal f.
  Milkman's f.
  Monteggia f.
  navicular f.
  nondisplaced f.
  nonunited f.
  oblique f.
  occult f.
  odontoid f.
  orbital f.
  pathological f.
  ping-pong f.
  Pott's f.
  Salter I f. (also Salter II fracture)
  Salter III f.
  Salter IV f.
  f. site
  spiral f.
  spontaneous f.
  sprain f.
  stellate f.
  stress f.
  subtrochanteric f.
  talar f.
  through-and-through f.
  torus f.
  trimalleolar f.
  undisplaced f.
  zygomatic f.

fragiform

fragilitas
  f. crinium
  f. unguium

fragility
  f. of blood
  erythrocyte f.
  mechanical f.
  osmotic f.

fragilocyte

fragilocytosis

fragment
  fracture f's

fragmentation

frame
  Stryker f.

Frankfort horizontal plane

freckling

freckle
  melanotic f. of Hutchinson

free air under the diaphragm

Freiberg's infraction

fremitus

frena (plural of frenum)

frenal

French (a unit of measurement of catheter diameter, preceded by a number)
  F. catheter
  F. pigtail catheter

French-American-British (FAB) classification

frenulum *pl.* frenula
  f. clitoridis
  f. labiorum pudendi
  f. linguae
  f. preputii penis
  f. veli medullaris superioris

frenum *pl.* frena

frequency
    supersonic f.
    ultrasonic f.

fretum *pl.* freta

Friedreich's ataxia

frog-leg view of the hips

frondose

frons

frontad

frontal

frontalis

frontipetal

frontomalar

frontomaxillary

fronto-occipital

frontoparietal

frontotemporal

frontozygomatic

frost
    urea f.

frostbite
    deep f.
    superficial f.

FSE
    fast spin echo
        FSEviews

Fuchs position

fumonisin

function
    motor f.

fundal

fundament

fundi (plural of fundus)

fundic

fundiform

fundus *pl.* fundi
    gastric f.
    f. gastricus
    f. meatus acustici interni
    f. of the stomach
    uterine f.
    f. uteri
    f. of the uterus
    f. vesicae biliaris
    f. vesicae felleae
    f. vesicae urinariae

fungal

fungiform

fungus *pl.* fungi

funicle

funicular

funiculus *pl.* funiculi
    f. anterior medullae spinalis
    f. lateralis medullae oblongatae
    f. lateralis medullae spinalis
    funiculi medullae spinalis
    f. posterior medullae spinalis
    f. separans
    f. spermaticus

funiform

funis

funnel

funnel-shaped

furcal

furfuraceous

furifosmin

furocoumarin

furosemide

furrow
    digital f.
    gluteal f.

furrow *(continued)*
    Sibson's f.
    skin f's

furuncle

furuncular

furunculoid

furunculosis

furunculus

fusi (plural of fusus)

fusiform

fusion
    interbody f.
    spinal f.

fusus *pl.* fusi
    cortical fusi
    fracture fusi

Futcher's line

gadolinium
  g. 153

gadolinium-pentetic acid

Gaisböck's disease

galactography

galactorrhea

galea
  g. aponeurotica

gallbladder (GB)
  g. bed
  folded fundus g.
  nonfunctioning g.
  porcelain g.
  g. series

gallium
  g. 67
  g. Ga 67 citrate

gallstone
  faceted g.
  laminated g's
  layered g's
  solitary g.

gamma camera

gammagram

gammopathy
  monoclonal g's
  monoclonal g., benign

Gamna's disease

Gandy
  G.-Gamna spleen
  G.-Nanta disease

ganglia (plural of ganglion)

gangliocytoma

ganglioglioma

ganglioma

ganglion *pl.* ganglia
  ganglia aorticorenalia
  g. autonomicum

ganglion *(continued)*
  basal ganglia
  g. cervicale inferioris
  g. cervicale medium
  g. cervicale superius
  g. ciliare
  ganglia coeliaca
  g. craniospinale sensorium
  ganglia encephalica
  Gasser's g.
  g. geniculatum nervi faci-
    alis
  g. geniculi nervi facialis
  g. impar
  g. inferius nervi glossopha-
    ryngei
  g. inferius nervi vagi
  ganglia intermedia
  Küttner's g.
  ganglia lumbalia
  ganglia lymphatica
  g. mesentericum inferius
  g. mesentericum superius
  g. parasympathicum
  ganglia pelvica
  ganglia phrenica
  ganglia plexuum autonomi-
    corum
  ganglia renalia
  g. sensorium nervi cranialis
  g. sensorium nervi spinalis
  g. spirale cochleae
  g. stellatum
  g. sublinguale
  g. superius nervi glosso-
    pharyngei
  g. superius nervi vagi
  g. sympathicum
  synovial g.
  g. terminale
  ganglia thoracica
  g. thoracicum splanchni-
    cum
  g. of trigeminal nerve
  g. trigeminale
  Troisier's g.
  ganglia trunci sympathetici

ganglion *(continued)*
    ganglia trunci sympathici
    g. tympanicum
    g. vertebrale
    g. vestibulare

ganglioneuroblastoma

ganglioneurofibroma

ganglioneuroma

gangrene
    Meleney's g.
    Meleney's synergistic g.
    progressive bacterial sy-
        nergistic g.
    progressive synergistic g.
    progressive synergistic
        bacterial g.

gantry
    CT g.

Gardner-Diamond syndrome

gas
    hemolytic g.
    laughing g.

Gasser
    G's ganglion
    G's syndrome

gaster

gastrectomy
    Billroth I g.
    Billroth II g.

gastrinoma

gastritis
    bile reflux g.
    chronic active hepatitis
    cirrhotic g.
    Crohn's g.
    emphysematous g.

gastrocardiac

gastroenteritis

gastroesophageal (GE)
    g. junction
    g. reflux

Gastrografin

gastrojejunostomy

gastrolienal

gastropneumonic

gastroptosis

gastropulmonary

gastroschisis

gastroscopy

gastrosplenic

gate

gating
    cardiac g.

Gaucher's disease

gauge

gavage

GB
    gallbladder
        GB series
        GB-GI series

GE
    gastroesophageal
        gastroesophageal junc-
            tion
        gastroesophageal re-
            flux

Geiger
    G. counter
    G.-Müller counter

Gelfoam torpedoes

gelatinous

gemcitabine hydrochloride

gemma
    g. gustatoria

Gemzar

gene
    suicide g.
    tumor suppressor g.

genicula (plural of geniculum)

geniculate

geniculum *pl.* genicula
    g. canalis facialis
    g. canalis nervi facialis
    g. nervi facialis

genital

genitalia
    external g.
    internal g.

genitocrural

genitofemoral

genitography

genitourinary

genodermatology

genodermatosis

genotoxic

Gensini
    G. catheter
    G. coronary catheter

genu *pl.* genua
    g. capsulae internae
    g. corporis callosi
    g. of facial canal
    g. of facial nerve, external
    g. nervi facialis
    g. valgum
    g. varum

genua (plural of genu)

genual

geode

geophagia

Gerbich blood group

Gerlach's tonsil

germ
    hair g.

germinoma
    pineal g.

geroderma

gerodermia

geromorphism
    cutaneous g.

Gerota's method

gestation

Ghon complex

GI
    gastrointestinal
    GI series
    GI series and small
        bowel follow-through

Gianotti-Crosti syndrome

Giardia

giardiasis

gibbus

Gierke's corpuscles

Gilbert's disease (zhēl-bārz′)

Gill lesion

Gimbernat
    lacunar ligament of G.
    G's ligament

gingiva

ginglymus

girdle
    pelvic g.
    shoulder g.

girth
    increased abdominal g.

glabella

glabellad

gladiate

gladiolus

gland
    absorbent g.
    accessory g.

gland *(continued)*
    acinar g.
    acinotubular g.
    acinous g.
    adrenal g's
    aggregate g's
    aggregated g's
    alveolar g.
    apocrine g.
    apocrine sweat g.
    axillary g's
    brachial g's
    Bruch's g's
    Brunner's g's
    celiac g's
    Cloquet's g.
    coil g.
    compound g.
    Cowper's g's
    conglobate g.
    cutaneous g's
    eccrine g.
    eccrine sweat g.
    endoepithelial g.
    excretory g.
    exocrine g.
    heterocrine g.
    holocrine g.
    intraepithelial g.
    jugular g.
    large sweat g.
    lenticular g's of tongue
    lymph g.
    lymphatic g.
    mammary g's
    lymph g's, extraparotid
    mammary g., accessory
    merocrine g.
    mesenteric g's
    mesocolic g's
    mixed g.
    molar g's
    muciparous g.
    mucous g.
    oil g.
    parathyroid g's
    parotid g.
    pectoral g's
    Peyer's g's

gland *(continued)*
    pineal g.
    pituitary g.
    Poirier's g's
    prostate g.
    racemose g's
    retromolar g's
    Rosenmüller's g.
    saccular g.
    salivary g.
    sebaceous g.
    seromucous g.
    serous g.
    Sigmund's g's
    simple g.
    solitary g's of large intestine
    solitary g's of small intestine
    Stahr's g.
    subauricular g's
    submaxillary g.
    substernal thyroid g.
    sudoriferous g.
    sudoriparous g.
    sweat g's
    thymus g.
    thyroid g.
    tubular g.
    tubuloacinar g.
    Virchow's g.
    Wölfler's g's

glanderous

glanders

glandes (plural of glans)

glandilemma

glandula *pl.* glandulae
    glandulae areolares
    glandulae areolares [Montgomerii]
    glandulae bronchiales
    g. bulbourethralis
    g. bulbourethralis [Cowperi]
    glandulae cervicales uteri
    glandulae ciliares conjunctivales

glandula *(continued)*
glandulae conjunctivales
glandulae cutis
glandulae ductus biliaris
glandulae ductus choledo-
chi
glandulae duodenales
glandulae duodenales
[Brunneri]
glandulae endocrinae
glandulae intestinales
g. lacrimalis
glandulae lacrimales acces-
soriae
glandulae laryngeales
glandulae linguales
g. mammaria
glandulae molares
g. mucosa
glandulae nasales
glandulae oesophageae
glandulae olfactoriae
glandulae palatinae
g. parathyroidea inferior
g. parathyroidea superior
g. parotidea accessoria
glandulae pharyngeales
g. pinealis
g. pituitaria
glandulae preputiales
g. sebacea
glandulae sebaceae palpe-
brarum
g. seminalis
g. seromucosa
g. serosa
g. sudorifera
g. suprarenalis
glandulae suprarenales ac-
cessoriae
glandulae tarsales
g. thyroidea
glandulae thyroideae ac-
cessoriae
glandulae tracheales
glandulae tubariae
glandulae urethrales ure-
thrae femininae

glandula *(continued)*
glandulae urethrales ure-
thrae masculinae
glandulae uterinae
g. vesiculosa
g. vestibularis major
glandulae vestibulares minores

glandulae (plural of glandula)

glandular

glandule

glandulous

glans *pl.* glandes
g. clitoridis
g. penis

glanular

Glanzmann's thrombasthenia

glass
Wood's g.

Gleason score

Glidewire

glioblastoma
g. multiforme

glioma
astrocytic g.
g. endophytum
ependymal g.
g. exophytum
ganglionic g.
mixed g.
nasal g.
optic g.
opticochiasmatic g.
peripheral g.
pontine g.
g. retinae

gliomatosis
cerebral g.
g. cerebri
g. peritonei

gliomatous

glioneuroma

gliosarcoma

gliosis

globi (plural of globus)

globin

globulin
  AC g.
  accelerator g.
  antihemophilic g.

globus *pl.* globi
  g. pallidus lateralis
  g. hystericus
  g. pallidus medialis

glomangioma

glomera (plural of glomus)

glomerate

glomeruli (plural of glomerulus)

glomerulonephritis

glomerulus *pl.* glomeruli
  renal glomeruli
  glomeruli renis

glomus *pl.* glomera
  g. caroticum
  g. choroideum

glossa

glossal

glossitis
  herpetic geometric g.

glottis *pl.* glottides

glucagon

glucagonoma

gluceptate

glucoheptonate

Glucoscan

glucose-6-phosphate dehydro-
  genase deficiency

gluteal

gluteofemoral

gluteoinguinal

glycerolize

glycohemoglobin

glycophorin

glycosuria

Goeckerman treatment

goiter
  exophthalmic g.
  intrathoracic g.
  multinodular g.
  substernal g.

gold
  g. Au 198
  colloidal g.

Golden
  disturbed motility of G.

gomphosis

gonad

gonadoblastoma

gonadotropinoma

gonarthritis

goniometer

gonorrhea

Goodpasture's syndrome

Gore-Tex graft

Gorlin
  G's syndrome
  G.-Goltz syndrome

goserelin
  g. acetate

Gottron's sign

Gougerot
  G.-Blum syndrome

Gougerot *(continued)*
    G.-Carteaud syndrome

gout

Gowers' solution

grade
    Gleason g.

gradient

graft
    aortofemoral bypass g.
        (AFBG)
    coronary artery bypass g.
        (CABG)
    Dacron g.
    femoropopliteal bypass g.
    Gore-Tex g.
    interbody bone g.
    Sauvage filamentous g. ma-
        terial
    skin g.
    tricortical bone g.

Graham Little syndrome

Graham's test

Gram's stain

Granger
    G. line
    G.'s sign

granular

granulatio *pl.* granulationes
    granulationes arachnoideae
    granulationes arachnoide-
        ales

granulation

granulationes (plural of granu-
    latio)

granule
    alpha g's
    azurophil g.
    basophil g.
    Birbeck g's
    bull's eye g.
    dense g.
    elementary g's

granule *(continued)*
    eosinophil g.
    Fordyce's g's
    gelatinase g.
    kappa g.
    keratohyalin g's
    lamellar g.
    Langerhans' g's
    membrane-coating g.
    trichohyalin g's
    vermiform g's
    primary g.
    monocytic g.
    neutrophil g.
    secondary g.
    specific g.

granuloblast

granulocyte
    band-form g.
    segmented g.

granulocytic

granulocytopathy

granulocytopenia

granulocytopoiesis

granulocytopoietic

granulocytosis

granuloma
    actinic g.
    g. annulare
    Candida g.
    foreign-body g.
    g. fungoides
    giant cell reparative g., cen-
        tral
    giant cell reparative g., pe-
        ripheral
    Hodgkin's g.
    lipoid g.
    lipophagic g.
    Majocchi's g.
    Miescher's g.
    monilial g.
    g. multiforme
    pseudopyogenic g.
    pyogenic g.

granuloma *(continued)*
    reticulohistiocytic g.
    swimming pool g.
    trichophytic g.
    g. trichophyticum
    zirconium g.

granulomatosis
    g. disciformis progressiva
        et chronica
    lymphomatoid g.
    Wegener's g.

granulomere

granulopenia

granulopoiesis

granulopoietic

granulopoietin

granulosis
    g. rubra nasi

GRASS
    gradient recalled acquisi-
        tion in a steady state
            GRASS images

gravel

Graves' disease

Grawitz's tumor

gray

GRE
    gradient recalled echo
        GRE images

Greene needle

Greulich-Pyle chart for bone
    age

grid
    crossed g.
    focused g.
    moving g.
    parallel g.
    Potter-Bucky g.
    stationary g.

groin

Grollman catheter

groove
    arterial g's
    basilar g. of occipital bone
    bicipital g.
    lateral g. for lateral sinus of
        occipital bone
    lateral g. for lateral sinus of
        parietal bone
    lateral g. for sigmoidal part
        of lateral sinus
    g. for middle temporal ar-
        tery
    nail g.
    occipital g.
    optic g.
    sagittal g.
    sigmoid g. of temporal
        bone
    venous g's

Groshong catheter

ground-glass

group
    blood g.
    platelet g.

grouping
    blood g.

Gruber
    petrosphenooccipital su-
        ture of G.

Gruentzig
    G. balloon catheter
    G. dilatation catheter

GSW
    gunshot wound

gubernacular

gubernaculum *pl.* gubernacula
    g. testis

guidewire
    flexible g.
    Bentson g.

Guillain-Barré syndrome

Günz's ligament

gut

gutter

Guyon's amputation

gynandroblastoma

gynecography

gynecologic

gynecomastia

gyrus *pl.* gyri
   gyri breves insulae
   cerebral gyri
   gyri cerebri
   g. cinguli
   cingulate g.
   g. dentatus
   g. fasciolaris
   g. frontalis inferior
   g. frontalis medialis
   g. frontalis superior

gyrus *(continued)*
   gyri insulae
   g. longus insulae
   g. occipitotemporalis lateralis
   g. occipitotemporalis medialis
   g. olfactorius lateralis
   g. olfactorius medialis
   g. parahippocampalis
   g. postcentralis
   precentral g.
   g. precentralis
   g. rectus
   g. supramarginalis
   g. temporalis inferior
   g. temporalis medius
   g. temporalis superior
   gyri temporales transversi
   g. temporalis transversus anterior
   g. temporalis transversus posterior

H

habena

habenula *pl.* habenulae

habenular

Habermann's disease

habitus
    asthenic h.

Hageman factor

Hagie pin

Hahn's clefts

Hailey-Hailey disease

hair
    bamboo h.
    beaded h.
    burrowing h.
    club h.
    exclamation point h.
    ingrown h.
    knotted h.
    moniliform h.
    pubic h.
    resting h.
    stellate h.
    terminal h.
    twisted h.
    vellus h.

Haldane effect

half-axial

half-life
    biological h.-l.
    effective h.-l.

half-time
    plasma iron clearance h.-t.

half-value

Hallé's point

Haller's arches

Hallopeau's acrodermatitis

hallux *pl.* halluces
    h. valgus

hallux *(continued)*
    h. varus

halodermia

halometer

halothane

Ham's test

hamartoblastoma

hamartoma
    pulmonary h.
    sclerosing epithelial h.

hamartomatosis

hamartomatous

hamate

Hamburger
    H. interchange
    H. phenomenon

Hamman-Rich syndrome

Hampson unit

Hampton
    H. line
    H. maneuver
    H. view

hamular

hamulus *pl.* hamuli
    h. lacrimalis
    h. laminae spiralis
    h. ossis hamati
    h. pterygoideus

hand
    h.-injection
    h.-instilled

Hand-Schüller-Christian disease

handle

hangnail

Hansen's disease

H antigen

harara

hardness

harmonia

Harrington rod

Harris lines

Hartmann's pouch

Hashimoto's disease

Hassall
    H's bodies
    H's corpuscles

Haudek
    H's niche
    H's sign

hauptganglion of Küttner

haustra (plural of haustrum)

haustration

haustrum *pl.* haustra
    haustra coli
    haustra of colon

Hawkins
    H. needle
    H. sign

Hayem
    H's solution
    H.-Widal syndrome

head
    h. of the barium column
    h. of the caudate nucleus
    h. of the femur
    humeral h.
    h. of the humerus
    medial h. of abductor hallu-
      cis
    h. of the pancreas
    radial h.
    h. of the spleen
    white h.

heart
    flask-shaped h.
    sabot h.
    water-bottle h.

heat
    prickly h.

heavy vascular calcification

Hebra's disease

Heckathorn's disease

HED

heel
    basketball h.
    black h.
    cracked h's

Hefke-Turner sign

Hegglin's anomaly

Heimlich maneuver

Heinig's projection

Heinz body anemias

Heister
    valve of H.

Helicobacter pylori

helicotrema

helix

heloma
    h. durum
    h. molle

helosis

helotomy

hemachrome

hemacyte

hemacytometer

hemacytometry

hemafacient

hemal

hemanalysis

hemangioameloblastoma

hemangioblastoma
    cerebellar h.

hemangioblastoma *(continued)*
  retinal h.
  spinal h.

hemangioblastomatosis

hemangioendothelioblastoma

hemangioendothelioma
  benign h.
  epithelioid h.
  infantile h.
  malignant h.
  vertebral h.

hemangioendotheliosarcoma

hemangioma
  ameloblastic h.
  capillary h.
  cavernous h.
  sclerosing h.
  strawberry h.
  venous h.

hemangiomatosis

hemangiopericytoma
  h. of kidney

hemangiosarcoma

hemapheresis

hemapoiesis

hemapoietic

hemarthrosis

hematal

hematemesis

hematherapy

hematic

hematidrosis

hematimeter

hematin

hematinic

hematinometer

hematoblast

hematocrit
  large vessel h.
  total body h.
  whole body h.

hematocyte

hematocytoblast

hematocytolysis

hematocytometer

hematocytopenia

hematogenesis

hematogenic

hematogenous

hematogone

hematohidrosis

hematohistioblast

hematoid

hematoidin

hematologist

hematology

hematolymphangioma

hematolysis

hematolytic

hematoma
  subdural h.
  subungual h.

hematometer

hematometry

hematopathology

hematopenia

hematophage

hematophagocyte

hematophilia

hematoplastic

hematopoiesis
  extramedullary h.

hematopoietic

hematopoietin

hematoporphyrin

hematospectroscope

hematospectroscopy

hematostatic

hematotherapy

hematotoxic

hematotoxicosis

hematotropic

hematoxic

hematuria

heme

hemendothelioma

Hemerocampa

hemiaxial

hemic

hemicanities

hemicolectomy

hemicranium

hemidesmosome

hemidiaphoresis

hemidiaphragm
  cusp of the h.
  domes of the h's
  elevated (right or left) h.
  eventration of the (left or
    right) h.

hemidrosis

hemigastrectomy

hemihidrosis

hemihyperidrosis

hemilaminectomy

hemilateral

hemiparesis

hemiplegia

hemisotonic

hemisphaerium

hemisphere

hemispherium
  h. cerebelli
  h. cerebri

hemithorax

hemivertebra

hemoblast
  lymphoid h. of Pappenheim

hemocatheresis

hemochromatosis

hemochrome

hemochromogen
  hemoglobin h.

hemoclasis

hemoclastic

Hemoclip

Hemoccult
  H.-negative stool
  H.-positive stool

hemoconcentration

hemoconia

hemoconiosis

hemocryoscopy

hemoculture

hemocyte

hemocytoblast

hemocytocatheresis

hemocytoma

hemocytometer

hemocytometry

hemocytopenia

hemocytophagia

hemocytophagic

hemocytopoiesis

hemocytotripsis

hemodialysis

hemodiapedesis

hemodilution

hemodystrophy

hemofuscin

hemogenesis

hemogenic

hemoglobin
  h. A
  h. A_{1c}
  h. A_2
  h. anti-Lepore
  h. Bart's
  h. C
  h. C disease
  h. Chesapeake
  h. Constant Spring
  crossover h.
  h. C–thalassemia disease
  h. D
  h. D disease
  deoxygenated h.
  h. disease
  h. E
  h. E disease
  h. E–thalassemia disease
  h. F
  fast h's
  fetal h.
  h. G
  glycated h.

hemoglobin *(continued)*
  glycosylated h.
  Gower h.
  h. Gower
  h. Gun Hill
  h. H
  h. H disease
  h. I
  h. Kansas
  h. Kenya
  h. Köln
  h. Lepore
  h. M
  mean corpuscular h.
  oxidized h.
  oxygenated h.
  h. Portland
  h. Rainier
  reduced h.
  h. S
  h. SC disease
  h. SD disease
  h. Seattle
  slow h's
  unstable h's
  h. Yakima

hemoglobinated

hemoglobinemia

hemoglobinolysis

hemoglobinometer

hemoglobinometry

hemoglobinopathy

hemoglobinopepsia

hemoglobinous

hemoglobinuria
  paroxysmal nocturnal h.

hemogram

hemohistioblast

hemology

hemolymph

hemolymphangioma

hemolysate

hemolysin
    bacterial h.
    heterophile h.
    hot-cold h.

hemolysis
    colloid osmotic h.
    contact h.
    venom h.

hemolytic

hemolyzable

hemolyzation

hemolyze

hemometer

hemometry

hemopathic

hemopathology

hemopathy

hemopexin

hemophage

hemophagocyte

hemophagocytosis

hemophagocytic

hemophilia
    h. A
    h. B
    h. B, Leyden
    h. C
    classical h.
    vascular h.

hemophiliac

hemophilic

hemophilioid

hemophthisis

hemoplastic

hemopneumothorax

hemopoiesis

hemopoietic

hemopoietin

hemoptysis

hemorheology

hemorrhage
    fibrinolytic h.
    intraventricular h.
    petechial h.
    punctate h.
    splinter h's

hemorrhagic

hemosiderosis

hemostasia

hemostasis

hemostat

hemostatic

hemostyptic

hemotherapeutics

hemotherapy

hemothorax

hemotoxic

hemotropic

hempa

HEMPAS

Henke
    H's space
    H's triangle

Henle
    H's band
    H's layer
    loops of H.

Henoch
    H's purpura
    H.-Schönlein purpura
    H.-Schönlein syndrome

hepar

heparin

heparinize

heparinization

hepaticopulmonary

hepatitis
   h. A
   h. B
   h. C
   halothane h.

hepatoblastoma

hepatobronchial

hepatocarcinogenesis

hepatocarcinogenic

hepatocarcinoma

hepatocholangiocarcinoma

hepatogram

hepatography

Hepatolite

hepatojugular

hepatolenticular

hepatolienal

hepatolienography

hepatoma
   fibrolamellar h.
   malignant h.

hepatomegaly

hepatonephric

hepatophlebography

hepatopleural

hepatopneumonic

hepatoptosis

hepatopulmonary

hepatorenal

hepatoscan

hepatosplenography

hepatosplenomegaly

heptoglobin

herpes
   h. blattae

hereditary

Herendeen phenomenon

Herlitz's disease

Hermansky-Pudlak syndrome

Hermodsson's projection

hernia
   Bochdalek h.
   diaphragmatic h.
   esophageal h.
   hiatal h.
   hiatus h.
   incarcerated h.
   incisional h.
   inguinal h.
   Morgagni h.
   paraesophageal hiatal h.
   short esophagus type hia-
      tal h.
   sliding hiatal h.
   strangulated h.
   tubular hiatal h.
   umbilical h.
   ventral h.

herniated intervertebral disk

herniation
   disc h.
   disk h.

herniorrhaphy

herpetiform

Herring tube

Herxheimer
   H's fibers
   H's spirals

Hesselbach's triangle

heterochiral

heteroeroticism

heterolateral

heterophil

heterophile

heterophilic

heterotopia

heterotopic bone formation

heterotrichosis
  h. superciliorum

Heublein method

hexachlorobenzene

Hexalen

hexamethylmelamine

hexamethylphosphoramide

hexobarbital
  h. sodium

Hey's ligament

Hh blood group

H1H catheter

hiatal

hiatus
  h. adductorius
  h. aorticus
  h. canalis nervi petrosi majoris
  h. canalis nervi petrosi minoris
  diaphragmatic esophageal h.
  esophageal h.
  h. leukemicus
  h. maxillaris
  h. of maxillary sinus
  h. oesophageus
  h. sacralis
  h. saphenus
  h. semilunaris
  subarcuate h.
  vena caval h.

hibernoma

Hickman catheter

HIDA

hidebound

hidradenitis
  h. axillaris
  h. suppurativa

hidradenocarcinoma
  clear cell h.

hidradenoma
  h. eruptivum
  nodular h.
  papillary h.
  h. papilliferum
  solid-cystic h.

hidroacanthoma
  h. simplex

hidroadenoma

hidrocystoma
  apocrine h.
  eccrine h.

hidropoiesis

hidropoietic

hidrosadenitis

hidroschesis

hidrotic

high-signal

hila (plural of hilum)

hilar
  h. shadows

hillock

hilum *pl.* hila
  h. glandulae suprarenalis
  h. lienale
  h. of lymph node
  h. nodi lymphatici
  h. lymphoglandulae
  h. nodi lymphoidei
  h. nuclei dentati
  h. nuclei olivaris inferioris

hilum *(continued)*
    h. ovarii
    h. pulmonis
    h. renale
    h. splenicum

hindfoot

hip

Hippel
    H's disease
    H.-Lindau disease

hippocampus

Hippuran

hirci (plural of hircus)

hircismus

hircus *pl.* hirci

Hirschsprung's disease

hirsute

hirsuties

hirsutism

hirudin

hirudinization

hirudinize

His
    bundle of H.

histiocyte
    wandering h.

histiocytic

histiocytoma
    benign fibrous h.
    h. cutis
    fibrous h.
    lipoid h.
    malignant fibrous h.

histiocytosis
    sinus h.
    sinus h. with massive lym-
        phadenopathy
    sinus h. with massive lym-
        phadenopathy

histiocytosis *(continued)*
    malignant h.

histocyte

histofluorescence

histology

histone
    h. nucleinate

histoplasmosis

Hitzelberger's sign

hive

hives

HN2 (mechlorethamine)

HNP
    herniated nucleus pulposus

hoarseness

Hodge's planes

Hodgkin
    H's cells
    H's disease
    H's granuloma
    H's lymphoma
    H's sarcoma

hole
    bur (burr) h's

hollow

holotopy

Holzknecht's space

Homans' sign

homeomorphous

homeostasis

Homer Mammalok needle

Homer Wright rosette

homing

homme
    h. rouge

homogeneity

homoglandular

homolateral

homologue

homotype

homotypic

honeycombing

Hong Kong foot

hook of the hamate bone

HOP
    hydroxydaunomycin (doxo-
        rubicin), Oncovin (vin-
        cristine), and prednisone

horizontal

horizontalis

hormone
    ectopic h.
    eutopic h.
    fibroblast growth h.
    pituitary growth h.

horn
    cicatricial h.
    cutaneous h.
    frontal h.
    h. of the lateral ventricle
    occipital h.

Horner's sign

hornification

horripilation

hot

Hounsfield unit

Howel-Evans' syndrome

Hughston
    H. view of the knee
    H's projection

humerus *pl.* humeri

humor
    h. aquosus

humor *(continued)*
    h. vitreus

humoral

hump
    Hampton's h.
    dowager's h.
    dromedary h.

Hunter
    H. balloon
    H's line
    H.-Sessions balloon

Hürthle
    H. cell carcinoma
    H. cell tumor

Hutchinson
    H's disease
    melanotic freckle of H.
    H's plaques

Hutchison syndrome

Huxley's membrane

HX bodies

hyal

hyalomere

Hycamtin

hydradenitis

hydradenoma

hydramnios

Hydrea

hydremia

hydroa
    h. estivale
    h. vacciniforme

hydrocele

hydrocephalic

hydrocephalus
    normal-pressure h.

hydrocephaly

hydrocystadenoma

hydrocytosis

hydrogen
   arseniuretted h.
   heavy h.

hydromyoma

hydronephrosis

hydronephrotic

hydropneumothorax

hydrosalpinx

hydrothorax

hydrotomy

hydroureter

hydroxyapatite

hydroxyheptadecatrienoic acid

hydroxyurea

hygiene
   radiation h.

hygroma
   cystic h.
   h. cysticum

hymen

hymenology

Hypaque

hypaxial

hyperacanthosis

hyperactivity

hyperaeration of the lungs

hyperaldosteronoma

hypercalcemia

hyperchlorhydria

hypercoagulability

hypercoagulable

hypercyanotic

hypercythemia

hypercytosis

hyperdense

hyperechoic

hyperemesis gravidarum

hyperemia

hypereosinophilia

hypererythrocythemia

hyperextension

hyperferremia

hyperferremic

hyperferricemia

hyperfibrinogenemia

hyperfractionation

hypergammaglobulinemia
   monoclonal h's

hyperhemoglobinemia

hyperheparinemia

hyperhidrosis
   axillary h.
   emotional h.
   h. unilateralis
   volar h.

hyperhidrotic

hyperidrosis

hyperinflation

hyperintense

hyperkeratinization

hyperkeratosis
   follicular h.
   h. follicularis in cutem pe-
      netrans
   h. follicularis et parafollicu-
      laris in cutem penetrans
   h. lenticularis perstans

hyperkeratosis *(continued)*
    h. of palms and soles
    h. penetrans
    progressive dystrophic h.
    h. subungualis

hyperleukocytosis

hyperlipidemia

hyperlucency

hypermotility

hypernatremia

hyperneocytosis

hypernephroid

hypernephroma

hyperonychia

hyperorthocytosis

hyperostosis
    diffuse idiopathic skeletal
        h. (DISH)
    h. frontalis interna
    infantile cortical h. (Caf-
        fey's disease)

hyperparathyroidism

hyperperistalsis

hyperplasia
    angiolymphoid h. with eo-
        sinophilia
    C-cell h.
    cutaneous lymphoid h.
    giant follicular h.
    giant lymph node h.
    gingival h.
    intravascular papillary en-
        dothelial h.
    lymphoid h.
    sebaceous h.
    verrucous h.

hyperplasmia

hyperpyrexia
    malignant h.

hyperreflexia

hypersecretion
    gastric h.

hypersegmentation
    hereditary h. of neutrophils

hypersensitivity
    contact h.

hypersplenia

hypersplenism

hypersteatosis

hyperstereoradiography

hyperstereoskiagraphy

hypertelorism

hypertension
    portal h.

hyperthermia
    h. of anesthesia
    malignant h.

hyperthrombinemia

hyperthymism

hyperthyroidism

hypertonia
    h. polycythaemica

hypertransfusion

hypertrichosis
    h. lanuginosa
    h. universalis

hypertrophy
    compensatory h.
    left ventricular h.
    prostatic h.

hyperventilation

hyperviscosity

hypervolemia
    h. of pregnancy

hypervolemic

hyphidrosis

hypnoanesthesia

hypoaeration of the lungs

hypochondria

hypochondriac

hypochondrium

hypochromotrichia

hypocoagulability

hypocoagulable

hypocythemia

hypocytosis

hypodense

hypoderm

hypodermatomy

hypodermis

hypodermosis

hypodiaphragmatic

hypoechoic

hypoeosinophilia

hypofibrinogenemia

hypogastric

hypogastrium

hypogranulocytosis

hypohidrosis

hypohidrotic

hypoidrosis

hypointense

hypokinesis

hypomelanosis
    idiopathic guttate h.
    h. of Ito

hypomotility

hyponatremia

hyponeocytosis

hyponychial

hyponychium

hyponychon

hypo-orthocytosis

hypoparathyroidism

hypoperistalsis

hypopharynx

hypophrenic

hypophrenium

hypophyseal

hypophysis
    pharyngeal h.
    h. pharyngealis

hypopigmentation

hypoplasia

hypoplastic

hypoprothrombinemia

hyposplenism

hypotension
    postural h.

hypothalamus

hypothenar

hypothrombinemia

hypothymism

hypothyroidism

hypotrichiasis

hypotrichosis

hypoventilation

hypovolemia

hypovolemic

hypoxia
    anemic h.

hypsiloid

hyrax
    tree h.

hysterectomy

hysterogram

hysterography

hysteromyoma

hysterosalpingography

hysterostat

hysterotubography

I

iatrogenic

I blood group

ichthyosiform

ichthyosis
    harlequin i.
    i. palmaris et plantaris
    i. simplex
    i. vulgaris

ichthyotic

icteric

icteroanemia

icterus
    chronic familial i.
    congenital familial i.
    congenital hemolytic i.

Idamycin

idarubicin hydrochloride

idiopathic

idiotopy

Ifex

ifosfamide

IHSS
    idiopathic hypertrophic
        subaortic stenosis

ileitis
    regional i.

ileocecostomy

ileostomy

ileum
    terminal i.

ileus
    adynamic i.
    paralytic i.
    reflex i.

ilia (plural of ilium)

iliohypogastric

ilioinguinal

iliolumbar

iliolumbocostoabdominal

iliopectineal

iliopelvic

iliopubic

ilium *pl.* ilia

ill-defined

illness
    radiation i.

IM
    intramuscular

ima

image
    axial and longitudinal i's
    diffusion weighted i's
        (DWI)
    dynamic i's
    fat saturated i's (*may be
        dictated* "fat sat")
    flip angle i's
    gradient i's
    magnetization transfer i's
    mirror i.
    proton density i's
    radioisotope i.
    redistribution i's
    spin echo i's
    TR i's

Imagent GI

imaging
    color flow Doppler i.
    echo planar i.
    gated cardiac blood pool i.
    hepatobiliary i.
    hot spot i.
    infarct avid i.
    magnetic resonance i.
        (MRI)
    magnetic resonance i.,
        gated

imaging *(continued)*
  myocardial i.
  myocardial perfusion i.
  nuclear magnetic resonance i.
  pyrophosphate i.
  real-time i.
  technetium Tc 99m pyrophosphate i.
  thallium i.
  thallium myocardial i.
  whole-body i.

Imerslund
  I. syndrome
  I.-Graesbeck syndrome

iminodiacetic acid

immobile

immobility

immortalization

immunochemotherapy

immunodermatology

immunoglobulinopathy
  monoclonal i's

immunohematology

immunolymphoscintigraphy

immunophenotype

immunoscintigraphy

immunosurveillance

immunotherapy
  adoptive i.
  adoptive cellular i.

impaction
  fecal i.

impar

impetiginization

impetiginous

impetigo
  Bockhart's i.
  i. bullosa

impetigo *(continued)*
  i. contagiosa
  i. contagiosa bullosa
  i. herpetiformis
  i. neonatorum
  staphylococcal i.
  streptococcal i.
  i. vulgaris
  bullous i.

impilation

impingement

impinging upon

implant
  penile i.
  silicone i's

impressio *pl.* impressiones
  i. cardiaca hepatis
  i. cardiaca pulmonis
  i. colica hepatis
  impressiones digitatae
  i. duodenalis hepatis
  i. gastrica hepatis
  i. ligamenti costoclavicularis
  i. meningealis
  i. oesophagea hepatis
  i. renalis hepatis
  i. suprarenalis hepatis
  i. trigeminalis ossis temporalis

impression
  meningeal i.

impressiones (plural of impressio)

incarnatio
  i. unguis

incisura *pl.* incisurae
  i. acetabuli
  i. angularis gastris
  i. anterior auriculae
  i. apicis cordis
  i. cardiaca gastris
  i. cardiaca pulmonis sinistri
  i. cardialis

incisura *(continued)*
   i. cartilaginis meatus acustici
   i. clavicularis sterni
   incisurae costales sterni
   i. ethmoidalis ossis frontalis
   i. fibularis tibiae
   i. frontalis
   i. interarytenoidea
   i. intertragica
   i. ischiadica major
   i. ischiadica minor
   i. jugularis ossis occipitalis
   i. jugularis ossis temporalis
   i. jugularis sterni
   i. lacrimalis maxillae
   i. ligamenti teretis
   i. mastoidea ossis temporalis
   i. nasalis maxillae
   i. pancreatis
   i. parietalis ossis temporalis
   i. preoccipitalis
   i. pterygoidea
   i. radialis ulnae
   i. scapulae
   i. sphenopalatina ossis palatini
   i. supraorbitalis
   i. tentorii cerebelli
   i. terminalis auricularis
   i. terminalis auris
   i. thyroidea inferior
   i. thyroidea superior
   i. trochlearis ulnae
   i. tympanica
   i. tympanica [Rivini]
   i. ulnaris radii
   i. vertebralis inferior
   i. vertebralis superior
incisurae (plural of incisura)
incisure
   ethmoidal i. of frontal bone
   falciform i. of fascia lata
   frontal i.
   parietal i. of temporal bone

incisure *(continued)*
   supraorbital i.
inclinatio
   i. pelvis
incoagulability
incoagulable
incontinence
incontinentia
   i. pigmenti achromians
incudiform
incus
indenization
indentation
index
   Arneth i.
   Broders' i.
   cardiothoracic i.
   erythrocyte indices
   red blood cell indices
   red cell indices
indicator
   radioactive i.
indium
   i. 111
   i. 113m
   i. In 111 chloride
   i. In 111 DTPA
   i. In 111 oxine
   i. In 111 oxyquinoline
   i. In 111 pentetreotide
   i. In 111 pentetate
   i. In 111 satumomab pendetide
Indocin
induction
   magnetic i.
induration
   phlebitic i.
indusium griseum
infarct
   ischemic i.

infarct *(continued)*
     lacunar i.
     watershed i.

infarction
     myocardial i.
     thalamic i.

infection
     nosocomial i.
     staph i.
     urinary tract i. (UTI

inferent

inferior

inferolateral

inferomedian

inferoposterior

inferosuperior

infiltrate
     lung i.
     patchy i.
     pneumonic i.

infiltration
     lymphocytic i. of skin
     paraneural i.
     perineural i.

inflammation

inflection, inflexion

infra-axillary

infraclavicular

infracortical

infracostal

infraction
     Freiberg's i.

infradiaphragmatic

infrahilar

infralevator

inframammillary

inframammary

inframarginal

infraorbital

infrapatellar

infrapulmonary

infrascapular

infrasternal

infratemporal

infratrochlear

infratubal

infraumbilical

infundibular

infundibuliform

infundibuloma

infundibulum *pl.* infundibula
     i. ethmoidale cavitatis nasi
     i. ethmoidale ossis ethmoi-
          dalis
     i. tubae uterinae
     i. neurohypophyseos
     i. lobi posterioris hypophy-
          seos

infusion

Infusaport catheter

ingestion

inguen *pl.* inguina

inguinal

inguinoabdominal

inguinocrural

inhaler
     ether i.

inhalation

inherent

inhibitor
     lupus i.
     α_2-plasmin i.
     plasminogen activator i.
     platelet i.

inhibitor *(continued)*
    protein C i.

inhomogeneity

iniac

iniad

inial

inion

initiation

injection
    anatomical i.
    bismuth i.
    bolus i.
    chymopapain i.
    coarse i.
    fine i.
    gaseous i.
    intravenous i.
    iobenguane I 123 i.
    iodinated I 131 albumin ag-
        gregated i.
    ipsilateral i.
    opacifying i.
    selective i.
    sodium radiochromate i.
    subarachnoid i.
    uneventful i.

injury
    contrecoup i.
    phrenic nerve i.

inlet
    pelvic i.
    thoracic i.

innidiation

innominatal

innominate

inosemia

inscriptio *pl.* inscriptiones

inscription

inscriptiones (plural of inscrip-
    tio)

insertio

insertion
    percutaneous cholecysto-
        tomy tube i.

in situ

insonate

inspiration
    shallow i.

inspiration and expiration
    views (*not* inspiration-expira-
    tion)

instability

instillation

instilled

insufficiency
    mitral i.
    renal i.

insufflation
    perirenal i.
    presacral i.

insula

insular

insulinoma

insuloma

intact

integument
    common i.

integumentary

integumentum
    i. commune

intensionometer

intensity
    signal i.
    i. of x-rays

interacinar

interacinous

interalveolar

interangular

interannular

intercanalicular

intercartilaginous

intercavernous

interchange
    Hamburger i.

interchondral

intercilium

interclavicular

intercolumnar

intercostal

intercostohumeral

intercristal

intercrural

interdigitation

interfascicular

interfemoral

interferon
    i.-α
    i. alfa-2a
    i. alfa-2b
    leukocyte i.

interfrontal

intergluteal

interior

interischiadic

interlabial

interleukin
    i.-6

interligamentary

interligamentous

interlobar

interlobular

intermammillary

intermammary

intermediate

intermediolateral

intermedius

intermural

intermuscular

internal

internal and external rotation
    views

internatal

internodal

internodular

internus

interoinferiorly

interorbital

interosseal

interosseous

interparietal

interpeduncular

interphalangeal (IP) joints

interposition
    i. of colon between the
      liver and diaphragm (Chi-
      laiditi's syndrome)

interpubic

interpupillary

interruption

interscapilium

interscapular

interscapulum

intersciatic

intersectio *pl.* intersectiones
    i. tendinea
    intersectiones tendineae
      musculi recti abdominis

intersection

intersectiones (plural of inter-
    sectio)

intersegment

intersegmental

interseptal

interseptum

interspaces

interstice

interstitial

interstitium

intertriginous

intertrigo

intertubercular

intertubular

interureteral

interureteric

intervalvular

interventricular

intestinal

intestine

intestinum
    i. crassum
    i. tenue

intima

intoxication
    roentgen i.

intra-abdominal

intra-acinous

intra-atrial

intra-articular

intracanalicular (*not* intracani-
    cular)

intracapsular

intracavitary

intracelial

intracerebellar

intracerebral

intracorporal

intracorporeal

intracorpuscular

intractable

intracutaneous

intrad

intradermal

intraductal

intradural

intraepidermal

intraerythrocytic

intrafascicular

intraglandular

intraglobular

intrajugular

intraleukocytic

intralobar

intralobular

intraluminal

intramammary

intramarginal

intramedullary

intramural

intramuscular (IM)

intraorbital

intraparenchymal

intraparietal

intrapelvic

intraperitoneal

intrasegmental

intrasplenic

intrathecal

intrathoracic

intratrabecular

intratubular

intravenous (IV)
    i. administration of con-
      trast material

intraventricular

intrinsic

introducer set

introflexion

introitus

Intron A

intubation

intumescentia
    i. cervicalis
    i. lumbosacralis
    i. tympanica

in utero

intussusception

invagination
    basilar i.

invasion

invasive

invasiveness

inversion
    nipple i.

inversus

invertor

invest

in vitro

in vivo

involution

iobenguane
    i. I 123
    i. I 131
    i. I 123 sulfate

iocetamic acid

iodide seeds

iodamide

iodine
    i. 123
    i. 125
    i. 131
    radioactive i. (RAI)

iodipamide
    i. meglumine
    i. methylglucamine
    i. sodium

iodixanol

iodochlorol

iodocholesterol I 131

iododerma

iodohippurate sodium
    i. s. I 123
    i. s. I 131

iodolography

iodomethylnorcholesterol

iodopanoic acid

iodophilia

iodophthalein sodium

iodopyracet

iodoventriculography

iodoxamic acid

iofetamine hydrochloride I 123

ioglycamic acid

iohexol

ionization
  avalanche i.
  Townsend i.

ionometer

ionotherapy

iontoquantimeter

iontoradiometer

iopamidol

iopanoic acid

iophendylate

iophenoxic acid

iopromide

ioseric acid

iosulamide meglumine

iothalamate
  i. meglumine
  i. sodium
  i. I 125 sodium

iothalamic acid

ioversol

ioxaglate

ioxaglic acid

ioxilan

IP
  interphalangeal
    IP joint

ipodate
  i. calcium
  i. sodium

iproplatin

ipsilateral

irides (plural of iris)

iridium
  i. Ir 192

iris *pl.* irides

iron
  i. 55
  i. 59

irradiate

irradiation
  extended field i.
  external beam i.
  hemibody i.
  interstitial i.
  inverted Y field i.
  involved field i.
  mantle field i.
  radical i.
  total body i.
  total lymphoid i.
  whole-body i.

irregularity

irrelevant

irrigation

irrigoradioscopy

irrigoscopy

irritant
  primary i.

irritation

irritative

ischemia
  focal i.
  myocardial i.
  stress-induced i.

ischemic

ischia

ischiadic

ischial

ischiatic

ischioanal

ischiobulbar

ischiococcygeus

ischiorectal

ischiovaginal

ischium

island
bone i.

isocenter

isodense

isodose

isoeffect

isoenzyme
Regan i.

isoeugenol

isoflurane

isointense

Isopaque

N-isopropyl-*p*-iodo-amphetamine

isothiazine hydrochloride

isotope
radioactive i.

Isovue
I. 200
I. 300
I. 370

isthmi (plural of isthmus)

isthmian

isthmic

isthmus *pl.* isthmi
i. aortae
aortic i.
i. cartilaginis auricularis
i. cartilaginis auris
i. faucium
i. glandulae thyroideae
i. gyri cinguli
i. prostatae
i. rhombencephali
thyroid i.
i. tubae auditivae
i. tubae auditoriae

isthmus *(continued)*
i. tubae uterinae
i. uteri

itch
bakers' i.
barbers' i.
clam diggers' i.
copra i.
dew i.
dhobie i.
dhobie mark i.
grain i.
grocers' i.
ground i.
jock i.
prairie i.
seven-year i.
straw i.
swimmers' i.
winter i.

itching

iter

iteral

I-131 therapy

Ito
nevus of I.

IUCD
intrauterine contraceptive device

IUD
intrauterine device

IUP
intrauterine pregnancy

IV
intravenous

IVC
intravenous cholangiogram

IVP
intravenous pyelogram

Ivy
I's method
I's test

Jacob's ulcer

Jacquet
 J's dermatitis
 J's erythema

Jadassohn
 nevus sebaceus of J.
 J's anetoderma
 J's sebaceous nevus
 J.-Lewandowsky syndrome
 J.-Pellizari anetoderma
 J.-Tièche nevus

Jamshidi needle

jaundice
 acholuric familial j.
 chronic acholuric j.
 congenital hemolytic j.
 familial acholuric j.
 hemolytic j.
 obstructive j.

jaw

Jefferson fracture

jejunoileal (JI)
 j. shunt

jejunoileostomy

jejunostomy

jejunum

Jewett nail

JI
 jejunoileal
  JI shunt

Johnson-Stevens disease

joint
 acromioclavicular j.
 ball and socket j.
 bleeder's j.
 bony j's
 carpometacarpal j.
 Charcot j.
 elbow j.

joint *(continued)*
 glenohumeral j.
 hemophilic j.
 humeral j.
 interphalangeal (IP) j.
 metacarpophalangeal
  (MP) j.
 metatarsophalangeal
  (MTP) j.
 mortise j.
 osseous j's
 patellofemoral j.
 peg-and-socket j.
 radiohumeral j.
 sacroiliac (SI) j's
 shoulder j.
 SI (sacroiliac) j's
 j. space narrowing
 sternoclavicular j.
 talonavicular j.
 talotibial j.
 temporomandibular j.
  (TMJ)
 trapeziometacarpal j.

Jones fracture

Jordans' anomaly

JRA
 juvenile rheumatoid arthritis

Judet view

Judkins
 J. coronary catheter
 J. pigtail left ventriculography catheter
 J. technique

juga (plural of jugum)

jugal

jugum *pl.* juga
 j. sphenoidale
 juga cerebralia

junctio
 j. anorectalis

junction
  atriocaval j.
  dermoepidermal j.
  costochondral j.
  gastroduodenal j.
  gastroesophageal (GE) j.
  lumbrosacral (LS) j.
  mucocutaneous j.
  rectosigmoid j.
  sternomanubrial j.
  sternochondral j.
  sternoclavicular j.
  thoracolumbar j.
  ureteropelvic j. (UPJ)
  ureterovesical j. (UVJ)

junctional

junctura *pl.* juncturae
  j. cartilaginea
  j. fibrosa
  juncturae cinguli pectoralis

junctura *(continued)*
  juncturae cinguli pelvici
  juncturae columnae verte-
    bralis
  juncturae cranii
  juncturae membri inferioris
  juncturae membri inferioris
    liberi
  juncturae membri superi-
    oris
  juncturae membri superi-
    oris liberi
  juncturae ossium
  j. ossea
  juncturae thoracis

juxta-articular

juxtaepiphyseal

juxtaposition

juxtaspinal

kabure

kallak

kallikrein
    plasma k.
    tissue k.

kallikreinogen

Kantor's sign

Kaposi
    K's sarcoma
    K's varicelliform eruption

Kartagener
    K's syndrome
    K's triad

Kasabach-Merritt syndrome

Kast's syndrome

Kehr's sign

Kelene

Kell blood group

keloid
    acne k.

keratinization

keratinize

keratinocyte

keratinosome

keratoacanthoma
    eruptive k.
    giant k.
    multiple k.
    solitary k.

keratoderma
    k. blennorrhagicum
    k. climactericum
    k. palmare et plantare
    palmoplantar k.
    palmoplantar k., diffuse

keratodermia

keratohyalin

keratolysis
    pitted k.
    k. plantare sulcatum

keratoma *pl.* keratomata
    k. hereditarium mutilans
    k. plantare sulcatum
    k. senile

keratomata (plural of keratoma)

keratomycosis
    k. nigricans

keratosis *pl.* keratoses
    actinic k.
    arsenic k.
    arsenical k.
    k. blennorrhagica
    k. follicularis
    k. follicularis contagiosa
    inverted follicular k.
    k. palmaris et plantaris
    k. pilaris
    k. punctata
    roentgen k.
    seborrheic k.
    k. seborrheica
    senile k.
    solar k.
    stucco k.
    tar k.

keratotic

Kerckring's folds

kerion

Kerley
    K. A lines
    K. B lines
    K. C lines
    K's lines

kerma

Kernig's sign

Ketaject

Ketalar

ketamine hydrochloride

Ketaset

ketosteroid
  17-k.

Kidd blood group

kidney
  Ask-Upmark k.
  ectopic k.
  k. failure
  floating k.
  fused k.
  horseshoe k's
  medullary sponge k.
  nonfunctioning k.
  pelvic k.
  Potter Type IV k.
  transplanted k.

Kiel classification

Kienböck
  K. unit
  K.-Adamson points

Kikuchi
  K's disease
  K's lymphadenitis
  K.-Fujimoto disease

kilocurie

Kimmelstiel-Wilson syndrome

Kimura's disease

Kinevac

kininogen
  high-molecular-weight k.
  low-molecular-weight k.

King syndrome

kinking

Kirschner wires

Klatskin's tumor

Klebsiella pneumonia

Kleihauer
  K. test
  K.-Betke test

Klemm's sign

Klinefelter's syndrome

Klippel-Feil syndrome

knee
  k. jerk reflex
  knock-k.
  "lover's k."
  prosthetic k. replacement

knife
  gamma k.

knob
  aortic k.
  surfers' k's

Knops blood group

knot
  surfers' k's

knuckle
  aortic k.

Koebner's phenomenon

Koenen's tumor

koilonychia

Kopans needle

Kostmann's syndrome

kraurosis
  k. vulvae

krebiozen

kringle

Kromayer's lamp

Krukenberg's tumor

krypton
  k. Kr 81m

KUB
  kidneys, ureters, bladder
  KUB film

Kulchitzky-cell carcinoma

Kupffer cell sarcoma

Kussmaul's sign

Küttner
    hauptganglion of K.
    K's ganglion

K wires

kymography
    roentgen k.

kyphosis

kyphoscoliosis

Kyrle's disease

Labbé's triangle

label
   radioactive l.

labeling
   l. abnormality
   l. of the isotope

labia (plural of labium)

labial

labially

labium *pl.* labia
   l. anterius ostii uteri
   l. externum cristae iliacae
   l. internum cristae iliacae
   l. laterale lineae asperae femoris
   l. limbi tympanicum
   l. limbi vestibulare
   l. majus pudendi
   l. medialis lineae asperae femoris
   l. minus pudendi
   l. posterius ostii uteri

labrum *pl.* labra
   l. acetabulare
   l. acetabuli
   l. articulare
   glenoid l.
   l. glenoidale

labyrinth
   bony l.
   cochlear l.
   ethmoid l.
   membranous l.
   vestibular l.

labyrinthitis

labyrinthus *pl.* labyrinthi
   l. cochlearis
   l. ethmoidalis
   l. membranaceus
   l. osseus
   l. vestibularis

lacertus
   l. fibrosus musculi bicipitis brachii
   l. musculi recti lateralis bulbi

lacteal

lactoferrin

lacuna *pl.* lacunae
   lacunae laterales
   l. of muscles
   l. musculorum
   lacunae urethrales
   vascular l.
   muscular l.
   l. vasorum

lacunar

lacune

lacunule

lacus
   l. lacrimalis

LAD
   left anterior descending
   LAD artery

Laënnec's cirrhosis

lageniform

lake
   vascular l.
   venous l.

Laki-Lorand factor

lambdoid

lambda

Lambert
   L.-Eaton myasthenic syndrome
   L.-Eaton syndrome

lame foliacée

lamella *pl.* lamellae
   cornoid l.

lamellar

lamelliform

lamina *pl.* laminae
- l. affixa
- l. alaris
- l. anterior vaginae musculi recti abdominis
- l. arcus vertebrae
- l. basalis choroideae
- l. basalis corporis ciliaris
- l. basilaris ductus cochlearis
- l. cartilaginis cricoideae
- l. cartilaginis lateralis tubae auditivae
- l. cartilaginis medialis tubae auditivae
- l. cartilaginis thyroideae dextra/sinistra
- l. choroidocapillaris
- l. cribrosa ossis ethmoidalis
- l. cribrosa sclerae
- l. dura
- l. episcleralis
- l. externa calvariae
- l. externa ossium cranii
- external l. of peritoneum
- l. fusca sclerae
- l. granularis externa
- l. granularis interna
- l. horizontalis ossis palatini
- l. interna calvariae
- l. interna cranii
- l. interna ossium cranii
- l. lateralis cartilaginis tubae auditivae
- l. lateralis cartilaginis tubae auditoriae
- l. lateralis processus pterygoidei
- l. limitans anterior corneae
- l. limitans posterior corneae
- l. medialis cartilaginis tubae auditivae
- l. medialis cartilaginis tubae auditoriae

lamina *(continued)*
- l. medialis processus pterygoidei
- l. medullaris externa corporis striati
- l. medullaris interna corporis striati
- l. medullaris lateralis corporis striati
- l. medullaris lateralis thalami
- l. medullaris medialis corporis striati
- l. medullaris medialis thalami
- l. membranacea tubae auditivae
- l. membranacea tubae auditoriae
- l. modioli
- l. molecularis
- l. multiformis
- l. muscularis mucosae
- l. muscularis mucosae gastris
- l. muscularis mucosae intestini crassi
- l. muscularis mucosae intestini tenuis
- l. muscularis mucosae oesophagi
- l. muscularis mucosae recti
- l. orbitalis ossis ethmoidalis
- l. papyracea
- l. parietalis pericardi serosi
- l. parietalis tunicae vaginalis propriae testis
- l. parietalis tunicae vaginalis testis
- l. perpendicularis ossis palatini
- l. posterior vaginae musculi recti abdominis
- l. pretrachealis fasciae cervicalis
- l. prevertebralis fasciae cervicalis

lamina *(continued)*
- l. profunda fasciae temporalis
- l. profunda musculi levatoris palpebrae superioris
- l. propria mucosae
- l. pyramidalis externa
- l. pyramidalis interna
- l. quadrigemina
- l. septi pellucidi
- l. spiralis ossea
- l. spiralis secundaria
- l. superficialis fasciae cervicalis
- l. superficialis fasciae temporalis
- l. superfiicalis musculi levatoris palpebrae superioris
- l. suprachorioidea
- l. tecti mesencephali
- l. terminalis hypothalami
- l. tragi
- l. tragica
- l. vasculosa chorioideae
- l. vasculosa choroideae
- l. visceralis pericardii serosi
- l. visceralis tunicae vaginalis testis

laminae *(plural of lamina)*

laminagram

laminagraph

laminagraphy

laminar

laminectomy
- lumbar l.

laminogram

laminography

lamp
- cold quartz l.
- germicidal l.
- high pressure mercury arc l.
- hot quartz l.
- Kromayer's l.

lamp *(continued)*
- low pressure mercury arc l.
- mercury arc l.
- mercury vapor l.
- quartz l.
- sun l.
- ultraviolet l.
- Wood's l.
- xenon arc l.

Lan blood group

lancet
- acne l.

landmark

Langenbeck's triangle

Langer's lines

Langerhans
- L's cells
- L's granules

lanugo

LAO
- left anterior oblique
- LAO view

laparoscopy

laparotomy
- staging l.

Larrey
- L's cleft
- L's spaces

Larsen's disease

larva
- l. currens
- l. migrans
- l. migrans, cutaneous

larynges *(plural of larynx)*

laryngogram

laryngography

laryngostat

larynx *pl.* larynges

laser

Lasix

laterad

lateral
l. flexion and extension views
l. masses
l. meniscus
l. projection
l. recess
l. recess stenosis
l. projection
l. ventricle

lateralis

lateroabdominal

laterodeviation

lateroflexion

lateroposition

lateroversion

latissimus

latus

Laurin's projection

lavage
gastric l.

Law's view

law
Bergonié-Tribondeau l.
Coutard's l.
Virchow's l.

layer
basal l.
basal l. of epidermis
clear l. of epidermis
cortical l.
deep l. of temporal fascia
germinative l.
germinative l. of epidermis
germinative l. of nail
granular l. of epidermis
half-value l.
Henle's l.

layer *(continued)*
horny l. of epidermis
horny l. of nail
Huxley's l.
malpighian l.
mucous l.
papillary l. of corium
papillary l. of dermis
prevertebral l. of cervical fascia
prickle cell l.
reticular l. of corium
reticular l. of dermis
second half-value l.
spinous l. of epidermis
superficial l. of temporal fascia

layering of contrast material

layering-out of pleural effusion

LE
lupus erythematosus

lead
bipolar l.
transvenous l.
unipolar l.

leaf of the diaphragm

leash

Leber's corpuscles

Le Fort procedure

leiodermia

leiomyoblastoma

leiomyofibroma

leiomyoma
bizarre l.
l. cutis
epithelioid l.
intraligamentous l.
intramural l.
parasitic l.
pedunculated l.
submucosal l.
subserosal l.
l. uteri

leiomyoma *(continued)*
    uterine l.
    vascular l.

leiomyomatosis
    l. peritonealis disseminata

leiomyosarcoma
    renal l.

leiomyosarcomatosis

lemniscus *pl.* lemnisci
    l. lateralis
    l. medialis
    l. spinalis
    l. trigeminalis

lengthening

Lennert's
    L. classification
    L. lymphoma

lens

lenticel

lenticular

lentiform

lentigines (plural of lentigo)

lentiginosis

lentiginous

lentigo *pl.* lentigines
    l. maligna
    nevoid l.
    senile l.
    l. senilis
    l. simplex
    solar l.

leontiasis

leper

lepidic

lepra

leprid

lepride

leprologist

leprology

leproma

lepromatous

leprosarium

leprosary

leprosy
    borderline l.
    borderline lepromatous l.
    borderline tuberculoid l.
    diffuse l. of Lucio
    dimorphous l.
    indeterminate l.
    intermediate l.
    lazarine l.
    lepromatous l.
    Lucio's l.
    murine l.
    rat l.
    reactional l.
    tuberculoid l.
    uncharacteristic l.

leprotic

leprous

leptocytosis

leptomeningioma

leptomeningitis
    sarcomatous l.

leptomeninx

Leriche's disease

Leser-Trélat sign

lesion
    angiocentric immunoproli-
      ferative l.
    angiodysplastic l.
    annular l.
    annular constricting l.
    blastic l.
    bull's-eye l.
    coin l. of the lung
    constricting l.
    destructive bone l.

lesion *(continued)*
    discrete l.
    enhancing l.
    exophytic l.
    expansile l.
    Gill l.
    herpetic l.
    hypervascular l.
    intracranial l.
    intraluminal l.
    intraspinal l.
    malignant l.
    mass l.
    mucosal l.
    multifocal l.
    neoplastic l.
    nodular l.
    occult l.
    osteoblastic l.
    polypoid l.
    precancerous l.
    premalignant l.
    primary l.
    punctate l.
    satellite l.
    target l.

Letterer-Siwe disease

leukapheresis

leukemia
    acute l.
    acute granulocytic l.
    acute lymphoblastic l.
    acute lymphoblastic l., B-cell type
    acute lymphoblastic l., Burkitt-like
    acute lymphoblastic l., common type
    acute lymphoblastic l., null cell type
    acute lymphoblastic l., pre-B-cell type
    acute lymphoblastic l., T-cell type
    acute lymphocytic l.
    acute megakaryoblastic l.
    acute megakaryocytic l.

leukemia *(continued)*
    acute monocytic l.
    acute myeloblastic l.
    acute myelocytic l.
    acute myelogenous l.
    acute myeloid l.
    acute myelomonocytic l.
    acute nonlymphocytic l.
    acute promyelocytic l.
    acute undifferentiated l.
    adult T-cell l.
    adult T-cell l./lymphoma
    aleukemic l.
    aleukocythemic l.
    basophilic l.
    blast cell l.
    chronic l.
    chronic granulocytic l.
    chronic lymphocytic l.
    chronic myelocytic l.
    chronic myelogenous l.
    chronic myeloid l.
    chronic myelomonocytic l.
    l. cutis
    eosinophilic l.
    granulocytic l.
    hairy cell l.
    hand mirror-cell l.
    hemoblastic l.
    hemocytoblastic l.
    histiocytic l.
    leukopenic l.
    lymphatic l.
    lymphoblastic l.
    lymphocytic l.
    lymphogenous l.
    lymphoid l.
    lymphosarcoma cell l.
    mast cell l.
    megakaryoblastic l.
    megakaryocytic l.
    micromyeloblastic l.
    monocytic l.
    myeloblastic l.
    myelocytic l.
    myelogenous l.
    myeloid granulocytic l.
    myelomonocytic l.

leukemia *(continued)*
    Naegeli's l.
    plasma cell l.
    plasmacytic l.
    prolymphocytic l.
    promyelocytic l.
    Rieder's cell l.
    Schilling's l.
    stem cell l.
    subleukemic l.
    undifferentiated cell l.

leukemic

leukemid

leukemogen

leukemogenesis

leukemogenic

leukemoid

Leukine

leukoblast

leukoblastosis

leukocrit

leukocytal

leukocyte
    agranular l.
    basophilic l.
    endothelial l.
    eosinophilic l.
    granular l.
    heterophilic l.
    mast l.
    motile l.
    neutrophilic l.
    nongranular l.
    nonmotile l.
    polymorphonuclear l.
    polynuclear neutrophilic l.

leukocythemia

leukocytic

leukocytogenesis

leukocytoid

leukocytology

leukocytolysis
    venom l.

leukocytolytic

leukocytoma

leukocytopenia

leukocytoplania

leukocytopoiesis

leukocytosis
    absolute l.
    agonal l.
    basophilic l.
    eosinophilic l.
    mononuclear l.
    neutrophilic l.
    pathologic l.
    physiologic l.
    pure l.
    relative l.
    terminal l.
    toxic l.

leukocytotactic

leukocytotaxis

leukocytotherapy

leukocytotoxicity

leukocytotropic

leukoderma
    l. acquisitum centrifugum
    l. colli
    occupational l.
    postinflammatory l.
    syphilitic l.

leukodermatous

leukodermia

leukodermic

leukoencephalopathy
    necrotizing l.

leukoerythroblastic

leukoerythroblastosis

leukokinesis

leukokinetic

leukokinetics

leukokraurosis

leukolymphosarcoma

leukolysis

leukolytic

leukon

leukonychia

leukopathia
  l. punctata reticularis sym-
    metrica
  l. unguium

leukopathy

leukopedesis

leukopenia
  basophil l.
  basophilic l.
  congenital l.
  malignant l.
  pernicious l.

leukopenic

leukoplakia
  atrophic l.
  speckled l.
  l. vulvae

leukopoiesis

leukopoietic

leukopoietin

leukosarcoma

leukosis

leukostasis

leukotactic

leukotaxis

leukotrichia

leuprolide acetate

Leustatin

levallorphan tartrate

levamisole hydrochloride

levator
  l. ani

levatores

LeVeen peritoneovenous shunt

level
  air-fluid l.
  aldosterone l.
  fat-fluid l.
  fluid-fluid l.
  parathormone l.

Levine tube

levocardia

levoscoliosis

Lewandowsky
  nevus elasticus of L.
  L.-Lutz disease

Lewis blood group

Leydig cell tumor

Li-Fraumeni syndrome

lichen
  l. amyloidosus
  l. corneus hypertrophicus
  l. fibromucinoidosus
  l. myxedematosus
  l. nitidus
  l. obtusus corneus
  l. pilaris
  l. planopilaris
  l. planus
  l. planus, bullous
  l. planus, vesiculobullous
  l. planus actinicus
  l. planus annularis
  l. planus atrophicus
  l. planus erythematosus
  l. planus follicularis
  l. planus hypertrophicus
  l. planus subtropicum
  l. planus tropicum
  l. planus verrucosus

lichen *(continued)*
 l. ruber moniliformis
 l. ruber planus
 l. sclerosus
 l. sclerosus et atrophicus
 l. scrofulosorum
 l. scrofulosus
 l. simplex chronicus
 l. spinulosus
 l. striatus
 l. syphiliticus
 l. tropicus
 l. urticatus

lichenification

lichenoid

lidocaine
 l. hydrochloride

lidofenin

lie
 transverse l.

lien
 l. accessorius
 l. mobilis

lienal

lienculus

lienitis

lienocele

lienography

lienomalacia

lienomedullary

lienomyelogenous

lienomyelomalacia

lienopancreatic

lienopathy

lienorenal

lienotoxin

lienunculus

life
 mean l.

lifetime

ligament
 accessory l.
 anococcygeal l.
 anterior longitudinal l.
 appendiculo-ovarian l.
 arcuate l., lateral
 arcuate l., medial
 arcuate l., median
 arcuate l. of diaphragm, external
 arcuate l. of diaphragm, internal
 arcuate l. of diaphragm, lateral
 Burns' l.
 caudal l. of common integument
 Clado's l.
 Cooper's l.
 cordiform l. of diaphragm
 costopericardiac l.
 cruciate l.
 false l.
 Gimbernat's l.
 Günz's l.
 Hey's l.
 inguinal l.
 inguinal l. of Cooper
 interosseous l.
 lacunar l.
 lacunar l. of Gimbernat
 longitudinal l. of abdomen
 nephrocolic l.
 obturator l. of pelvis
 pectineal l.
 petroclinoid l's
 pterygospinous l.
 rhomboid l.
 serous l.
 sutural l.
 l. of Treitz
 triangular l. of linea alba
 umbilical l., lateral
 umbilical l., median
 umbilical l., middle
 vesical l., lateral
 vesicoumbilical l.

ligamenta (plural of ligamentum)

ligamentous

ligamentum *pl.* ligamenta
l. acromioclaviculare
ligamenta alaria
l. anococcygeum
l. anulare radii
l. anulare stapediale
ligamenta anularia tracheae
l. apicis dentis
l. arcuatum laterale
l. arcuatum mediale
l. arcuatum medianum
l. arteriosum
l. atlantooccipitale laterale
ligamenta auricularia
l. auriculare anterius
l. auriculare posterius
l. auriculare superius
l. bifurcatum
l. calcaneocuboideum
l. calcaneocuboideum plantare
l. calcaneofibulare
l. calcaneonaviculare
l. calcaneonaviculare plantare
l. capitis costae intraarticu-
lare
l. capitis costae radiatum
l. capitis femoris
l. capitis fibulae anterius
l. capitis fibulae posterius
l. capituli costae interarti-
culare
ligamenta capsularia
l. carpi radiatum
ligamenta carpometacarpa-
lia dorsalia
ligamenta carpometacarpa-
lia palmaria
l. caudale integumenti communis
l. ceratocricoideum

ligamentum *(continued)*
ligamenta collateralia arti-
culationum interphalan-
gealium manus
ligamenta collateralia arti-
culationum interphalan-
gealium pedis
ligamenta collateralia arti-
culationum metacarpo-
phalangealium
ligamenta collateralia arti-
culationum metatarso-
phalangealium
l. collaterale carpi radiale
l. collaterale carpi ulnare
l. collaterale fibulare
l. collaterale laterale articulationis talocruralis
l. collaterale mediale articulationis talocruralis
l. collaterale radiale
l. collaterale tibiale
l. collaterale ulnare
l. conoideum
l. coracoacromiale
l. coracoclaviculare
l. coracohumerale
l. coronarium hepatis
l. costoclaviculare
l. costotransversarium
l. costotransversarium laterale
l. costotransversarium superius
ligamenta costoxiphoidea
l. cricoarytenoideum
l. crico-arytenoideum posterius
l. cricopharyngeum
l. cricothyroideum me-
dianum
l. cricotracheale
l. cruciatum anterius genus
l. cruciatum posterius genus
l. cruciforme atlantis
l. cuboideonaviculare dorsale

ligamentum *(continued)*
- l. cuboideonaviculare plantare
- l. cuneocuboideum dorsale
- l. cuneocuboideum interosseum
- l. cuneocuboideum plantare
- ligamenta cuneometatarsalia interossea
- ligamenta cuneonavicularia dorsalia
- ligamenta cuneonavicularia plantaria
- l. deltoideum articulationis talocruralis
- l. denticulatum
- l. epididymidis inferius
- l. epididymidis superius
- ligamenta extracapsularia
- l. falciforme hepatis
- ligamenta flava
- l. flavum
- l. fundiforme penis
- l. gastrocolicum
- l. gastrolienale
- l. gastrophrenicum
- l. gastrosplenicum
- ligamenta glenohumeralia
- ligamenta hepatis
- l. hepatocolicum
- l. hepatoduodenale
- l. hepatogastricum
- l. hepatorenale
- l. hyoepiglotticum
- l. iliofemorale
- l. iliolumbale
- l. incudis posterius
- l. incudis superius
- l. inguinale
- l. inguinale reflexum
- ligamenta intercarpalia dorsalia
- ligamenta intercarpalia interossea
- ligamenta intercarpalia palmaria
- l. interclaviculare

ligamentum *(continued)*
- ligamenta intercuneiformia dorsalia
- ligamenta intercuneiformia interossea
- ligamenta intercuneiformia plantaria
- l. interfoveolare
- ligamenta interspinalia
- ligamenta intertransversaria
- ligamenta intracapsularia
- l. ischiofemorale
- l. lacunare
- l. lacunare [Gimbernati]
- l. laterale articulationis temporomandibularis
- l. latum uteri
- l. lienorenale
- l. longitudinale anterius
- l. longitudinale posterius
- l. lumbocostale
- l. mallei anterius
- l. mallei laterale
- l. mallei superius
- l. mediale articulationis temporomandibularis
- l. meniscofemorale anterius
- l. meniscofemorale posterius
- ligamenta metacarpalia dorsalia
- ligamenta metacarpalia interossea
- ligamenta metacarpalia palmaria
- l. metacarpale transversum profundum
- l. metacarpale transversum superficiale
- ligamenta metatarsalia dorsalia
- ligamenta metatarsalia interossea
- ligamenta metatarsalia plantaria
- l. metatarsale transversum profundum

ligamentum *(continued)*
l. metatarsale transversum
superficiale
l. nuchae
ligamenta ossiculorum au-
ditoriorum
ligamenta ossiculorum au-
ditus
l. ovarii proprium
ligamenta palmaria articu-
lationum interphalangeal-
ium manus
ligamenta palmaria articu-
lationum metacarpophal-
angealium
l. palpebrale laterale
l. palpebrale mediale
l. patellae
l. pectinatum anguli iridocornealis
l. pectineale
l. pectineum
l. phrenicocolicum
l. pisohamatum
l. pisometacarpeum
ligamenta plantaria articu-
lationum interphalangeal-
ium pedis
ligamenta plantaria articu-
lationum metatarsophal-
angealium
l. plantare longum
l. popliteum arcuatum
l. popliteum obliquum
l. pterygospinale
l. pubicum inferius
l. pubicum superius
l. pubofemorale
l. puboprostaticum
l. pubovesicale
l. pulmonale
l. quadratum
l. radiocarpale dorsale
l. radiocarpale palmare
l. sacrococcygeum anterius
l. sacrococcygeum dorsale
profundum
l. sacrococcygeum dorsale
superficiale

ligamentum *(continued)*
l. sacrococcygeum laterale
l. sacrococcygeum poster-
ius profundum
l. sacrococcygeum poster-
ius superficiale
l. sacrococcygeum ventrale
l. sacroiliacum anterius
l. sacroiliacum dorsalis
l. sacroiliacum interosseum
l. sacroiliacum posterius
l. sacroiliacum ventralis
l. sacrospinale
l. sacrotuberale
l. serosum
l. sphenomandibulare
l. spirale cochleae
l. spirale ductus cochlearis
l. splenorenale
l. sternoclaviculare anterius
l. sternoclaviculare posterius
l. sternocostale intraarticu-
lare
ligamenta sternocostalia radiata
ligamenta sternopericardi-
aca
l. stylohyoideum
l. stylomandibulare
l. supraspinale
l. suspensorium clitoridis
ligamenta suspensoria
mammae
ligamenta suspensoria
mammaria
l. suspensorium ovarii
l. suspensorium penis
l. talocalcaneare mediale
l. talocalcaneum interos-
seum
l. talocalcaneum laterale
l. talocalcaneum mediale
l. talofibulare anterius
l. talofibulare posterius
l. talonaviculare
ligamenta tarsi
ligamenta tarsi dorsalia

ligamentum *(continued)*
    ligamenta tarsi interossea
    ligamenta tarsi plantaria
    ligamenta tarsometarsalia
      dorsalia
    ligamenta tarsometatarsalia
      plantaria
    l. teres hepatis
    l. teres uteri
    l. thyroepiglotticum
    l. thyrohyoideum laterale
    l. thyrohyoideum me-
      dianum
    l. tibiofibulare anterius
    l. tibiofibulare posterius
    ligamenta trachealia
    l. transversum acetabuli
    l. transversum atlantis
    l. transversum genus
    l. transversum perinei
    l. transversum scapulae in-
      ferius
    l. transversum scapulae su-
      perius
    l. trapezoideum
    l. triangulare dextrum he-
      patis
    l. triangulare sinistrum he-
      patis
    l. ulnocarpale palmare
    l. umbilicale laterale
    l. umbilicale mediale
    l. umbilicale medianum
    l. venosum
    l. vestibulare
    l. vocale
light
    Wood's l.
lignocaine
limb
    pectoral l.
    pelvic l.
    thoracic l.
limbal
limbi (plural of limbus)
limbic

limbus *pl.* limbi
    l. acetabuli
    l. anterior palpebrae
    l. corneae
    l. fossae ovalis
    l. palpebralis anterior
    l. palpebralis posterior
    l. posterior palpebrae
    l. spiralis
lime
    barium hydroxide l.
    soda l.
limen *pl.* limina
    l. insulae
    l. nasi
limit
    quantum l.
limitation of motion
Lindau
    L's disease
    L's tumor
    L.-von Hippel disease
line
    abdominal l.
    anococcygeal l., white
    anterior humeral l.
    arcuate l. of occipital bone,
      external superior
    arcuate l. of occipital bone,
      highest
    arcuate l. of occipital bone,
      inferior
    arcuate l. of occipital bone,
      superior
    arcuate l. of occipital bone,
      supreme
    arcuate l. of sheath of rec-
      tus abdominis muscle
    axillary l.
    axillary l., median
    axillary l., posterior
    Blumensaat's l.
    Cameron's l's
    central venous pressure
      (CVP) l.
    clavicular l.

line *(continued)*
   cleavage l's
   Correra's l.
   costoclavicular l.
   costophrenic septal l's
   cricoclavicular l.
   cruciate l.
   curved l. of occipital bone,
     highest
   curved l. of occipital bone,
     inferior
   curved l. of occipital bone,
     superior
   curved l. of occipital bone,
     supreme
   Daubenton's l.
   l. of Douglas
   dynamic l's
   epiphyseal l.
   l's of expression
   Futcher's l.
   Granger l.
   grid l's
   Hampton l.
   Harris l's
   Hunter's l.
   infracostal l.
   infrascapular l.
   iliopectineal l.
   intermediate l. of iliac crest
   interspinal l.
   intertuberal l.
   intertubercular l.
   isoeffect l's
   Kerley's l's
   Kerley A l's
   Kerley B l's
   Kerley C l's
   Langer's l's
   lower lung l.
   mammillary l.
   median l.
   median l., anterior
   median l., posterior
   medioclavicular l.
   midaxillary l.
   midclavicular l.
   l's of minimal tension
   Monro's l.

line *(continued)*
   Monro-Richter l.
   Morgan's l.
   Moyer's l.
   Nélaton's l.
   nipple l.
   nuchal l.
   nuchal l., highest
   nuchal l., inferior
   nuchal l., median
   nuchal l., middle
   nuchal l., superior
   nuchal l., supreme
   oblique l.
   omphalospinous l.
   orthostatic l's
   papillary l.
   pararectal l.
   parasternal l.
   paravertebral l.
   postaxillary l.
   Poupart's l.
   properitoneal fat l.
   preaxillary l.
   radiocapitellar l.
   relaxed skin tension l's
   Richter-Monro l.
   Robson's l.
   Rolando's l.
   Roser's l.
   scapular l.
   Schoemaker's l.
   Schon dual l.
   semicircular l's, supreme
   semicircular l. of Douglas
   semicircular l. of frontal
     bone
   semicircular l. of occipital
     bone, highest
   semicircular l. of occipital
     bone, middle
   semicircular l. of occipital
     bone, superior
   semicircular l. of parietal
     bone, inferior
   semicircular l. of parietal
     bone, superior
   semilunar l.
   Shenton's l.

line *(continued)*
    Skinner's l.
    Spieghel's l.
    spigelian l.
    Spigelius' l.
    sternal l.
    sternal l., lateral
    subclavian l.
    subcostal l.
    supracrestal l.
    supracristal l.
    supraorbital l.
    suture l.
    sylvian l.
    temporal l., inferior
    temporal l., superior
    temporal l. of frontal bone
    temporal l. of parietal
      bone, inferior
    temporal l. of parietal
      bone, superior
    umbilicoiliac l.
    vertebral l.
    Voigt's l.
    white l.
    white l. of ischiococcygeal
      muscle
    Z-l.

linea *pl.* lineae
    l. alba
    l. alba abdominis
    l. alba cervicalis
    l. arcuata ossis ilii
    l. arcuata vaginae musculi
      recti abdominis
    l. aspera
    lineae atrophicae
    l. axillaris
    l. axillaris anterior
    l. axillaris media
    l. axillaris posterior
    l. epiphysialis
    l. glutea anterior
    l. glutea inferior
    l. glutea posterior
    l. intercondylaris
    l. intercondyloidea
    l. intermedia cristae iliacae
    l. intertrochanterica

linea *(continued)*
    l. mammillaris
    l. mediana anterior
    l. mediana posterior
    l. medio-axillaris
    l. medioclavicularis
    l. musculi solei
    l. nuchae inferior
    l. nuchae superior
    l. nuchae suprema
    l. nuchalis inferior
    l. nuchalis superior
    l. nuchalis suprema
    l. obliqua cartilaginis thyro-
      ideae
    l. pararectalis
    l. parasternalis
    l. paravertebralis
    l. pectinea
    l. postaxillaris
    l. preaxillaris
    l. scapularis
    l. semicircularis [Douglasi]
    l. semilunaris
    l. semilunaris [Spigeli]
    l. sternalis
    l. supracondylaris lateralis
    l. supracondylaris medialis
    l. temporalis inferior ossis
      parietalis
    l. temporalis ossis frontalis
    l. temporalis superior ossis
      parietalis
    l. terminalis pelvis
    lineae transversae ossis
      sacri
    l. trapezoidea
    l. vertebralis

lineae (plural of linea)

lingua *pl.* linguae

lingula *pl.* lingulae
    l. cerebelli
    l. pulmonis sinistri
    l. of sphenoid
    l. sphenoidalis

lingulae (plural of lingula)

lingular

linitis
    l. plastica

linoleate
    ethyl l.

Linsman's water test

liothyronine
    l. I 125

lip

Lipiodol

lipoadenoma

lipoblastoma

lipoblastomatosis

lipochondroma

lipofibroma

lipogranuloma

lipogranulomatous

lipohemarthrosis

lipoma
    l. annulare colli
    l. arborescens
    atypical l.
    l. capsulare
    l. cavernosum
    l. fibrosum
    intermuscular l.
    intradural l.
    intramedullary l.
    intramuscular l.
    intraspinal l.
    l. myxomatodes
    l. ossificans
    ossifying l.
    pleomorphic l.
    l. sarcomatodes
    spindle cell l.
    telangiectatic l.
    l. telangiectodes

lipomatoid

lipomatosis

lipomatous

lipomyohemangioma

lipomyoma

lipomyxoma

liposarcoma
    dedifferentiated l.
    myxoid l.
    pleomorphic l.
    round cell l.
    well-differentiated l.

Lippes loop

lipping

liquor
    l. cerebrospinalis

liquores

Lisfranc fracture

lithiasis

lithotripsy
    extracorporeal shock
      wave l.

livedo
    l. racemosa
    l. reticularis
    l. reticularis, idiopathic
    l. reticularis, symptomatic
    l. telangiectatica

livedoid

liver

lobar

lobate

lobation
    renal l.

lobe
    caudate l.
    frontal l.
    lingular l.
    parietal l.
    quadrate l. of the liver

lobe *(continued)*
    Riedel's l.
    spigelian l.
    superior parietal l.
    temporal l.
    l's of thymus

lobectomy

lobi (plural of lobe)

lobite

lobular

lobulated

lobulation
    fetal l.

lobule
    superior parietal l.
    l's of thymus

lobuli (plural of lobulus)

lobulose

lobulous

lobulus *pl.* lobuli
    l. ansiformis
    l. auriculae
    l. auricularis
    l. biventer
    l. centralis cerebelli
    lobuli epididymidis
    lobuli glandulae mammariae
    lobuli glandulae thyroideae
    l. gracilis cerebelli
    lobuli hepatis
    l. paracentralis
    l. paramedianus cerebelli
    l. parietalis inferior
    l. parietalis superior
    l. quadrangularis anterior cerebelli
    l. quadrangularis posterior cerebelli
    l. simplex cerebelli
    lobuli testis
    lobuli thymi
    lobuli semilunares

lobulus *(continued)*
    l. semilunaris inferior
    l. semilunaris superior

lobus *pl.* lobi
    l. anterior hypophyseos
    l. caudatus hepatis
    l. caudatus [Spigeli]
    l. cerebelli anterior
    l. cerebelli posterior
    lobi cerebri
    l. flocculonodularis
    l. frontalis
    lobi glandulae mammariae
    l. glandulae thyroideae
    l. hepatis dexter
    l. hepatis sinister
    l. inferior pulmonis dextri
    l. inferior pulmonis sinistri
    l. insularis
    l. limbicus
    l. medius prostatae
    l. medius pulmonis dextri
    l. nervosus neurohypophyseos
    l. occipitalis
    l. parietalis
    l. posterior hypophysis
    lobi prostatae dexter et sinister
    l. pyramidalis glandulae thyroideae
    l. quadratus hepatis
    lobi renales
    l. superior pulmonis dextri
    l. superior pulmonis sinistri
    l. temporalis
    l. thymi

localization
    needle l. of breast lesion
    l. purposes

localizer

loci (plural of locus)

locomotorium

locular

loculate

loculated

loculation

loculus *pl.* loculi

locus *pl.* loci
  l. caeruleus
  l. ceruleus

Loeffler's syndrome

Löfgren's syndrome

loin

lomustine (CCNU)

Longdwell needle

longilineal

longimanous

longipedate

longissimus

longitudinal

longitudinalis

longitypical

longstanding

longus

loop
  afferent l.
  l. of bowel
  duodenal l.
  l. distribution
  efferent l.
  l's of Henle
  Lippes l.
  sentinel l.

loopogram

loosening of the prosthesis

lordosis

lordotic
  l. curve

Louis' angle

"lover's knee"

low-signal

LS
  lumbosacral
    LS junction
    LS spine

L-shaped

lucency

lucent

Lucio's phenomenon

lucotherapy

Ludwig
  L's angle
  L's plane

lues

luetic

Lukes-Collins Classification

lumbar
  l. disk herniation

lumbarization

lumboabdominal

lumbocostal

lumbocrural

lumbodorsal

lumboiliac

lumboinguinal

lumbosacral (LS)

lumbus

lumen *pl.* lumina
  appendiceal l.

luminal

luminalis

lunate

Lund-Browder classification

Lunderquist
  L. catheter

Lunderquist *(continued)*
    L. wire

lung
    artificial l.
    honeycomb l.
    l. perfusion

lunula *pl.* lunulae
    l. of nail
    l. unguis
    lunulae valvularum semilu-
        narium valvae aortae
    lunulae valvularum semilu-
        narium valvae trunci pul-
        monalis

lunulae (plural of lunula)

lupiform

lupoid

Lupron

lupus
    chilblain l.
    l. erythematosus (LE)
    l. erythematosus, chilblain
    l. hypertrophicus
    l. miliaris disseminatus fa-
        ciei
    l. pernio
    systemic l. erythematosus
        (SLE)
    l. tumidus
    l. vulgaris

Luschka
    foramen of L.
    glandular foveae of L.
    joints of L.
    L's tonsil

Lutembacher's disease

luteoma

Lutheran blood group

Lyell
    L's disease
    L's syndrome

lymph
    aplastic l.

lymph *(continued)*
    corpuscular l.
    euplastic l.
    fibrinous l.
    intercellular l.
    intravascular l.
    tissue l.

lympha

lymphaden

lymphadenectomy
    retroperitoneal l.

lymphadenitis
    cervical l.
    cervical l., tuberculous
    histiocytic necrotizing l.
    Kikuchi's l.
    subacute necrotizing l.
    tuberculous l.

lymphadenocele

lymphadenocyst

lymphadenogram

lymphadenography

lymphadenoid

lymphadenoleukopoiesis

lymphadenoma

lymphadenopathy
    dermatopathic l.
    hilar l.
    mediastinal l.

lymphadenosis

lymphadenovarix

lymphangeitis

lymphangial

lymphangiectasia
    intestinal l.

lymphangiectasis

lymphangiitis

lymphangioadenography

lymphangioendothelioma

lymphangiofibroma

lymphangiogram

lymphangiography
    bipedal l.
    pedal l.

lymphangiology

lymphangioma
    capillary l.
    l. cavernosum
    cavernous l.
    l. circumscriptum
    cystic l.
    l. cysticum
    fissural l.
    simple l.
    l. simplex

lymphangiomyomatosis

lymphangion

lymphangiosarcoma

lymphangitic
    l. spread of carcinoma

lymphangitis
    l. carcinomatosa

lymphatic

lymphatitis

lymphatogenous

lymphatology

lymphatolysis

lymphatolytic

lymphectasia

lymphedema
    l. praecox

lymphepithelioma

lymphization

lymphnoditis

lymphoblastoma

lymphoblastosis

lymphocele

lymphocinesia

lymphocyst

lymphocyte
    plasmacytoid l.
    Rieder's l.
    tumor-infiltrating l's

lymphocytoma
    l. cutis

lymphoduct

lymphoepithelioma

lymphogenesis

lymphogenous

lymphoglandula

lymphogram

lymphogranuloma
    l. malignum

lymphogranulomatosis
    l. cutis

lymphography
    bipedal l.

lymphohistiocytosis
    erythrophagocytic l.
    hemophagocytic l.

lymphoid

lymphoidocyte

lymphokinesis

lymphology

lymphoma
    adult T-cell l.
    adult T-cell leukemia/l.
    African l.
    B-cell l.
    B-cell monocytoid l.
    Burkitt's l.
    centrocytic l.
    l. cutis
    diffuse l.

lymphoma *(continued)*
   diffuse, large cell l.
   diffuse, mixed small and
     large cell l.
   diffuse, small cleaved cell l.
   follicular l.
   follicular center cell l.
   follicular, mixed small
     cleaved and large cell l.
   follicular, predominantly
     large cell l.
   follicular, predominantly
     small cleaved cell l.
   giant follicle l.
   giant follicular l.
   granulomatous l.
   histiocytic l.
   Hodgkin's l.
   Ki-1 l.
   large cell l.
   large cell, immunoblastic l.
   large cleaved cell l.
   large noncleaved cell l.
   Lennert's l.
   lymphoblastic l.
   lymphocytic l., intermedi-
     ate
   lymphocytic l., intermedi-
     ately differentiated
   lymphocytic l., plasmacy-
     toid
   lymphocytic l., poorly dif-
     ferentiated
   lymphocytic l., small
   lymphocytic l., well differ-
     entiated
   malignant l.
   MALT l.
   mantle cell l.
   mantle zone l.
   marginal zone l.
   Mediterranean l.
   mixed lymphocytic-histio-
     cytic l.
   nodular l.
   non-Hodgkin's l.
   plasmacytoid l.
   pleomorphic l.
   primary effusion l.

lymphoma *(continued)*
   primary central nervous
     system l.
   small B-cell l.
   small cleaved cell l.
   small noncleaved cell l.
   T-cell l's
   T-cell l., convoluted
   T-cell l., cutaneous
   T-cell l., small lymphocytic
   U-cell l.
   undefined l.
   undifferentiated l.

lymphomatoid

lymphomatosis

lymphomatous

lymphomyxoma

lymphonodi

lymphonoduli

lymphonodulus
   lymphonoduli splenici

lymphonodus

lymphopathia

lymphopathy

lymphoplasia
   cutaneous l.

lymphoplasmapheresis

lymphopoiesis

lymphopoietic

lymphoproliferative

lymphoreticulosis

lymphorrhagia

lymphorrhea

lymphosarcoma

lymphoscintigraphy
   radiocolloid l.

lymphostasis

lymphotism

lymphotrophy

lymphotropic

lymphous

lyra

lyre

lysis of adhesions

lysokinase

MAA

Macalister
  triangular fascia of M.

Macewen's triangle

Mach
  M. effect
  M. phenomenon

McLeod
  M. phenotype
  M. syndrome

McNeer classification

macroadenoma

macrocephalic

macrocephaly

macrocythemia

macrocytosis

macroglobulinemia
  Waldenström's m.

macronychia

macrophage
  fixed m.
  . free m.
  inflammatory m.

macrophagocyte

macroprolactinoma

Macrotec

Macrozamia

macrozamin

macula *pl.* maculae
  maculae atrophicae
  maculae ceruleae
  maculae cribrosae
  m. cribrosa inferior
  m. cribrosa media
  m. cribrosa superior
  mongolian m.
  m. luteae
  m. sacculi

macula *(continued)*
  m. utriculi

maculae (plural of macula)

macular

maculate

macule
  ash-leaf m.
  lance-ovate m.

maculopapular

maculovesicular

madarosis

Madelung's disease

magenblase

Magendie
  foramen of M.

magnetization
  longitudinal m.
  transverse m.

Magnevist

magnification factor

magnum

MAI
  *Mycobacterium avium intra-
    cellulare*

Majocchi
  M's disease
  M's granuloma
  M's purpura

mal
  m. de Meleda
  m. perforant du pied

malaise

malalignment

malformation
  Arnold-Chiari m.
  arteriovenous m. (AVM)

Malherbe's calcifying epithelioma

Malibu disease

malignancy

malignant

malleolus *pl.* malleoli
    m. lateralis
    medial m.
    m. medialis

malleus *pl.* mallei

Mallinckrodt catheter

Mallorca acne

Mallory
    M.-Weiss syndrome
    M.-Weiss tear

malocclusion

malpighian
    m. cell
    m. corpuscles of spleen

malposition

malrotation

MALToma

malunion

mamelon

mamma *pl.* mammae
    m. accessoria
    m. masculina
    supernumerary m.
    m. virilis

mammae (plural of mamma)

mammary

mammiform

mammilla

mammillary

mammillated

mammillation

mammilliform

mammogram
    diagnostic m.

mammography
    screening m.

mammoplasty
    augmentation m.
    reduction m.

mammose

Manan needle

mandible

mandibular

maneuver
    Adson's m.
    Hampton m.
    Heimlich m.
    Mendelson m.
    Müller's m.
    Valsalva m.

Mani cerebral catheter

manikin

manipulation and application of plaster

mantle
    cerebral m.

manual reduction

manubrium *pl.* manubria
    m. mallei
    m. of malleus
    m. sterni
    m. of sternum

manus

Marcaine

Marchiafava-Micheli syndrome

Marcus Gunn syndrome

Marfan's syndrome

margaritoma

margin
    anterior m. of parietal bone
    anterior m. of spleen
    arcuate m. of saphenous hiatus

margin *(continued)*
    coronal m. of frontal bone
    coronal m. of parietal bone
    crenate m. of spleen
    cristate m. of spleen
    disc m's
    disk m's
    falciform m. of fascia lata
    falciform m. of saphenus
      hiatus
    free m. of nail
    frontal m. of parietal bone
    gingival m.
    hidden m. of nail
    indistinct m's
    inferior m. of spleen
    irregular m's
    lambdoid m. of occipital
      bone
    lambdoid m. of parietal
      bone
    lateral m. of nail
    mammillary m.
    mastoid m. of occipital
      bone
    mastoid m. of parietal bone
    obtuse m. of spleen
    occipital m. of parietal
      bone
    occipital m. of temporal
      bone
    parietal m. of frontal bone
    parietal m. of occipital
      bone
    parietal m. of parietal bone
    parietal m. of squamous
      part of temporal bone
    periarticular m's
    posterior m. of petrous
      part of temporal bone
    posterior m. of spleen
    sagittal m. of parietal bone
    sphenoidal m. of parietal
      bone
    sphenoidal m. of squamous
      part of temporal bone
    sphenotemporal m. of pari-
      etal bone

margin *(continued)*
    squamous m. of parietal
      bone
    superior m. of parietal
      bone
    superior m. of petrous part
      of temporal bone
    superior m. of spleen
    temporal m. of parietal
      bone

marginal

margination

margines (plural of margo)

margo *pl.* margines
    m. acetabuli
    m. anterior fibulae
    m. anterior splenis
    m. anterior corporis pan-
      creatis
    m. anterior corporis pan-
      creatis
    m. anterior pulmonis
    m. anterior radii
    m. anterior testis
    m. anterior tibiae
    m. anterior ulnae
    m. arcuatus hiatus sapheni
    m. ciliaris iridis
    m. dexter cordis
    m. falciformis fasciae latae
    m. falciformis hiatus sa-
      pheni
    m. fibularis pedis
    m. frontalis alae majoris
    m. frontalis ossis parietalis
    m. inferior hepatis
    m. inferior lienis
    m. inferior corporis pan-
      creatis
    m. inferior corporis pan-
      creatis
    m. inferior pulmonis
    m. inferior splenis
    m. inferolateralis hemi-
      spherii cerebri
    m. inferomedialis hemi-
      spherii cerebri

margo *(continued)*
- m. infraorbitalis corporis maxillae
- m. infraorbitalis corporis maxillae
- m. infraorbitalis orbitae
- m. interosseus fibulae
- m. interosseus radii
- m. interosseus tibiae
- m. interosseus ulnae
- m. lacrimalis maxillae
- m. lambdoideus ossis occipitalis
- m. lateralis antebrachii
- m. lateralis humeri
- m. lateralis orbitae
- m. lateralis pedis
- m. lateralis renis
- m. lateralis scapulae
- m. lateralis unguis
- m. liber ovarii
- m. liber unguis
- m. linguae
- m. mastoideus ossis occipitalis
- m. medialis antebrachii
- m. medialis glandulae suprarenalis
- m. medialis humeri
- m. medialis orbitae
- m. medialis pedis
- m. medialis renis
- m. medialis scapulae
- m. medialis tibiae
- m. mesovaricus ovarii
- m. nasalis ossis frontalis
- m. occipitalis ossis parietalis
- m. occipitalis ossis temporalis
- m. occultus unguis
- m. orbitalis
- m. parietalis alae majoris
- m. parietalis ossis frontalis
- m. parietalis partis squamosae ossis temporalis
- m. parietalis squamae temporalis
- m. posterior fibulae

margo *(continued)*
- m. posterior splenis
- m. posterior partis petrosae ossis temporalis
- m. posterior radii
- m. posterior testis
- m. posterior ulnae
- m. pupillaris iridis
- m. radialis antebrachii
- m. sagittalis ossis parietalis
- m. sphenoidalis partis squamosae ossis temporalis
- m. sphenoidalis squamae temporalis
- m. squamosus alae majoris
- m. squamosus ossis parietalis
- m. superior corporis pancreatis
- m. superior hemispherii cerebri
- m. superior glandulae suprarenalis
- m. superior lienis
- m. superior partis petrosae ossis temporalis
- m. superior scapulae
- m. superior splenis
- m. supraorbitalis orbitae
- m. supraorbitalis ossis frontalis
- m. tibialis pedis
- m. ulnaris antebrachii
- m. uteri
- m. zygomaticus alae majoris

Marjolin's ulcer

mark
- beauty m.
- birth m.
- pock m.
- Pohl-Pinkus m.
- port-wine m.

marker
- metallic m.

marker *(continued)*
    needle m.
    nipple m.
    tumor m.

marking
    convolutional m's
    haustral m's
    increased lung m's
    interstitial m's
    peribronchial m's

Marlex mesh

Marogen

marrow
    depressed m.
    gelatinous m.

mask
    full-face m.
    m. of pregnancy

masoprocol

mass
    abdominopelvic m.
    adrenal m.
    dominant m.
    m. effect
    hilar m.
    injection m.
    intrasellar m.
    lateral m's
    m. lesion
    mediastinal m.
    mulberry-like m.
    pelvic m.
    posterior mediastinal m.
    pulsating m.
    tubo-ovarian m.

massa *pl.* massae
    m. lateralis atlantis

mastectomy
    radical m.

mastitis
    cystic m.
    mastectomy m.

mastoccipital

mastoid

mastoidectomy

mastoiditis
    coalescent m.

masto-occipital

mastoparietal

mastopexy

matching
    cross m.

maté

material
    coffee-grounds m.
    fecal m.
    gas and fecal m.
    impacted fecal m.
    particulate m.
    semisolid fecal m.
    tissue equivalent m.

matrix
    hair m.
    nail m.
    m. unguis

matter
    gray m.
    white m.

maxilla *pl.* maxillae

maximal

May-Hegglin anomaly

Mayer
    M. position
    M. view

maytansine

mayweed

MCI/MI

meal
    Boyden m.

meal *(continued)*
 fatty m.
 opaque m.

measurement
 pelvic m's

meatal

meatus
 m. acusticus externus
 m. acusticus externus carti-
  lagineus
 m. acusticus internus
 auditory m.
 internal auditory m.
 m. nasopharyngeus
 m. nasi inferior
 m. nasi medius
 m. nasi superior

mebrofenin

meCCNU (semustine)

mechanism
 swallowing m.

mechlorethamine hydrochloride

mecobalamine

Meckel
 M.'s cave
 internal zygomatic foramen
  of M.
 M.'s plane

media

mediad

medial

medialis

median

medianus

mediastina

mediastinal

mediastinogram

mediastinography

mediastinoscopy

mediastinum
 m. anterius
 m. inferius
 m. medium
 m. posterius
 m. superius
 m. superius
 m. testis

medicine
 nuclear m.

medifrontal

medioccipital

mediolateral

Medi Omni II catheter

medisect

Mediterranean
 M. anemia
 M. disease
 M. lymphoma

medium
 contrast m.
 radiolucent m.
 radiopaque m.
 Wickersheimer's m.

medius

medronate

medulla *pl.* medullae
 m. glandulae suprarenalis
 m. of lymph node
 m. nodi lymphatici
 m. nodi lymphoidei
 m. oblongata
 m. ossium
 m. ossium flava
 m. ossium rubra
 m. ovarii
 m. renalis
 m. spinalis
 m. thymi

medullae (plural of medulla)

medullation

medulloblastoma

medulloepithelioma

megabecquerel

megacaryoblast

megacaryocyte

Megace

megacolon

megacurie

megaesophagus

megakaryoblast

megakaryocyte

megakaryocytopoiesis

megakaryocytosis

megalobulbus

megalocytosis

megalokaryocyte

megalonychia

Megalopyge

megalosplenia

megalothymus

megaloureter

megaureter

megavoltage

megestrol acetate

Méglin's point

meglumine
   m. diatrizoate
   m. iothalamate

Meigs
   M's syndrome
   M.-Salmon syndrome

Meirowsky phenomenon

melanemia

melanoacanthoma

melanoameloblastoma

melanoblastoma

melanocarcinoma

melanocyte
   dendritic m.

melanocytic

melanocytoma
   compound m.
   dermal m.
   m. of optic disk

melanocytosis
   oculodermal m.

melanoderma
   parasitic m.
   senile m.

melanodermatitis
   m. toxica lichenoides

melanoleukoderma
   m. colli

melanoma
   acral-lentiginous m.
   amelanotic m.
   benign juvenile m.
   intraocular m.
   juvenile m.
   lentigo maligna m.
   malignant m.
   mucosal m.
   nodular m.
   nontumorigenic m.
   ocular m.
   ocular malignant m.
   subungual m.
   superficial spreading m.
   tumorigenic m.
   uveal m.
   uveal malignant m.

melanomatosis

melanomatous

melanonychia

melanosis
  circumscribed precancer-
    ous m. of Dubreuilh
  neurocutaneous m.
  oculocutaneous m.
  Riehl's m.
  tar m.
  transient neonatal pustu-
    lar m.

melanosome

melanotrichia

melasma

Meleda disease

melena

Meleney
  M's chronic undermining
    ulcer
  M's gangrene
  M's synergistic gangrene
  M's ulcer

melengestrol acetate

melenic (*not* melanotic)

melorheostosis

melphalan

member

memberment

membra (plural of membrum)

membrana *pl.* membranae
  m. adventitia
  m. atlantooccipitalis ante-
    rior
  m. atlantooccipitalis poste-
    rior
  m. fibroelastica laryngis
  m. fibrosa capsulae articu-
    laris
  m. intercostalis externa
  m. intercostalis interna
  m. interossea antebrachii
  m. interossea antibrachii
  m. interossea cruris

membrana *(continued)*
  m. obturatoria
  m. obturatrix
  m. perinei
  m. pupillaris
  m. quadrangularis
  m. reticularis organi spir-
    alis
  m. reticulata
  m. serosa
  m. spiralis ductus coch-
    learis
  m. stapedialis
  m. stapedis
  m. statoconiorum macu-
    larum
  m. sterni
  m. suprapleuralis
  m. synovialis capsulae arti-
    cularis
  m. tectoria
  m. tectoria ductus coch-
    learis
  m. thyrohyoidea
  m. tympani
  m. tympanica
  m. tympani secundaria
  m. vestibularis ductus
    cochlearis
  m. vitrea

membranaceous

membranae (plural of mem-
  brana)

membranate

membrane
  glassy m.
  Huxley's m.
  hyaline m.
  keratogenous m.
  limiting m.
  mucous m.
  obturator m.
  platelet demarcation m.
  serous m.
  submucous m.
  vascular m. of viscera
  vitreous m.

membraniform

membranocartilaginous

membranoid

membranous

membrum *pl.* membra
  m. inferius
  m. superius

Mendelson
  M. maneuver
  M.'s syndrome

Ménétrier's disease

Meniere's syndrome

meninges (plural of meninx)

meningioma
  angioblastic m.
  cerebellopontine angle m.
  clival m.
  convexity m's
  cystic m.
  falcine m.
  falx m.
  fibroblastic m.
  fibrous m.
  meningotheliomatous m.
  m. of the olfactory groove
  parasagittal m.
  posterior fossa m.
  psammomatous m.
  m. of the sphenoid ridge
  suprasellar m.
  syncytial m.
  tentorial m.
  transitional m.
  m. of the tuberculum sellae

meningiomatosis

meningismus

meningitis
  m. carcinomatosa
  carcinomatous m.
  neoplastic m.

meningofibroblastoma

meningoma

meningomyelocele

meningothelioma

meninx *pl.* meninges

meniscal

menisci (plural of meniscus)

meniscectomy

meniscocytosis

meniscus *pl.*
  m. articularis
  lateral m.
  m. lateralis articulationis
    genus
  m. medialis articulationis
    genus

mentalis

mentolabial

mentum

meperidine hydrochloride

mepivacaine hydrochloride

MER

mercaptopurine

Mercedes-Benz sign

Merchant's projection

mercury
  m. 197
  m. 203
  m. tip of the Dobbhoff tube

meridian

meridianus *pl.* meridiani
  meridiani bulbi oculi

meridional

Merkel
  M. cell carcinoma
  M. cell tumor
  M.-Ranvier cells

mertiatide

MES
   meconium aspiration syndrome

mesad

mesencephalon

mesenchyma

mesenchymal

mesenchymoma
   benign m.
   malignant m.

mesenteric

mesenterium

mesentery

mesepithelium

mesh
   Marlex m.
   tantalum m.

mesiad

mesien

mesion

mesna

mesoappendix

mesocolon
   m. ascendens
   m. descendens
   m. sigmoideum
   m. transversum

mesocortex

mesomelic

mesometrium

meson

mesonephroi

mesonephroma

mesophryon

mesosalpinx

mesotendineum

mesotendon

mesotenon

mesothelial

mesothelioma
   benign fibrous m.
   diffuse m.
   localized fibrous m.
   malignant m.
   peritoneal m.
   pleural m.
   m. of testis
   m. of tunica vaginalis

mesotropic

mesovarium

metabolism

metacarpus

metachondroplasia

metadiaphyseal

metadiaphysis

metahemoglobin

metallic
   m. cage
   m. debris
   m. distal end of tube
   m. foreign body
   m. marker
   m. needle
   m. pointer
   m. staples
   m. surgical clips
   m. sutures
   m. track of bullet

metamyelocyte

metaphysis *pl.* metaphyses

metaplasia
   myeloid m.
   myeloid m., agnogenic
   myeloid m., primary
   myeloid m., secondary

metaplasia *(continued)*
　　nephrogenic m.

metaplastic

metarubricyte

metastasectomy

metastases

metastasis *pl.* metastases
　　metaplastic m.
　　osseous m's
　　pleural m's

metastasize

metastasized

metastatic

Metastron

metatarsus

metathalamus

metathrombin

metatypic

metatypical

metencephalon

meter
　　dosage m.
　　rate m.

methanal

methemalbuminemia

metheme

methemoglobin

methemoglobinemia
　　acquired m.
　　toxic m.
　　congenital m.
　　hereditary m.

methemoglobinemic

methiodal sodium

methionine
　　m. C 11

method
　　acid hematin m.
　　Clauss m.
　　Coutard's m.
　　Duke's m.
　　Fahraeus m.
　　fibrinogen, m. for
　　Gerota's m.
　　Heublein m.
　　Ivy's m.
　　Nikiforoff's m.
　　point source m.
　　radioactive balloon m.
　　Sahli's m.
　　suspension m.
　　template m.
　　Westergren m.
　　Wintrobe m.

methohexital
　　m. sodium

methotrexate
　　m. sodium

methoxyflurane

methylazoxymethanol

methylchloroisothiazolinone

3-methylcholanthrene

methylisothiazolinone

methyl methacrylate

methylene blue

metopic

metopion

metrizamide

metrizoate sodium

metrofibroma

metrography

metrosalpingography

metrotubography

Mexate

Mexican hat sign

Meyer's organ

Mibelli
   angiokeratoma of M.
   porokeratosis of M.

MIBI (sestamibi)

Michaelis' rhomboid

Mickulicz' syndrome

microabscess
   Munro m.
   Pautrier's m.

microadenoma

microaerotonometer

microaggregate

microangiopathy
   thrombotic m.

microblast

microcalcification

microcephaly

microcurie

microcurie-hour

microcythemia

microcytosis

microdrepanocytic

microdrepanocytosis

microfracture

microglioma

microgliomatosis

microhematocrit

microinvasion

microinvasive

microleukoblast

Microlite

micrometastasis

micrometastatic

micronychia

Micropaque

microphage

microphagocyte

microprolactinoma

microradiogram

microradiography

microrefractometer

microroentgen

microscler

microscopy
   epiluminescent m.

microspherocytosis

microsplenia

microsplenic

microsporosis
   m. nigra

microthelia

microviscosimeter

midaxilla

midazolam
   m. maleate

midbody

midfrontal

midoccipital

midplane

midriff

midsection

Miescher
   M's granuloma
   M's granulomatous cheilitis

migraine

migration
   m. of leukocytes

migratory

Mikity-Wilson syndrome

Mikulicz syndrome

milia (plural of milium)

miliaria
  m. alba
  apocrine m.
  m. crystallina
  m. profunda
  m. rubra

miliary

militate against

milium *pl.* milia
  cold m.

milk of calcium bile

Milkman
  M's fracture
  M's syndrome

Miller-Abbott tube

millicurie

millicurie-hour

millimicrocurie

millirad

millirem

milliroentgen

milphosis

Milton's disease

mineralization

minimal

minimum

Minkowski-Chauffard syndrome

Minnesota tube

Minor's triangle

Minot-von Willebrand syndrome

minute
  m. amount
  double m's

misonidazole

mithramycin

mitocarcin

mitocromin

mitolactol

mitomalcin

mitomycin

mitosper

mitotane

mitoxantrone hydrochloride

mitralization

Mittelschmerz

mivacurium chloride

Mivacron

mixture
  barium m.

MNSs blood group

modeling

model

modifier
  biologic response m.

modioliform

modiolus

modulation
  biochemical m.

modulus of the skull

Mohrenheim
  M's fossa
  M's space
  M's triangle

Mohs
  M. chemotherapy

Mohs *(continued)*
    M's technique

moiety

molar
    unerupted m.

molding of the fetal cranial
  bones

mole
    hydatidaform m.
    invasive m.
    malignant m.
    pigmented m.
    m. on the skin

molluscous

molluscum
    m. contagiosum

Molnar disk

monarthritis

monarticular

monilated

monilethrix

moniliasis

moniliform

moniliid

monitoring equipment

monoarthritis

monoblast

monoblastoma

monocyte

monocytic

monocytoid

monocytopenia

monocytopoiesis

monocytosis

monodermal

monodermoma

monomer
    fibrin m.

monomorphous

mononucleosis

monooctanoin

monopenia

monophyletic

monophyletism

monophyletist

monopoiesis

monostotic

Monro
    M's line
    M.-Richter line

mons *pl.* montes
    m. pubis
    m. veneris

Monteggia fracture

monticulus

Moore prosthesis

MOPP
    mechlorethamine, Oncovin
      (vincristine), procarba-
      zine, and prednisone

morbilliform

morbus
    m. moniliformis

more apparent than real

Morgagni
    foramen of M. hernia
    M. hernia

Morgan's line

Morison's pouch

morphea
    generalized m.
    guttate m.
    linear m.
    m. linearis

morphine

morphology

Morquio's disease

mortise of the ankle

Morton
    M's foot
    M's neuroma
    M's plane

mosaicism
    erythrocyte m.

Moschcowitz's disease

Mosher bag

Mosler's sign

Mosse's syndrome

"moth-eaten" appearance

motion
    m. on the films
    limitation of m.
    paradoxical m. of the dia-
        phragm
    passive range of m.
    patient m.
    respiratory m.

motility
    disturbed m. of Golden

Mott
    M. bodies
    M. cell

mottling

mouse
    joint m.

mouth

movement

Moyer's line

MP
    metacarpophalangeal
        MP joint

MPI DMSA Kidney Reagent

MPI MDP

MPI Pyrophosphate

MPI Tc 99m DTPA

MRA
    magnetic resonance angi-
        ography

MRI
    magnetic resonance imag-
        ing

MTP
    metatarsophalangeal
        MTP joint

Mucha
    M's disease
    M.-Habermann disease

mucinosis
    follicular m.
    papular m.

mucocele

mucocutaneous

mucoepidermoid

mucoperichondrial

mucoperichondrium

mucoperiosteal

mucoperiosteum

mucormycosis
    cutaneous m.

mucosa
    buccal m.
    gastric m.

mucosal

mucosocutaneous

mucous

mucro

mucronate

mucroniform

Mucuna

mucus

MUGA
multiple gated acquisition
MUGA scan

Muir-Torre syndrome

Müller
M.'s experiment
M.'s maneuver

multicapsular

multicystic

multidentate

multifid

multifidus

multiglandular

multilobar

multilobular

Munro
M. abscess
M. microabscess

mural

murmur
holosystolic m.
systolic m.

Murphy's sign

muscle
anconeus m.
agonistic m.
antagonistic m.
arrector m. of hair
bipennate m.
Braune's m.
congenerous m's

muscle *(continued)*
cricopharyngeus m.
cruciate m.
cutaneous m.
deltoideus m.
diaphragmatic m.
dilator m.
dorsal m's
emergency m's
epicranial m.
extrinsic m.
fixation m's
fixator m's
fusiform m.
gastrocnemius m.
gluteus maximus m.
hamstring m's
hypaxial m's
iliacus m.
iliococcygeal m.
iliopsoas m.
inspiratory m's
intrinsic m.
involuntary m.
latissimus dorsi m.
levator ani m.
multipennate m.
mylohyoid m.
nonstriated m.
oblique m. of abdomen, external
oblique m. of abdomen, internal
occipitofrontal m.
orbicular m.
organic m.
m's of pelvic diaphragm
pectoralis major m.
pectoralis minor m.
pennate m.
perineal m's
m's of perineum
penniform m.
platysma m.
pleuroesophageal m.
popliteus m.
procerus m.
psoas m.
pubococcygeal m.

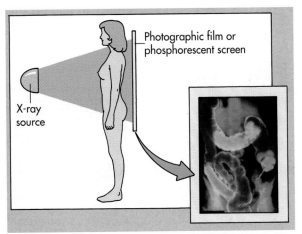

Radiography, or x-ray photography. (From Thibodeau, GA, Patton, KT: Anatomy & Physiology, 4th ed. St. Louis, Mosby, Inc., 1999.)

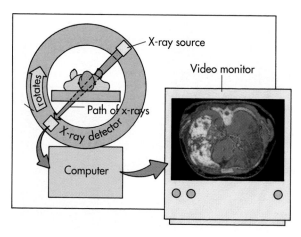

Computed tomography (CT). (From Thibodeau, GA, Patton, KT: Anatomy & Physiology, 4th ed. St. Louis, Mosby, Inc., 1999.)

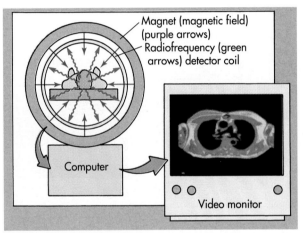

Magnetic resonance imaging (MRI). (From Thibodeau, GA, Patton, KT: Anatomy & Physiology, 4th ed. St. Louis, Mosby, Inc., 1999.)

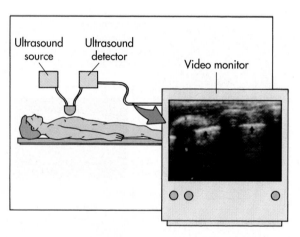

Ultrasonography. (From Thibodeau, GA, Patton, KT: Anatomy & Physiology, 4th ed. St. Louis, Mosby, Inc., 1999.)

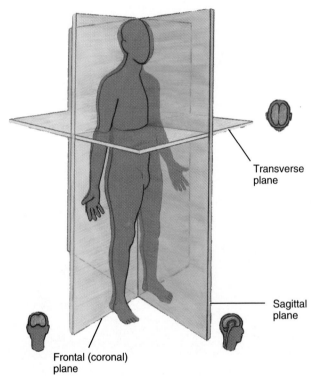

Traverse, sagittal, and frontal planes of the body. (From Applegate, E: The Anatomy and Physiology Learning System, 2nd ed. Philadelphia, W. B. Saunders Company, 2000.)

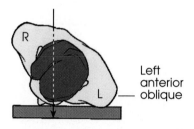

Left
anterior
oblique

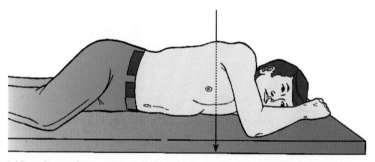

LAD radiographic position of the chest results in a PA oblique projection.
(From Ballinger, PW, Frank ED: Merrill's Atlas of Radiographic Positions and
Radiologic Procedures, 9th ed. St. Louis, Mosby, Inc., 1999.)

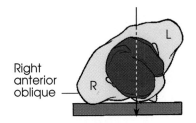

Right anterior oblique

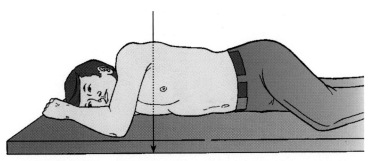

RAD radiographic position of the chest results in a PA oblique projection. (From Ballinger, PW, Frank ED: Merrill's Atlas of Radiographic Positions and Radiologic Procedures, 9th ed. St. Louis, Mosby, Inc., 1999.)

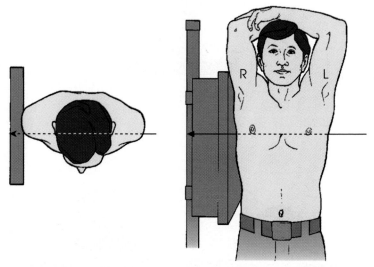

Right lateral radiographic position of the chest results in a lateral projection. (From Ballinger, PW, Frank ED: Merrill's Atlas of Radiographic Positions and Radiologic Procedures, 9th ed. St. Louis, Mosby, Inc., 1999.)

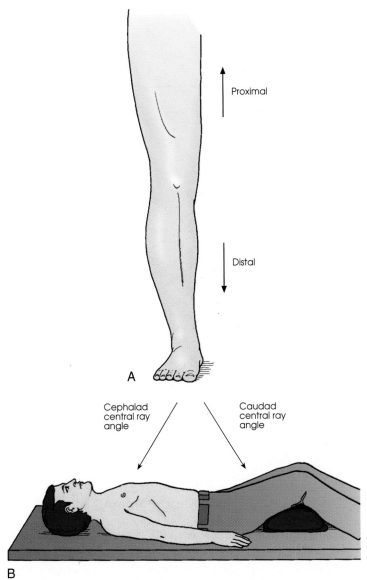

A, Use of the common radiology terms proximal and distal. *B,* Use of the common radiology terms caudad angle and cephalad angle. (From Ballinger, PW, Frank ED: Merrill's Atlas of Radiographic Positions and Radiologic Procedures, 9th ed. St. Louis, Mosby, Inc., 1999.)

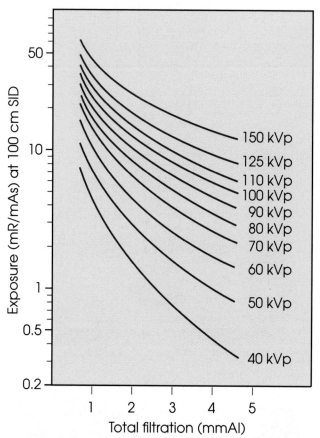

A nomogram estimates the radiation intensity from a single-phase radiographic unit. (From Ballinger, PW, Frank ED: Merrill's Atlas of Radiographic Positions and Radiologic Procedures, 9th ed. St. Louis, Mosby, Inc., 1999.)

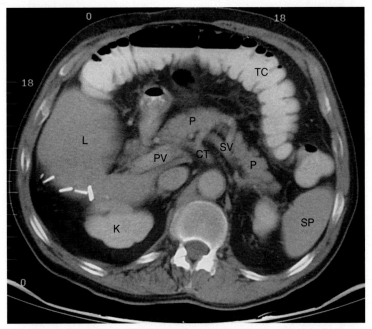

Abdominal image demonstrating transverse colon (TC) with air-fluid levels; the liver (L), pancreas (P), spleen (SP), kidney (K), portal vein (PV), celiac trunk (CT), and splenic veins (SV) are demonstrated with contrast medium. Surgical clips are seen in posterior liver. (From Ballinger, PW, Frank ED: Merrill's Atlas of Radiographic Positions and Radiologic Procedures, 9th ed. St. Louis, Mosby, Inc., 1999.)

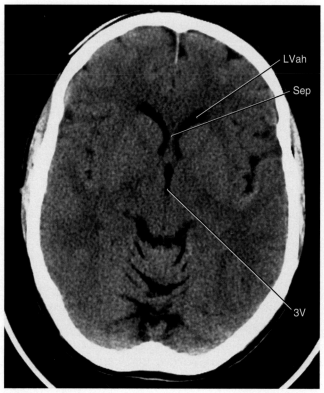

Axial CT scan of lateral ventricles (LVah), septum (Sep), and third ventricle (3V). (From Kelley, LL, Peterson, CM: Sectional Anatomy for Imaging Professionals. St. Louis, Mosby-Yearbook, Inc., 1997.)

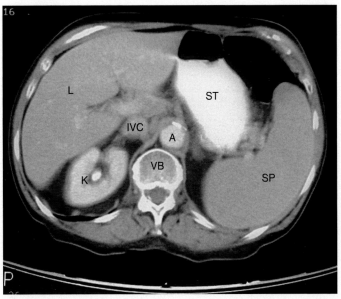

Axial image of abdomen demonstrating liver (L), stomach (ST), spleen (SP), aorta (A), inferior vena cava (IVC), vertebral body of thoracic spine (VB), and kidney (K). (From Ballinger, PW, Frank ED: Merrill's Atlas of Radiographic Positions and Radiologic Procedures, 9th ed. St. Louis, Mosby, Inc., 1999.)

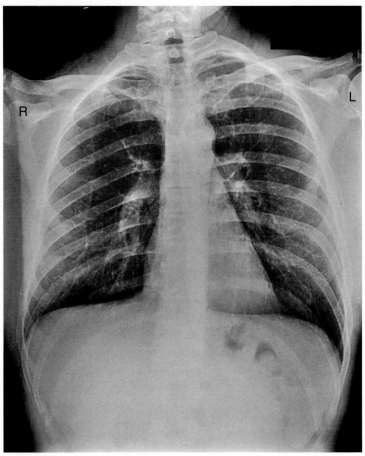

Anteroposterior (AP) projection of the chest. Note the patient's left side is on your right, as though the patient were facing you. (From Ballinger, PW, Frank ED: Merrill's Atlas of Radiographic Positions and Radiologic Procedures, 9th ed. St. Louis, Mosby, Inc., 1999.)

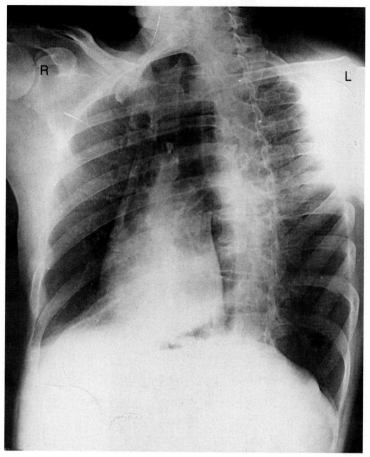

Posteroanterior (PA) oblique chest radiograph is placed on the illuminator with the anatomy in the anatomic position. Note that the patient's left side is on your right, as though the patient were facing you. (From Ballinger, PW, Frank ED: Merrill's Atlas of Radiographic Positions and Radiologic Procedures, 9th ed. St. Louis, Mosby, Inc., 1999.)

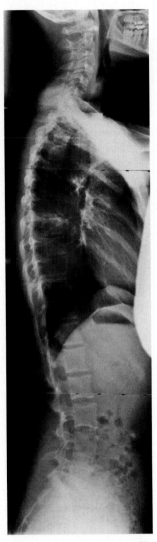

Standing full spine radiography, lateral projection. Note the breast shielding. (From Ballinger, PW, Frank ED: Merrill's Atlas of Radiographic Positions and Radiologic Procedures, 9th ed. St. Louis, Mosby, Inc., 1999.)

muscle *(continued)*
    puborectal m.
    pyramidal m.
    pyriformis m.
    quadrate m.
    rectococcygeal m.
    ribbon m's
    scalenus anticus m.
    Sibson's m.
    semipennate m.
    semispinalis capitis m.
    smooth m.
    soleus m.
    sphincter m.
    sternocleidomastoid m.
    strap m's
    striated m.
    striped m.
    stylohyoideus m.
    subvertebral m's
    synergic m's
    synergistic m's
    temporoparietal m.
    teres minor m.
    Theile's m.
    transverse abdominal m.
    transverse m. of neck
    transverse perineal m.,
      deep
    transverse perineal m., su-
      perficial
    triangular m.
    trapezius m.
    unipennate m.
    unstriated m.
    visceral m.
    voluntary m.
    yoked m's

muscular

muscularis
    m. mucosae

musculature

musculi (plural of musculus)

musculocutaneous

musculodermic

musculointestinal

musculophrenic

musculospiral

musculus *pl.* musculi
    musculi abdominis
    m. abductor digiti minimi
      manus
    m. abductor digiti minimi
      pedis
    m. abductor hallucis
    m. abductor pollicis brevis
    m. abductor pollicis longus
    m. adductor brevis
    m. adductor hallucis
    m. adductor longus
    m. adductor magnus
    m. adductor minimus
    m. adductor pollicis
    m. anconeus
    m. antitragicus
    m. arrector pili
    m. articularis cubiti
    m. articularis genus
    m. arytenoideus obliquus
    m. arytenoideus transver-
      sus
    m. auricularis anterior
    m. auricularis posterior
    m. auricularis superior
    m. biceps brachii
    m. biceps femoris
    m. bipennatus
    m. brachialis
    m. brachioradialis
    m. bronchooesophageus
    m. buccinator
    m. bulbospongiosus
    musculi capitis
    m. ceratocricoideus
    musculi cervicis
    m. chondroglossus
    m. ciliaris
    m. coccygeus
    musculi colli
    m. constrictor pharyngis
      inferior
    m. constrictor pharyngis
      medius

musculus *(continued)*
    m. constrictor pharyngis superior
    m. coracobrachialis
    m. corrugator supercilii
    m. cremaster
    m. cricoarytenoideus lateralis
    m. cricoarytenoideus posterior
    m. cricopharyngeus
    m. cricothyroideus
    m. cruciatus
    m. cutaneus
    m. dartos
    m. depressor septi nasi
    m. depressor supercilii
    m. detrusor vesicae
    musculi diaphragmatis pelvis
    m. digastricus
    m. dilatator
    m. dilatator pupillae
    musculi dorsi
    m. epicranius
    m. erector spinae
    m. extensor carpi radialis brevis
    m. extensor carpi radialis longus
    m. extensor carpi ulnaris
    m. extensor digiti minimi
    m. extensor digitorum
    m. extensor digitorum brevis
    m. extensor digitorum longus
    m. extensor hallucis brevis
    m. extensor hallucis longus
    m. extensor indicis
    m. extensor pollicis brevis
    m. extensor pollicis longus
    musculi externi bulbi oculi
    musculi faciales
    musculi faciei
    m. fibularis brevis
    m. fibularis longus
    m. fibularis tertius

musculus *(continued)*
    m. flexor accessorius
    m. flexor carpi radialis
    m. flexor carpi ulnaris
    m. flexor digiti minimi brevis manus
    m. flexor digiti minimi brevis pedis
    m. flexor digitorum brevis
    m. flexor digitorum longus
    m. flexor digitorum profundus
    m. flexor digitorum superficialis
    m. flexor hallucis brevis
    m. flexor hallucis longus
    m. flexor pollicis brevis
    m. flexor pollicis longus
    m. fusiformis
    m. gastrocnemius
    m. gemellus inferior
    m. gemellus superior
    m. genioglossus
    m. geniohyoideus
    m. gluteus maximus
    m. gluteus medius
    m. gluteus minimus
    m. gracilis
    m. helicis major
    m. helicis minor
    m. hyoglossus
    m. iliacus
    m. iliococcygeus
    m. iliocostalis
    m. iliocostalis cervicis
    m. iliocostalis colli
    m. iliocostalis lumborum
    m. iliopsoas
    m. incisurae terminalis
    musculi infrahyoidei
    m. infraspinatus
    musculi intercostales externi
    musculi intercostales interni
    musculi intercostales intimi
    musculi interossei dorsales manus

musculus *(continued)*
- musculi interossei dorsales pedis
- musculi interossei palmares
- musculi interossei plantares
- musculi interspinales
- musculi interspinales cervicis
- musculi interspinales colli
- musculi interspinales lumborum
- musculi interspinales thoracis
- musculi intertransversarii
- musculi intertransversarii anteriores cervicis
- musculi intertransversarii anteriores colli
- musculi intertransversarii laterales lumborum
- musculi intertransversarii mediales lumborum
- musculi intertransversarii posteriores laterales cervicis
- musculi intertransversarii posteriores laterales colli
- musculi intertransversarii thoracis
- m. ischiocavernosus
- musculi laryngis
- m. latissimus dorsi
- m. levator ani
- musculi levatores costarum
- musculi levatores costarum breves
- musculi levatores costarum longi
- m. levator glandulae thyroideae
- m. levator labii superioris alaeque nasi
- m. levator palpebrae superioris
- m. levator prostatae
- m. levator scapulae
- m. levator veli palatini

musculus *(continued)*
- musculi linguae
- musculi linguales
- m. longissimus
- m. longissimus capitis
- m. longissimus cervicis
- m. longissimus colli
- m. longissimus thoracis
- m. longitudinalis inferior linguae
- m. longitudinalis superior linguae
- m. longus capitis
- m. longus cervicis
- m. longus colli
- musculi lumbricales manus
- musculi lumbricales pedis
- m. masseter
- musculi masticatorii
- musculi membri inferioris
- musculi membri superioris
- m. mentalis
- musculi multifidi
- m. multipennatus
- m. mylohyoideus
- m. nasalis
- m. obliquus auriculae
- m. obliquus auricularis
- m. obliquus capitis inferior
- m. obliquus capitis superior
- m. obliquus externus abdominis
- m. obliquus inferior bulbi
- m. obliquus internus abdominis
- m. obliquus superior bulbi
- m. obturatorius externus
- m. obturatorius internus
- m. occipitofrontalis
- m. omohyoideus
- m. opponens digiti minimi
- m. opponens pollicis
- m. orbicularis
- m. orbicularis oculi
- m. orbitalis
- musculi ossiculorum auditoriorum

musculus *(continued)*
  musculi palati mollis et fau-
    cium
  m. palatoglossus
  m. palatopharyngeus
  m. palmaris brevis
  m. palmaris longus
  musculi papillares
  m. papillaris anterior ven-
    triculi dextri
  m. papillaris anterior ven-
    triculi sinistri
  m. papillaris posterior ven-
    triculi dextri
  m. papillaris posterior ven-
    triculi sinistri
  musculi pectinati atrii dex-
    tri
  musculi pectinati atrii sinis-
    tri
  m. pectineus
  m. pectoralis major
  m. pectoralis minor
  m. pennatus
  musculi perineales
  musculi perinei
  m. peroneus brevis
  m. peroneus longus
  m. peroneus tertius
  musculi pharyngis
  m. piriformis
  m. plantaris
  m. pleurooesophageus
  m. popliteus
  m. procerus
  m. pronator quadratus
  m. pronator teres
  m. psoas major
  m. psoas minor
  m. pterygoideus lateralis
  m. pterygoideus medialis
  m. pubococcygeus
  m. puboprostaticus
  m. puborectalis
  m. pubovaginalis
  m. pubovesicalis
  m. pyramidalis
  m. pyramidalis auriculae
  m. pyramidalis auricularis

musculus *(continued)*
  m. quadratus
  m. quadratus femoris
  m. quadratus lumborum
  m. quadratus plantae
  m. quadriceps femoris
  m. rectococcygeus
  m. rectourethralis
  m. rectouterinus
  m. rectovesicalis
  m. rectus abdominis
  m. rectus capitis anterior
  m. rectus capitis lateralis
  m. rectus capitis posterior
    major
  m. rectus capitis posterior
    minor
  m. rectus femoris
  m. rectus inferior bulbi
  m. rectus lateralis bulbi
  m. rectus medialis bulbi
  m. rectus superior bulbi
  m. rhomboideus major
  m. rhomboideus minor
  m. risorius
  musculi rotatores
  musculi rotatores cervicis
  musculi rotatores lum-
    borum
  musculi rotatores thoracis
  m. salpingopharyngeus
  m. sartorius
  m. scalenus anterior
  m. scalenus medius
  m. scalenus minimus
  m. scalenus posterior
  m. semimembranosus
  m. semipennatus
  m. semispinalis
  m. semispinalis capitis
  m. semispinalis cervicis
  m. semispinalis thoracis
  m. semitendinosus
  m. serratus anterior
  m. serratus posterior infe-
    rior
  m. serratus posterior supe-
    rior
  musculi skeleti

musculus *(continued)*
- m. soleus
- m. sphincter
- m. sphincter ampullae hepatopancreaticae
- m. sphincter ani externus
- m. sphincter ani internus
- m. sphincter ductus biliaris
- m. sphincter ductus choledochi
- m. sphincter pupillae
- m. sphincter pyloricus
- m. spinalis
- m. spinalis capitis
- m. spinalis cervicis
- m. spinalis thoracis
- m. splenius capitis
- m. splenius cervicis
- m. stapedius
- m. sternalis
- m. sternocleidomastoideus
- m. sternohyoideus
- m. sternothyroideus
- m. styloglossus
- m. stylohyoideus
- m. stylopharyngeus
- m. subclavius
- musculi subcostales
- musculi suboccipitales
- m. subscapularis
- m. supinator
- musculi suprahyoidei
- m. supraspinatus
- m. suspensorius duodeni
- m. tarsalis inferior
- m. tarsalis superior
- m. temporalis
- m. temporoparietalis
- m. tensor fasciae latae
- m. tensor tympani
- m. tensor veli palatini
- m. teres major
- m. teres minor
- musculi thoracis
- m. thyroarytenoideus
- m. thyrohyoideus
- m. thyropharyngeus
- m. tibialis anterior
- m. tibialis posterior

musculus *(continued)*
- m. trachealis
- m. tragicus
- musculi transversospinales
- m. transversus abdominis
- m. transversus auriculae
- m. transversus auricularis
- m. transversus linguae
- m. transversus nuchae
- m. transversus perinei profundus
- m. transversus perinei superficialis
- m. transversus thoracis
- m. trapezius
- m. triangularis
- m. triceps brachii
- m. triceps surae
- m. unipennatus
- m. uvulae
- m. vastus intermedius
- m. vastus lateralis
- m. vastus medialis
- m. verticalis linguae
- m. vocalis
- m. zygomaticus major
- m. zygomaticus minor

mustard
- nitrogen m.
- L-phenylalanine m.
- uracil m.

Mustargen

Mutamycin

M-VAC
- methotrexate, vinblastine, doxorubicin, and cisplatin myalgia

myasthenia gravis

mycid

Mycobacterium avium intracellulare (MAI)

mycoderma

mycobacterium
- avian intracellular m.

mycodermatitis

Mycoplasma pneumonia

mycosis
    m. fungoides
    m. fungoides d'emblée
    splenic m.

myelemia

myelencephalon

myelinization

myeloablation

myeloablative

myeloblast

myeloblastemia

myeloblastoma

myeloblastomatosis

myeloblastosis

myelocyte

myelocythemia

myelocytic

myelocytoma

myelocytosis

myelodysplasia

myelodysplastic

myelofibrosis

myelogenesis

myelogenic

myelogenous

myelogone

myelogram
    lumbar m.

myelography
    oxygen m.

myeloid

myelokentric

myelolipoma

myeloma
    giant cell m.
    indolent m.
    localized m.
    multiple m.
    plasma cell m.
    sclerosing m.
    solitary m.

myelomalacia

myelomatoid

myelomatosis

myelomeningocele

myelomonocytic

myelopathy

myelophthisic

myelophthisis

myeloplast

myelopoiesis

myelopoietic

myeloproliferative

myelosarcoma

myelosarcomatosis

myelosclerosis

myelosis
    aleukemic m.
    chronic nonleukemic m.
    erythremic m.
    nonleukemic m.

myelosuppression

myelosuppressive

myelotoxic

myelotoxicity

myiasis
    creeping m.
    cutaneous m.
    dermal m.
    m. linearis

Myleran

myoblastoma
    granular cell m.

myoblastomyoma

myocardiopathy

myocarditis

myocardium

myoclonus
    opsoclonus-m.

myocytoma

myoepithelioma

myofascial

myofibroma

myography

myolipoma

myology

myoma *pl.* myomata
    m. previum
    m. striocellulare
    uterine m.

myomagenesis

myomata (plural of myoma)

myomatosis

myomatous

myomectomy

myometrium

myonymy

myopathy

myosarcoma

myoschwannoma

myositis
    m. ossificans
    proliferative m.

myosteoma

myotomy

myovascular

Myoview

myxadenoma

myxedema
    papular m.

myxoblastoma

myxochondrofibrosarcoma

myxochondroma

myxochondrosarcoma

myxocystoma

myxoenchondroma

myxoendothelioma

myxofibroma
    odontogenic m.

myxofibrosarcoma

myxoglioma

myxolipoma

myxoma
    atrial m.
    cystic m.
    enchondromatous m.
    m. fibrosum
    lipomatous m.
    odontogenic m.
    m. sarcomatosum
    vascular m.

myxomatosis

myxomatous

myxomyoma

myxopapilloma

myxosarcoma
    odontogenic m.

myxosarcomatous

N

Naegeli's leukemia

nail
  eggshell n.
  gamma n.
  ingrown n.
  Jewett n.
  parrot beak n.
  pitted n's
  racket n.
  reedy n.
  Rush intramedullary n.
  Smith-Petersen n.
  spoon n.
  turtle-back n.
  watch-crystal n.

nailing
  hip n.

nanocurie

nape

napex

naphthylamine

narcosis
  basal n.

narcotic

narcotize

naris *pl.* nares

narrowing
  arteriolar n.
  circumferential n.
  concentric n.
  disk space n.
  eccentric n.
  joint space n.
  luminal n.

nasal

nasioiniac

nasion

nasociliary

nasopharyngeal

nasopharynx

nasus

natal

nates

navel

Navelbine

navicula
  bipartite n.
  carpal n.
  tarsal n.

navicular

nebularine

NEC
  necrotizing enterocolitis

neck
  bull n.
  n. of hair follicle
  n. of the humerus
  Madelung's n.
  radial n.
  surgical n.

necklace
  Casal's n.

necrobiosis
  n. lipoidica
  n. lipoidica diabeticorum

necrolysis
  toxic epidermal n.

necrosis
  radiation n.
  aseptic n.
  avascular n.
  irradiation n.

needle
  butterfly n.
  Chiba n.
  fine n.
  fine n. biopsy

needle *(continued)*
    Greene n.
    Hawkins n.
    Homer Mammalok n.
    Jamshidi n.
    Kopans n.
    large bore n.
    n. localization of breast lesion
    Longdwell n.
    Manan n.
    n. marker
    metallic n.
    percutaneous n. biopsy
    scalp vein n.
    Seldinger n.
    skinny n.
    thin-walled n.
    Tru-Cut n.

Neer prosthesis

negatron

Nélaton
    N's line
    N's tumor

Nembutal

neoadjuvant

neoantigen

neocerebellum

neocortex

neocytosis

neonatal

neoplasia
    cervical intraepithelial n.
    gestational trophoblastic n.
    lobular n.
    multiple endocrine n.
    multiple endocrine n., type I
    multiple endocrine n., type II
    multiple endocrine n., type IIA
    multiple endocrine n., type IIB

neoplasia *(continued)*
    multiple endocrine n., type III
    prostatic intraepithelial n.

neoplasm
    colonic n.
    pancreatic n.
    primary n.

neoplastic

neoplastigenic

Neoscan

neovascularity

nephradenoma

nephrectomy

nephritic

nephritis *pl.* nephritides

nephroabdominal

nephroblastoma

nephroblastomatosis

nephrocalcinosis

nephrocardiac

nephrocolic

nephroerysipelas

nephrogastric

nephrogram

nephrography

nephroid

nephrolithiasis

nephrolithotomy

nephroma
    congenital mesoblastic n.
    embryonal n.

nephropyelography

nephrosonography

nephrostomy
    percutaneous n.

nephrotomogram

nephrotomography

nerve
  acoustic n.
  n. distribution
  n. root
  olfactory n.
  optic n.
  parasympathetic n's
  phrenic n.
  sciatic n.
  vagus n.

nervus *pl.* nervi
  n. abducens
  n. accessorius
  n. alveolaris inferior
  nervi alveolares superiores
  n. ampullaris anterior
  n. ampullaris lateralis
  n. ampullaris posterior
  nervi anales inferiores
  n. anococcygeus
  nervi auriculares anteriores
  n. auricularis magnus
  n. auricularis posterior
  n. auriculotemporalis
  n. autonomicus
  n. axillaris
  n. buccalis
  n. canalis pterygoidei
  n. cardiacus cervicalis inferior
  n. cardiacus cervicalis medius
  n. cardiacus cervicalis superior
  nervi caroticotympanici
  nervi carotici externi
  n. caroticus internus
  nervi cavernosi clitoridis
  nervi cavernosi penis
  nervi cervicales
  nervi ciliares breves
  nervi ciliares longi
  nervi clunium inferiores
  nervi clunium medii
  nervi clunium superiores

nervus *(continued)*
  n. coccygeus
  n. cochlearis
  nervi craniales
  n. cutaneus antebrachii lateralis
  n. cutaneus antebrachii medialis
  n. cutaneus antebrachii posterior
  n. cutaneus brachii lateralis inferior
  n. cutaneus brachii lateralis superior
  n. cutaneus brachii medialis
  n. cutaneus brachii posterior
  n. cutaneus dorsalis intermedius
  n. cutaneus dorsalis lateralis
  n. cutaneus dorsalis medialis
  n. cutaneus perforans
  n. cutaneus femoris lateralis
  n. cutaneus femoris posterior
  n. cutaneus surae lateralis
  n. cutaneus surae medialis
  nervi digitales dorsales nervi radialis
  nervi digitales dorsales nervi ulnaris
  nervi digitales dorsales pedis
  nervi digitales palmares communes nervi mediani
  nervi digitales palmares communes nervi ulnaris
  nervi digitales palmares proprii nervi mediani
  nervi digitales palmares proprii nervi ulnaris
  nervi digitales plantares communes nervi plantaris lateralis

nervus *(continued)*
  nervi digitales plantares communes nervi plantaris medialis
  nervi digitales plantares proprii nervi plantaris lateralis
  nervi digitales plantares proprii nervi plantaris medialis
  n. dorsalis clitoridis
  n. dorsalis penis
  n. dorsalis scapulae
  n. ethmoidalis anterior
  n. ethmoidalis posterior
  n. facialis
  n. femoralis
  n. fibularis communis
  n. fibularis profundus
  n. fibularis superficialis
  n. frontalis
  n. genitofemoralis
  n. glossopharyngeus
  n. gluteus inferior
  n. gluteus superior
  n. hypogastricus
  n. hypoglossus
  n. iliohypogastricus
  n. ilioinguinalis
  n. iliopubicus
  n. infraorbitalis
  n. infratrochlearis
  nervi intercostales
  nervi intercostobrachiales
  n. intermedius
  n. interosseus antebrachii anterior
  n. interosseus antebrachii posterior
  n. interosseus cruris
  n. ischiadicus
  n. jugularis
  nervi labiales anteriores
  nervi labiales posteriores
  n. lacrimalis
  n. laryngeus recurrens
  n. laryngeus superior
  n. lingualis
  nervi lumbales

nervus *(continued)*
  n. mandibularis
  n. massetericus
  n. maxillaris
  n. meatus acustici externi
  n. medianus
  n. mentalis
  n. mixtus
  n. motorius
  n. musculi obturatorii interni
  n. musculi piriformis
  n. musculi quadrati femoris
  n. musculi tensoris tympani
  n. musculi tensoris veli palatini
  n. musculocutaneus
  n. mylohyoideus
  n. nasociliaris
  n. nasopalatinus
  n. obturatorius
  n. obturatorius accessorius
  n. occipitalis major
  n. occipitalis minor
  n. occipitalis tertius
  n. oculomotorius
  n. olfactorius
  n. ophthalmicus
  n. opticus
  n. palatinus major
  nervi palatini minores
  n. pectoralis lateralis
  n. pectoralis medialis
  nervi perineales
  n. peroneus communis
  n. peroneus profundus
  n. peroneus superficialis
  n. petrosus major
  n. petrosus minor
  n. petrosus profundus
  n. pharyngeus
  n. phrenicus
  nervi phrenici accessorii
  n. plantaris lateralis
  n. plantaris medialis
  n. presacralis
  n. pterygoideus lateralis
  n. pterygoideus medialis

nervus *(continued)*
n. pudendus
n. radialis
nervi rectales inferiores
n. saccularis
nervi sacrales
nervi sacrales et n. coccygeus
n. saphenus
nervi scrotales anteriores
nervi scrotales posteriores
n. sensorius
nervi spinales
n. spinosus
n. splanchnicus imus
nervi splanchnici lumbales
n. splanchnicus major
n. splanchnicus minor
nervi splanchnici sacrales
n. stapedius
n. subclavius
n. subcostalis
n. sublingualis
n. suboccipitalis
nervi subscapulares
nervi supraclaviculares
nervi supraclaviculares intermedii
nervi supraclaviculares laterales
nervi supraclaviculares mediales
n. supraorbitalis
n. suprascapularis
n. supratrochlearis
n. suralis
nervi temporales profundi
n. terminalis
nervi thoracici
n. thoracicus longus
n. thoracodorsalis
n. tibialis
n. transversus cervicalis
n. transversus colli
n. trigeminus
n. trochlearis
n. tympanicus
n. ulnaris
n. utricularis

nervus *(continued)*
n. utriculoampullaris
nervi vaginales
n. vagus
nervi vasorum
n. vertebralis
n. vestibularis
n. vestibulocochlearis
n. zygomaticus

Nesacaine

nesidioblastoma

nest
junctional n.

net

Netherton's syndrome

network
lymphocapillary n.
peritarsal n.

Neupogen

neuralgia

neurilemmoma

neurilemoma
acoustic n.

neurinoma
acoustic n.

neuroacanthocytosis

neuroastrocytoma

neuroblastoma
olfactory n.

neurocranial

neurocranium
cartilaginous n.
membranous n.

neurocytoma

neurodermatitis
circumscribed n.
disseminated n.
exudative n.
localized n.
nummular n.

neuroepithelioma

neurofibra *pl.* neurofibrae
neurofibrae afferentes
neurofibrae autonomicae
neurofibrae efferentes
neurofibrae postganglioni-
cae
neurofibrae preganglioni-
cae
neurofibrae somaticae
neurofibrae tangentiales

neurofibroma
cutaneous n.
dermal n.
plexiform n.
solitary n.

neurofibrosarcoma

neurogliocytoma

neuroglioma
n. ganglionare

neurogliomatosis

neurogliosis

neurohypophysis

neuroimaging

neuroleptanalgesia

neuroleptanalgesic

neuroleptanesthesia

neuroleptanesthetic

neurolipomatosis
n. dolorosa

Neurolite

neuroma
acoustic n.
amyelinic n.
n. cutis
ganglionar n.
ganglionated n.
ganglionic n.
medullated n.
Morton's n.

neuroma *(continued)*
multiple n.
myelinic n.
nevoid n.
plexiform n.
n. telangiectodes
true n.
Verneuil's n.

neuromatosis

neuromyopathy
carcinomatous n.

neuronevus

neuro-oncology

neuropathy
paraneoplastic n.

neuroradiology

neuroroentgenography

neurosarcoma

neurospongioma

neurotomography

neutrino

neutrocyte

neutron
epithermal n.
fast n.
intermediate n.
slow n.
thermal n.

neutropenia
chronic benign n.
chronic familial n.
chronic hypoplastic n.
congenital n.
cyclic n.
drug-induced n.
familial benign chronic n.
hypersplenic n.
idiopathic n.
Kostmann's n.
malignant n.
neonatal n., alloimmune
neonatal n., isoimmune

neutropenia *(continued)*
    periodic n.
    peripheral n.
    primary splenic n.
    severe congenital n.

neutrophil
    band n.
    juvenile n.
    polymorphonuclear n.
    rod n.
    stab n.

neutrophilia

neutrotaxis

nevi (plural of nevus)

nevoblast

nevocellular

nevocyte

nevocytic

nevoid

nevolipoma

nevoxanthoendothelioma

nevus *pl.* nevi
    achromic n.
    acquired n.
    amelanotic n.
    n. anemicus
    n. araneus
    balloon cell n.
    bathing trunk n.
    Becker's n.
    blue n.
    blue rubber bleb n.
    cellular n.
    cellular blue n.
    n. comedonicus
    compound n.
    congenital n.
    connective tissue n.
    n. depigmentosus
    dermal n.
    dysplastic n.
    n. elasticus

nevus *(continued)*
    n. elasticus of Lewandowsky
    epidermal n.
    epithelial n.
    fatty n.
    n. flammeus
    n. fuscoceruleus acromiodeltoideus
    n. fuscoceruleus ophthalmomaxillaris
    giant congenital pigmented n.
    giant hairy n.
    giant pigmented n.
    hair follicle n.
    halo n.
    intradermal n.
    n. of Ito
    Jadassohn's sebaceous n.
    Jadassohn-Tièche n.
    junction n.
    junctional n.
    n. lipomatosus
    n. lipomatosus cutaneus superficialis
    melanocytic n.
    neural n.
    neuroid n.
    nevocellular n.
    nevocytic n.
    n. cell n.
    nuchal n.
    organoid n.
    n. of Ota
    Ota's n.
    pigmented n.
    n. pigmentosus
    pigmented hairy epidermal n.
    port-wine n.
    sebaceous n.
    n. sebaceus
    n. sebaceus of Jadassohn
    spider n.
    n. spilus
    n. spilus tardus
    spindle and epithelioid cell n.

nevus *(continued)*
 Spitz n.
 stellar n.
 Sutton's n.
 n. unius lateris
 Unna's n.

NG
 nasogastric
  NG tube

niche
 Barclay's n.
 Haudek's n.
 ulcer n.

nickel
 n. carbonyl

nifedipine

NIH catheter

Nikiforoff's method

Nikolsky's sign

Nilandron

nilutamide

Nimbex

Nipent

nipple
 supernumerary n.

Nissen fundoplication procedure

nitrilotriacetic acid

nitrogen
 n. 13
 n. mustards
 nonprotein n.
 rest n.

nitroglycerin

2-nitropropane

nitrosamine

N-nitrosodimethylamine

N-nitrosodiphenylamine

nitrosourea

nocardiosis

nodal

node
 abdominal lymph n's, parietal
 abdominal lymph n's, visceral
 accessory lymph n's
 anorectal lymph n's
 n. of anterior border of epiploic foramen
 aortic lymph n's
 aortic lymph n's, lateral
 apical lymph n's
 appendicular lymph n's
 axillary lymph n's
 axillary lymph n's, apical
 axillary lymph n's, anterior
 axillary lymph n's, central
 axillary lymph n's, lateral
 axillary lymph n's, pectoral
 axillary lymph n's, posterior
 axillary lymph n's, subscapular
 azygous n.
 brachial lymph n's
 bronchopulmonary lymph n's
 buccal lymph n.
 buccinator lymph n.
 caval lymph n's, lateral
 celiac lymph n's
 central lymph n's
 cervical lymph n's, anterior
 cervical lymph n's, anterior superficial
 cervical lymph n's, deep anterior
 cervical lymph n's, deep lateral
 cervical lymph n's, inferior deep
 cervical lymph n's, prelaryngeal

node *(continued)*

cervical lymph n's, superficial lateral

cervical lymph n's, superior deep

Cloquet's n.

n. of Cloquet

colic lymph n's, right/middle/left

colic lymph n's, terminal

cubital lymph n's

cystic lymph n.

Delphian n.

deltoideopectoral lymph n's

deltopectoral lymph n's

diaphragmatic lymph n's

epicolic lymph n's

epigastric lymph n's, inferior

n. of epiploic foramen

epitrochlear lymph n's

Ewald's n.

facial lymph n's

fibular lymph n.

foraminal lymph n.

gastric lymph n's, right/left

gastroepiploic lymph n's, right/left

gastro-omental lymph n's, right/left

gluteal lymph n's, inferior

gluteal lymph n's, superior

hepatic lymph n's

hilar n's

hilar lymph n's

ileocolic lymph n's

iliac lymph n's, circumflex

iliac lymph n's, common

iliac lymph n's, external

iliac lymph n's, intermediate common

iliac lymph n's, intermediate external

iliac lymph n's, internal

iliac lymph n's, lateral common

iliac lymph n's, lateral external

node *(continued)*

iliac lymph n's, medial common

iliac lymph n's, medial external

iliac lymph n's, promontory common

iliac lymph n's, subaortic common

infraclavicular lymph n's

infrahyoid lymph n's

inguinal lymph n's

inguinal lymph n's, deep

inguinal lymph n's, inferior superficial

inguinal lymph n's, superficial

inguinal lymph n's, superolateral superficial

inguinal lymph n's, superomedial superficial

intercostal lymph n's

interiliac lymph n's

interpectoral lymph n's

intrapulmonary lymph n's

jugular lymph n's, anterior

jugular lymph n's, lateral

jugulodigastric n.

jugulodigastric lymph n.

jugulo-omohyoid lymph n.

juxtaintestinal lymph n's

lacunar lymph n., intermediate

lacunar lymph n., lateral

lacunar lymph n., medial

lymph n. of ligamentum arteriosum

lumbar lymph n's

lumbar lymph n's, intermediate

lumbar lymph n's, left

lumbar lymph n's, right

lymph n.

lymph n. of arch of azygos vein

lymph n's of upper limb, deep

lymph n's of upper limb, superficial

node (*continued*)

malar lymph n.
mandibular lymph n.
mastoid lymph n's
mediastinal lymph n's, anterior
mediastinal lymph n's, posterior
mesenteric lymph n's
mesenteric lymph n's, central superior
mesenteric lymph n's, inferior
mesenteric lymph n's, justaintestinal
mesenteric lymph n's, superior
mesocolic lymph n's
nasolabial lymph n.
n. of neck of gallbladder
obturator lymph n's
occipital lymph n's
pancreatic lymph n's
pancreatic lymph n's, inferior
pancreatic lymph n's, superior
pancreaticoduodenal lymph n's, inferior
pancreaticoduodenal lymph n's, superior
para-aortic n's
paracardial lymph n's
paracolic lymph n's
paramammary lymph n's
pararectal lymph n's
parasternal lymph n's
paratracheal lymph n's
parauterine lymph n's
paravaginal lymph n's
paravesicular lymph n's
parietal lymph n's
parotid lymph n's, deep
parotid lymph n's, infra-auricular deep
parotid lymph n's, intraglandular deep
parotid lymph n's, preauricular deep

node (*continued*)

parotid lymph n's, superficial
pectoral lymph n's
pelvic lymph n's, parietal
pelvic lymph n's, visceral
periaortic lymph n's
pericardial lymph n's, lateral
peroneal lymph n.
phrenic lymph n's, inferior
phrenic lymph n's, superior
popliteal lymph n's
popliteal lymph n's, deep
popliteal lymph n's, superficial
postaortic lymph n's
postcaval lymph n's
postvesicular lymph n's
preaortic lymph n's
preauricular n's
precaval lymph n's
prececal lymph n's
prelaryngeal n.
prepericardial lymph n's
pretracheal n.
pretracheal lymph n's
prevertebral lymph n's
prevesicular lymph n's
pulmonary juxtaesophageal lymph n's
pulmonary lymph n's
pyloric lymph n's
rectal lymph n's, superior
retroaortic lymph n's
retroauricular lymph n's
retrocaval lymph n's
retrocecal lymph n's
retropharyngeal lymph n's
retropyloric n's
retrovesicular lymph n's
Rosenmüller's n.
Rotter's n's
n. of Rouvière
sacral lymph n's
sentinel n.
shotty (*not* shoddy) lymph n's

node *(continued)*
    sigmoid lymph n's
    signal n.
    splenic lymph n's
    subcarinal lymph n's
    submandibular lymph n's
    submental lymph n's
    subpyloric n's
    subscapular lymph n's
    supraclavicular lymph n's
    suprapyloric lymph n.
    supratrochlear lymph n's
    thyroid lymph n's
    tibial n., anterior
    tibial n., posterior
    tracheal lymph n's
    tracheobronchial lymph n's, inferior
    tracheobronchial lymph n's, superior
    Troisier's n.
    vesicular lymph n's, lateral
    Virchow's n.
    visceral lymph n's
    xiphisternal n.

nodi (plural of nodus)

nodose

nodosity

nodulated

nodulation

nodule
    accessory thymic n's
    aggregate n's
    Brenner n's
    "cold" n.
    cortical n's
    discrete n.
    lymphatic n.
    lymphatic n's of large intestine, solitary
    lymphatic n's of small intestine, solitary
    lymphatic n's of stomach
    lymphoid n's of large intestine, solitary

nodule *(continued)*
    lymphoid n's of small intestine, aggregated
    lymphoid n's of small intestine, solitary
    lymphoid n's of vermiform appendix, aggregated
    primary n.
    Schmorl's n.
    Sister Mary Joseph's n.
    solitary n.
    surfers' n's

noduli (plural of nodulus)

nodulous

nodulus *pl.* noduli
    noduli lymphatici aggregati processus vermiformis
    n. cerebelli
    n. lymphaticus
    noduli lymphatici aggregati intestini tenuis
    noduli lymphatici aggregati [Peyeri]
    noduli lymphatici bronchiales
    noduli lymphatici conjunctivales
    noduli lymphatici gastrici
    noduli lymphatici laryngei
    noduli lymphatici recti
    noduli lymphatici solitarii
    noduli lymphatici solitarii intestini crassi
    noduli lymphatici solitarii intestini tenuis
    noduli lymphatici vaginales
    noduli lymphatici vesicales
    n. lymphoideus
    noduli lymphoidei aggregati intestini tenuis
    noduli lymphoidei aggregati appendicis vermiformis
    noduli lymphoidei lienales
    noduli lymphoidei solitarii
    noduli lymphoidei splenici
    noduli lymphoidei tonsillae pharyngealis

nodulus *(continued)*
    noduli lymphoidei tonsillae
      lingualis
    noduli thymici accessorii
    noduli valvularum semilu-
      narium valvae aortae
    n. vermis
    noduli valvularum semilu-
      narium valvae trunci pul-
      monalis

nodus *pl.* nodi
    n. atrioventricularis
    n. lymphaticus
    n. lymphaticus buccalis
    nodi lymphatici hilares
    nodi lymphatici jugulares
      laterales
    nodi lymphatici retroce-
      cales
    n. lymphoideus
    nodi lymphoidei abdominis
      parietales
    nodi lymphoidei abdominis
      viscerales
    nodi lymphoidei accessorii
    nodi lymphoidei anorecta-
      les
    nodi lymphoidei aortici la-
      terales
    n. lymphoideus arcus ve-
      nae azygos
    nodi lymphoidei appendi-
      culares
    nodi lymphoidei axillares
    nodi lymphoidei axillares
      anteriores
    nodi lymphoidei axillares
      apicales
    nodi lymphoidei axillares
      centrales
    nodi lymphoidei axillares
      laterales
    nodi lymphoidei axillares
      pectorales
    nodi lymphoidei axillares
      posteriores
    nodi lymphoidei axillares
      subscapulares

nodus *(continued)*
    nodi lymphoidei brachiales
    nodi lymphoidei broncho-
      pulmonales
    n. lymphoideus bucci-
      natorius
    nodi lymphoidei cavales la-
      terales
    nodi lymphoidei cervicales
      anteriores
    nodi lymphoidei cervicales
      anteriores profundi
    nodi lymphoidei cervicales
      anteriores superficiales
    nodi lymphoidei cervicales
      laterales profundi
    nodi lymphoidei cervicales
      laterales superficiales
    nodi lymphoidei cervicales
      laterales profundi infe-
      riores
    nodi lymphoidei cervicales
      laterales profundi supe-
      riores
    nodi lymphoidei coeliaci
    nodi lymphoidei colici dex-
      tri/medii/sinistri
    nodi lymphoidei cubitales
    n. lymphoideus cysticus
    nodi lymphoidei deltopec-
      torales
    nodi lymphoidei epigastrici
      inferiores
    nodi lymphoidei faciales
    n. lymphoideus fibularis
    n. lymphoideus foraminalis
    nodi lymphoidei gastrici
      dextri/sinistri
    nodi lymphatici gastroepi-
      ploici dextri/sinistri
    nodi lymphoidei gastroom-
      entales dextri/sinistri
    nodi lymphoidei gluteales
      inferiores
    nodi lymphoidei gluteales
      superiores
    nodi lymphoidei hepatici
    nodi lymphoidei ileocolici

nodus *(continued)*

nodi lymphoidei iliaci communes

nodi lymphoidei iliaci communes intermedii

nodi lymphoidei iliaci communes laterales

nodi lymphoidei iliaci communes mediales

nodi lymphoidei iliaci communes promontorii

nodi lymphoidei iliaci communes subaortici

nodi lymphoidei iliaci externi

nodi lymphoidei iliaci externi intermedii

nodi lymphoidei iliaci externi laterales

nodi lymphoidei iliaci externi mediales

nodi lymphoidei iliaci interni

nodi lymphoidei infraclaviculares

nodi lymphoidei infrahyoidei

nodi lymphoidei inguinales superficiales inferiores

nodi lymphoidei inguinales profundi

nodi lymphoidei inguinales superficiales

nodi lymphoidei inguinales superficiales superolaterales

nodi lymphoidei inguinales superficiales superomediales

nodi lymphoidei intercostales

nodi lymphoidei interiliaci

nodi lymphoidei interpectorales

nodi lymphoidei intrapulmonales

nodi lymphoidei jugulares anteriores

nodus *(continued)*

n. lymphoideus jugulodigastricus

n. lymphoideus juguloomohyoideus

nodi lymphoidei juxtaoesophageales

n. lymphoideus lacunaris intermedius

n. lymphoideus lacunaris lateralis

n. lymphoideus lacunaris medialis

nodi lymphoidei lienales

n. lymphoideus ligamenti arteriosi

nodi lymphoidei linguales

nodi lymphoidei lumbales dextri

nodi lymphoidei lumbales intermedii

nodi lymphoidei lumbales sinistri

nodi lymphatici lumbares dextri

nodi lymphatici lumbares intermedii

nodi lymphatici lumbares sinistri

n. lymphoideus malaris

n. lymphoideus mandibularis

nodi lymphoidei mastoidei

nodi lymphatici mediastinales anteriores

nodi lymphatici mediastinales posteriores

nodi lymphoidei membri superioris profundi

nodi lymphoidei membri superioris superficiales

nodi lymphoidei mesenterici

nodi lymphoidei mesenterici inferiores

nodi lymphoidei mesenterici juxtaintestinales

nodi lymphoidei mesenterici superiores

nodus *(continued)*
    nodi lymphoidei mesenter-
      ici superiores centrales
    nodi lymphoidei mesocolici
    n. lymphoideus nasolabi-
      alis
    nodi lymphoidei obturato-
      rii
    nodi lymphoidei occipitales
    nodi lymphoidei pancrea-
      tici
    nodi lymphoidei pancrea-
      tici inferiores
    nodi lymphoidei pancrea-
      tici superiores
    nodi lymphoidei pancreati-
      coduodenales inferiores
    nodi lymphoidei pancreati-
      coduodenales superiores
    nodi lymphoidei paracolici
    nodi lymphoidei paramam-
      marii
    nodi lymphoidei pararecta-
      les
    nodi lymphoidei paraster-
      nales
    nodi lymphoidei paratra-
      cheales
    nodi lymphoidei parauter-
      ini
    nodi lymphoidei paravagin-
      ales
    nodi lymphoidei paravesi-
      cales
    nodi lymphatici paravesicu-
      lares
    nodi lymphoidei parietales
    nodi lymphoidei parotidei
      profundi
    nodi lymphoidei parotidei
      profundi infraauriculares
    nodi lymphoidei parotidei
      profundi intraglandulares
    nodi lymphoidei parotidei
      profundi preauriculares
    nodi lymphoidei parotidei
      superficiales
    nodi lymphoidei pelvis pa-
      rietales

nodus *(continued)*
    nodi lymphoidei pelvis vis-
      cerales
    nodi lymphoidei pericardi-
      aci laterales
    nodi lymphoidei pericardi-
      ales laterales
    nodi lymphoidei phrenici
      inferiores
    nodi lymphoidei phrenici
      superiores
    nodi lymphoidei poplite-
      ales
    nodi lymphoidei poplite-
      ales profundi
    nodi lymphoidei poplite-
      ales superficiales
    nodi lymphoidei poplitei
    nodi lymphoidei poplitei
      profundi
    nodi lymphoidei poplitei
      superficiales
    nodi lymphoidei postaor-
      tici
    nodi lymphoidei postcava-
      les
    nodi lymphoidei postvesi-
      cales
    nodi lymphatici postvesicu-
      lares
    nodi lymphoidei preaortici
    nodi lymphoidei precae-
      cales
    nodi lymphoidei precavales
    nodi lymphoidei prececales
    nodi lymphoidei prelaryn-
      geales
    nodi lymphoidei prelaryn-
      gei
    nodi lymphoidei preperi-
      cardiaci
    nodi lymphoidei preperi-
      cardiales
    nodi lymphoidei pretra-
      cheales
    nodi lymphoidei preverte-
      brales
    nodi lymphoidei prevesi-
      cales

nodus *(continued)*
    nodi lymphatici prevesiculares
    nodi lymphoidei profundi membri superioris
    nodi lymphoidei pulmonales
    nodi lymphoidei pylorici
    nodi lymphoidei rectales superiores
    nodi lymphoidei retroaortici
    nodi lymphatici retroauriculares
    nodi lymphoidei retrocaecales
    nodi lymphoidei retrocavales
    nodi lymphoidei retropharyngeales
    nodi lymphoidei retropylorici
    nodi lymphoidei retrovesicales
    nodi lymphoidei sacrales
    nodi lymphoidei sigmoidei
    nodi lymphoidei splenici
    nodi lymphoidei submandibulares
    nodi lymphoidei submentales
    nodi lymphoidei subpylorici
    nodi lymphoidei superficiales membri superioris
    nodi lymphoidei superiores centrales
    nodi lymphoidei supraclaviculares
    n. lymphoideus suprapyloricus
    nodi lymphoidei supratrochleares
    nodi lymphoidei thyroidei
    n. lymphoideus tibialis anterior
    n. lymphoideus tibialis posterior

nodus *(continued)*
    nodi lymphatici tracheales
    nodi lymphoidei tracheobronchiales inferiores
    nodi lymphoidei tracheobronchiales superiores
    nodi lymphoidei vesicales laterales
    nodi lymphatici vesiculares laterales
    nodi lymphoidei viscerales
    n. sinuatrialis

nogalamycin

nomen
    nomina generalia

nomenclature

nomotopic

nononcogenic

nonhomogeneous

nonopaque

nonsecretor

nonrotation

nonunion
    bony n. (frequently dictated "non-bony union")

nonvisualization

Norcuron

norma
    n. anterior
    n. basilaris
    n. basalis
    n. facialis
    n. frontalis
    n. inferior
    n. lateralis
    n. occipitalis
    n. posterior
    n. sagittalis
    n. superior
    n. temporalis
    n. ventralis
    n. verticalis

normoblast
    acidophilic n.
    basophilic n.
    early n.
    eosinophilic n.
    intermediate n.
    late n.
    orthochromatic n.
    oxyphilic n.
    polychromatic n.
    polychromatophilic n.

normoblastic

normoblastosis

normochromasia

normochromia

normochromic

normocyte

normocytic

normocytosis

normoerythrocyte

normo-orthocytosis

normoskeocytosis

normotensive

normovolemia

normovolemic

nose

nosegay
    Riolan's n.

notch
    ethmoidal n. of frontal
      bone
    frontal n.
    intercondylar n.
    nasal n. of frontal bone
    parietal n. of temporal
      bone
    semilunar n.
    sternal n.
    supraorbital n.

notch *(continued)*
    suprasternal n.
    trigeminal n.

notching
    rib n.

notochordoma

notum

Novantrone

Novocain

NP-59

nucha

nucleon

nucleonic

nucleonics

nucleus *pl.* nuclei
    nuclei accessorii nervi ocu-
      lomotorii
    n. accumbens
    n. ambiguus
    n. amygdalae centralis
    n. amygdalae corticalis
    n. amygdalae lateralis
    n. amygdalae medialis
    n. ansae lenticularis
    n. anterior hypothalami
    nuclei anteriores thalami
    n. anterodorsalis thalami
    n. anterolateralis medullae
      spinalis
    n. anteromedialis medullae
      spinalis
    n. anteromedialis nervi
      oculomotorii
    n. anteromedialis thalami
    n. anteroventralis thalami
    n. arcuatus hypothalami
    n. arcuatus medullae ob-
      longatae
    n. basalis telencephali
    nuclei basales
    n. caeruleus
    n. campi dorsalis
    n. campi medialis
    nuclei campi perizonalis

nucleus *(continued)*

    n. campi ventralis
    caudate n.
    n. caudatus
    n. centralis lateralis thal-
        ami
    n. centralis medullae spina-
        lis
    n. centralis medialis thal-
        ami
    n. centromedianus thalami
    nuclei cerebelli
    n. cervicalis lateralis
    nuclei cochleares
    n. cochlearis anterior
    n. cochlearis posterior
    nuclei colliculi inferioris
    n. commissuralis nervi vagi
    n. commissuralis rhomboi-
        dalis
    n. commissurae posterioris
    nuclei corporis geniculati
        medialis
    n. cuneatus
    n. cuneatus accessorius
    n. cuneiformis
    n. dentatus
    n. dorsalis corporis genicu-
        lati lateralis
    n. dorsalis corporis genicu-
        lati medialis
    n. dorsalis hypothalami
    n. dorsalis lateralis thalami
    n. dorsalis nervi oculomo-
        torii
    n. dorsalis nervi vagi
    nuclei dorsales thalami
    n. dorsomedialis hypothal-
        amicae intermediae
    drumstick n.
    n. emboliformis
    n. endopeduncularis
    n. fastigii
    n. globosus
    n. gigantocellularis
    n. gracilis
    n. habenularis lateralis
    n. habenularis medialis

nucleus *(continued)*

    herniated n. pulposus
        (HNP)
    n. hypothalamicus anterior
    n. infundibularis
    n. intercalatus
    n. intermediolateralis me-
        dullae spinalis
    n. intermediomedialis me-
        dullae spinalis
    n. interpeduncularis
    n. interpositus anterior
    n. interpositus posterior
    n. interstitialis
    nuclei intralaminares thal-
        ami
    n. lateralis cerebelli
    n. lateralis posterior thal-
        ami
    nuclei lemnisci lateralis
    lentiform n.
    n. lentiformis
    n. lentis
    n. linearis intermedius
    n. linearis inferioris
    n. linearis superior
    n. mammillaris lateralis
    n. mammillaris medialis
    n. medialis cerebelli
    n. medialis magnocellularis
        corporis geniculati medi-
        alis
    nuclei mediales thalami
    nuclei mediani thalami
    n. mediodorsalis thalami
    n. mesencephalicus nervi
        trigemini
    n. motorius nervi trigemini
    n. nervi abducentis
    n. nervi accessorii
    n. nervi cranialis
    n. nervi facialis
    n. nervi hypoglossi
    n. nervi oculomotorii
    n. nervi phrenici
    n. nervi pudendi
    n. nervi trochlearis
    n. olfactorius anterior

nucleus *(continued)*
- n. olivaris accessorius medialis
- n. olivaris accessorius posterior
- nuclei olivares inferiores
- n. olivaris superior
- n. originis
- nuclei parabrachiales
- n. parabrachialis lateralis
- n. parabrachialis medialis
- n. paracentralis thalami
- n. parafascicularis thalami
- n. paragigantocellularis lateralis
- n. parasolitarius
- nuclei parasympathici sacrales
- n. parataenialis thalami
- n. paraventricularis anterior thalami
- n. paraventricularis hypothalami
- n. paraventricularis posterior thalami
- n. periventricularis posterior
- nuclei paraventriculares thalami
- nuclei perihypoglossales
- nuclei pontis
- n. pontinus nervi trigeminalis
- n. posterior hypothalami
- n. posterior nervi vagi
- nuclei posteriores thalami
- n. posterolateralis medullae spinalis
- n. posteromedialis medullae spinalis
- n. pregeniculatus
- n. preopticus lateralis
- n. preopticus medialis
- n. preopticus medianus
- n. preopticus periventricularis
- n. prepositus
- nuclei pretectales

nucleus *(continued)*
- n. principalis nervi trigemini
- n. proprius
- n. pulposus disci intervertebralis
- nuclei pulvinares thalami
- n. paramedianus posterior
- nuclei raphes
- n. raphes magnus
- n. raphes medianus
- n. raphes obscurus
- n. raphes pallidus
- n. raphes pontis
- n. raphes posterior
- nuclei reticulares
- n. reticularis intermedius medullae oblongatae
- n. reticularis lateralis medullae oblongatae
- n. reticularis paramedianus
- n. reticularis parvocellularis
- n. reticularis pontis rostralis
- n. reticularis tegmenti pontis
- n. reticularis thalami
- n. retroambiguus
- n. retrofacialis
- n. retroposterolateralis medullae spinalis
- n. reuniens
- n. rhomboidalis
- n. ruber
- n. salivatorius inferior
- n. salivatorius superior
- n. semilunaris
- n. septalis lateralis
- n. septalis medialis
- n. spinalis nervi trigemini
- n. striae terminalis
- n. subcaeruleus
- n. subcuneiformis
- n. subparabrachialis
- n. subthalamicus
- n. suprachiasmaticus
- n. supraopticus

nucleus *(continued)*
    nuclei tegmentales ante-
      riores
    n. tegmentalis pedunculo-
      pontinus
    n. tegmentalis posterolater-
      alis
    n. terminationis
    n. thoracicus dorsalis
    n. thoracicus posterior
    nuclei tractus solitarii
    n. triangularis septi
    nuclei tuberales laterales
    n. ventralis anterior thal-
      ami
    n. ventralis corporis genic-
      ulati lateralis
    n. ventralis corporis genic-
      ulati medialis
    n. ventralis intermedius
      thalami
    nuclei ventrales laterales
      thalami
    nuclei ventrales mediales
      thalami
    n. ventralis posterolateralis
      thalami

nucleus *(continued)*
    n. ventralis posteromedi-
      alis thalami
    nuclei ventrales thalami
    nuclei ventrobasales thal-
      ami
    n. ventromedialis hypothal-
      ami
    nuclei vestibulares
    n. vestibularis inferior
    n. vestibularis lateralis
    n. vestibularis medialis
    n. vestibularis superior

nuclide
    radioactive n.

number
    CT n's

numbness

Nupercainal

Nupercaine

nutrition
    total parenteral n. (TPN)

oak
  poison o.

OAP
  Oncovin (vincristine), ara-C
  (cytarabine), and prednisone

obeliac

obeliad

obelion

obese

obesity
  morbid o.

obex

oblique
  external o.
  internal o.

obliquity

obliquus

obliteration

obstipation

obstruction
  bladder outlet o.
  gastric outlet o.
  incomplete o.
  intestinal o.
  outlet o.
  ureteral o.

obturator

occipital

occipitalis

occipitoatloid

occipitoaxoid

occipitobasilar

occipitobregmatic

occipitocalcarine

occipitocervical

occipitofacial

occipitofrontal

occipitofrontalis

occipitomastoid

occipitomental

occipitoparietal

occipitotemporal

occiput

occlusion
  coronary o.

occlusive

OCG
  oral cholecystogram

ochronosis

Octreoscan

ocular

oculus *pl.* oculi

Oddi
  sphincter of O.

Odland body

odontoameloblastoma

odontoblastoma

odontoid

odontoma
  o. adamantinum
  ameloblastic o.
  composite o.
  composite o., complex
  composite o., compound
  coronal o.
  coronary o.
  dilated o.
  embryoplastic o.
  mixed o.
  radicular o.

odontoradiograph

oil
    bhilawanol o.
    chloriodized o.
    ethiodized o.
    iodized o.

odynophagia

olecranon

oleoperitoneography

oligemia

oligoastrocytoma

oligodendroblastoma

oligodendroglioma

oligohemia

oliguria

oliguric

oliva

olivopontine

Ollier's disease

Omenn's syndrome

omentoportography

omentum
    greater o.
    lesser o.
    o. majus
    o. minus

Omnipaque
    O. oncosis

Omniscint

omphalic

omphaloma

omphaloncus

omphalus

oncocyte

oncocytic

oncocytoma
    renal o.

oncocytosis

oncogene
    viral o.

oncogenesis

oncogenetic

oncogenic

oncogenicity

oncogenous

oncolipid

oncology

oncolysate

oncolysis

oncolytic

oncoma

OncoScint CR/OV

oncosis
    Omnipaque o.

oncotherapy

oncothlipsis

oncotropic

Oncovin

on-end

onychatrophia

onychatrophy

onychauxis

onychectomy

onychia

onychitis

onychoclasis

onychocryptosis

onychodystrophy

onychogenic

onychogryphosis

onychogryposis

onychoheterotopia

onycholysis

onychomadesis

onychomalacia

onychomycosis
dermatophytic o.

onychopathic

onychopathology

onychopathy

onychoptosis

onychorrhexis

onychoschizia

onychosis

onychotomy

onyx

onyxis

oophorectomy

oophoroma
o. folliculare

opacification

opacity

opaque

opaque end of Dobbhoff tube

open reduction and internal fixation (ORIF)

opening
aortic o. in diaphragm
caval o.
esophageal o. in diaphragm
inferior o. of thorax
superior o. of thorax
thoracic o., inferior
thoracic o., lower
thoracic o., superior
thoracic o., upper

operating room (OR)

operation
Blalock-Taussig o.
Cotting's o.
pull-through o.

opercula

opercular

operculum
o. frontale
o. parietale
o. temporale

ophiasis

Ophthaine

ophthalmoplegia

Ophthetic

opisthiobasial

opisthion

opisthionasial

opium
o. pulveratum

opponens

opposing

opsoclonus
o.-myoclonus

optimal

optimum

OR
operating room

ora
o. serrata retinae

orad

orae

Oragrafin

oral

orbiculi

orbiculus
    o. ciliaris

orbit

orbita *pl.* orbitae

orbital

orchidoncus

orchioblastoma

orchioncus

orchis

organ
    critical o.
    extraperitoneal o.
    genital o's
    genital o's, external
    genital o's, internal
    Meyer's o.
    reproductive o's
    retroperitoneal o.
    vestigial o.

organa (plural of organum)

organization

organography

organoid

organology

organon

organum *pl.* organa
    o. extraperitoneale
    organa genitalia
    organa genitalia feminina
      externa
    organa genitalia feminina
      interna
    organa genitalia masculina
      externa
    organa genitalia masculina
      interna
    o. gustatorium
    o. gustus
    o. olfactorium

organum *(continued)*
    o. olfactus
    o. retroperitoneale
    organa sensoria
    organa sensuum
    o. spirale
    o. subcommissurale
    o. subfornicale
    organa uropoëtica
    o. vestibulocochleare
    o. vomeronasale

Oriental ringworm

ORIF
    open reduction and internal fixation

orifice
    pilosebaceous o's

orificia

orificial

orificium

origin
    o's of the brachiocephalic
      vessels
    neurogenic o.

Ornidyl

orthochromatic

orthochromia

orthochromic

orthocytosis

orthoiodohippurate

orthostereoscope

orthovoltage

oropharyngeal

oropharynx

Oroya fever

orthopedic (also orthopaedic)
    o. surgeon

orthopedist

os *pl.* ossa
    o. breve
    o. calcis
    o. capitatum
    ossa carpalia
    ossa carpi
    o. centrale
    o. coccygis
    o. costae
    o. costale
    o. coxae
    ossa cranialia
    ossa cranii
    o. cuboideum
    o. cuneiforme intermedium
    o. cuneiforme laterale
    o. cuneiforme mediale
    ossa digitorum manus
    ossa digitorum pedis
    o. ethmoidale
    o. fabella
    o. femoris
    ossa fonticulorum
    o. frontale
    o. hamatum
    o. hyoideum
    o. ilii
    o. ilium
    o. incae
    o. incisivum
    o. interparietale
    o. irregulare
    o. ischii
    o. lacrimale
    o. longum
    o. lunatum
    ossa manus
    ossa membri inferioris
    ossa membri superioris
    ossa metacarpalia
    o. metacarpale tertium
    ossa metacarpi
    o. metacarpi tertium
    ossa metatarsalia
    ossa metatarsi
    o. nasale

os *(continued)*
    o. naviculare
    o. occipitale
    o. in o.
    o. palatinum
    o. parietale
    ossa pedis
    o. pisiforme
    o. planum
    o. pneumaticum
    o. pubis
    o. pelvicum
    o. sacrum
    o. scaphoideum
    ossa sesamoidea manus
    ossa sesamoidea pedis
    o. sphenoidale
    o. subfibulare
    ossa suprasternalia
    o. suturale
    ossa tarsalia
    ossa tarsi
    o. temporale
    ossa thoracis
    o. trapezium
    o. trapezoideum
    o. trigonum
    o. triquetrum
    ossa Wormi
    o. zygomaticum

Osbil

oscheoma

oscheoncus

osculum

Osgood-Schlatter disease

Osler
    O's disease
    O.-Vaquez disease

osmidrosis

ossa (plural of os)

ossature

osseous

ossicle
    Andernach's o's
    epactal o's
    intercalcar o's
    Riolan's o's
    wormian o's

ossicula (plural of ossiculum)

ossicular

ossiculum *pl.* ossicula
    ossicula auditoria
    ossicula auditus

ossification

ossiform

osteal

osteitis
    o. condensans ilii
    o. deformans
    o. pubis

osteoarthritis

osteoarthropathy
    hypertrophic o., idiopathic
    hypertrophic o., primary

osteoblastoma

osteochondritis
    o. dissecans
    o. ischiopubica

osteochondrofibroma

osteochondroma
    fibrosing o.

osteochondromatosis
    multiple o.

osteochondromyxoma

osteochondrosarcoma

osteoclastoma

osteodentin

osteodermia

osteodystrophy

osteoenchondroma

osteofibroma

osteogenesis
    o. imperfecta
    o. imperfecta tarda

osteogenic

osteolipochondroma

osteolipoma

Osteolite

osteologia

osteolytic

osteoma
    cavalryman's o.
    compact o.
    o. cutis
    o. durum
    o. eburneum
    giant osteoid o.
    ivory o.
    o. medullare
    osteoid o.
    o. spongiosum
    spongy o.
    trabecular o.

osteomalacia
    oncogenic o.
    oncogenous o.

osteomatoid

osteomatosis

osteomyelitis

osteomyelography

osteomyxochondroma

osteopetrosis

osteophyte

osteophytosis

osteoporosis

osteoradionecrosis

osteosarcoma
    chondroblastic o.

osteosarcoma *(continued)*
 classical o.
 extraosseous o.
 fibroblastic o.
 gnathic o.
 high-grade surface o.
 intracortical o.
 intraosseous low-grade o.
 o. of jaw
 juxtacortical o.
 multicentric o.
 osteoblastic o.
 parosteal o.
 periosteal o.
 small-cell o.
 telangiectatic o.

osteosarcomatosis

osteosarcomatous

osteosclerosis

osteosis
 o. cutis

osteotomy

ostia (plural of ostium)

ostial

ostiomeatal

ostium *pl.* ostia
 o. abdominale tubae uterinae
 o. aortae
 o. appendicis vermiformis
 o. atrioventriculare dextrum
 o. atrioventriculare sinistrum
 o. cardiacum
 o. ileale
 o. pharyngeum tubae auditivae
 o. pharyngeum tubae auditoriae
 o. pyloricum
 o. sinus coronarii
 o. trunci pulmonalis
 o. tympanicum tubae auditivae

ostium *(continued)*
 o. tympanicum tubae auditoriae
 o. ureteris
 o. urethrae externum femininae
 o. urethrae externum masculinae
 o. urethrae internum
 o. uteri
 o. uterinum tubae uterinae
 o. vaginae
 o. venae cavae inferioris
 o. venae cavae superioris
 ostia venarum pulmonal-
  ium

Ota
 nevus of O.

otitis
 o. externa
 o. media

otorhinolaryngology

Otto pelvis

outlet
 pelvic o.
 thoracic o.

outpocketing

outpouching

output
 cardiac o.
 exposure o. rate

ova (plural of ovum)

oval in shape

ovalocytosis

ovarium

ovarian

ovary

overlapping of the fracture fragments

overlying
 o. bowel content

overlying *(continued)*
    o. bowel gas
    o. bowel shadows

overriding of the fracture fragments

overtransfusion

ovular

ovule

ovum *pl.* ova
    blighted o.

Owren's disease

oxide
    diethyl o.
    nitrous o.

oxidronate

oximeter
    CO-o.
    ear o.

oximeter *(continued)*
    finger o.
    pulse o.
    whole blood o.

oximetry

oxirane

oxygen
    o. 15

oxygenator
    bubble o.
    disk o.
    film o.
    membrane o.
    rotating disk o.
    screen o.

oxyheme

oxyhemochromogen

oxyhemoglobin

ozonophore

PA
  posteroanterior
  PA view

pacemaker
  bipolar p.
  p. battery pack
  permanent p.

pachycheilia

pachyderma

pachydermatocele

pachydermatous

pachydermic

pachydermoperiostosis

pachygyria

pachymeninx

pachyonychia
  p. congenita

paclitaxel

pad
  fat p.
  knuckle p's
  pericardial fat p.

Paget
  P's carcinoma
  P's cell
  P's disease of the bone
  P's disease of the breast
  P's disease, extramammary
  P's disease, vulvar

pagetic

pagetoid
  p. cell

pagoplexia

pain
  exquisite p.
  flank p.
  phantom limb p.
  pleuritic p.

pair
  ion p.

palata (plural of palatum)

palate
  hard p.
  soft p.

palatine

palatum *pl.* palata
  p. durum
  p. molle
  p. osseum

paleocerebellum

paleocortex

palliation

palliative

pallium

palm
  tripe p.

palma

palmaris

palpable

palpation

palpebra
  p. inferior
  p. superior

palsy
  Bell's p.

pamidronate

L-PAM (melphalan)

Pancoast's syndrome

pancreas
  p. accessorium
  accessory p.
  p. divisum

pancreaticosplenic

pancreatic pseudocyst

pancreatitis
  acute necrotizing p.

pancreatoblastoma

pancreatogram

pancreatography
  endoscopic retrograde p.

pancuronium bromide

pancytopenia
  congenital p.
  Fanconi's p.

panhematopenia

Panizza's plexuses

panmyeloid

panmyelopathia

panmyelopathy
  constitutional infantile p.
  Fanconi's p.

panmyelophthisis

panniculalgia

panniculitis
  lobular p.
  nodular nonsuppurative p.
  relapsing febrile nodular
    nonsuppurative p.
  subacute nodular migrato-
    ry p.
  Weber-Christian p.

panniculus
  p. adiposus
  p. carnosus

pannus
  p. formation

Panorex
  P. views

pansinusitis

Pantopaque

panus

Pap smear

Papanicolaou smear

papilla *pl.* papillae
  p. corii
  p. of corium
  p. dermatis
  p. dermis
  p. duodeni major
  p. duodeni minor
  papillae filiformes
  papillae foliatae
  papillae fungiformes
  hair p.
  p. ilealis
  p. lacrimalis
  papillae linguales
  p. mammae
  p. mammaria
  mammary p.
  p. pili
  p. renalis
  skin p.
  papillae vallatae

papillae (plural of papilla)

papillary

papillate

papilledema

papilliferous

papilliform

papilloadenocystoma

papillocarcinoma

papilloma
  choroid plexus p.
  cutaneous p.
  fibroepithelial p.
  hirsutoid p's of penis
  intracystic p.
  intraductal p.
  inverted p.
  inverted ductal p.
  inverted schneiderian p.
  squamous p.

papilloma *(continued)*
    villous p.

papillomatosis
    confluent and reticulate p.

papillomatous

papular

papulation

papule
    Gottron's p's
    moist p.
    mucous p.
    pearly penile p's
    prurigo p.
    split p's

papuloerythematous

papuloid

papulopustular

papulosis
    bowenoid p.
    lymphomatoid p.
    malignant atrophic p.

papulosquamous

papulovesicular

para-adventitial

paracentesis

paracentral

paracervix

paradidymis

paraflocculus
    p. ventralis

paraganglioma
    medullary p.
    nonchromaffin p.

paragranuloma

parahemophilia

parakeratosis
    p. ostracea

parakeratosis *(continued)*
    p. scutularis
    p. variegata

parallel

paralogy

paralysis
    Erb's p.
    phrenic nerve p.

parameatal

paramedian

paramesial

parameter

parametrium

paraneoplastic

paranephroma

paraomphalic

Paraplatin

paraplegia

paraplegic

paraproteinemia

parapsoriasis
    acute p.
    atrophic p.
    chronic p.
    p. guttata
    guttate p.
    large plaque p.
    p. lichenoides
    p. en plaques
    poikilodermic p.
    poikilodermatous p.
    retiform p.
    small plaque p.
    p. variegata
    p. varioliformis acuta
    p. varioliformis chronica

parapyramidal

parasinoidal

parasplenic

parathyroidoma

paratracheal

paraumbilical

paraungual

paravariceally
paravertebral

paravisceral

paraxial

pareleidin

parenchyma
breast p.
hepatic p.
lung p.
p. of prostatae
renal p.
p. of testis

parenteral

paries *pl.* parietes
p. anterior gastris
p. anterior vaginae
p. caroticus cavitatis tympanicae
p. caroticus cavitatis tympani
p. externus ductus cochlearis
p. inferior orbitae
p. jugularis cavitatis tympanicae
p. jugularis cavitatis tympani
p. labyrinthicus cavitatis tympanicae
p. labyrinthicus cavitatis tympani
p. lateralis orbitae
p. mastoideus cavitatis tympanicae
p. mastoideus cavitatis tympani
p. medialis orbitae
p. membranaceus cavitatis tympanicae

paries *(continued)*
p. membranaceus cavitatis tympani
p. membranaceus tracheae
p. posterior gastris
p. posterior vaginae
p. superior orbitae
p. tegmentalis cavitatis tympanicae
p. tegmentalis cavitatis tympani
p. tympanicus ductus cochlearis
p. vestibularis ductus cochlearis

parietal

parietes (plural of paries)

parietofrontal

parietography
gastric p.

parieto-occipital

parietosphenoid

parietosplanchnic

parietosquamosal

parietotemporal

parietovisceral

Parkinson's disease

parkinsonism

paroccipital

paronychia

paronychial

paroöphoron

parophthalmoncus

parotitis

parrot-beak tear of the medial
meniscus

pars *pl.* partes
  p. abdominalis aortae
  p. abdominalis ductus thoracici
  p. abdominalis musculi pectoralis majoris
  p. abdominalis oesophagi
  p. abdominalis ureteris
  p. alaris musculi nasalis
  p. anterior commissurae anterioris
  p. anterior commissurae rostralis
  p. anterior dorsi linguae
  p. anterior faciei diaphragmaticae hepatis
  p. anterior fornicis vaginae
  p. anterior lobuli quadrangularis anterioris
  p. anularis vaginae fibrosae digitorum manus
  p. anularis vaginae fibrosae digitorum pedis
  p. aryepiglottica musculi arytenoidei obliqui
  p. ascendens aortae
  p. ascendens duodeni
  p. atlantica arteriae vertebralis
  p. autonomica systematis nervosi peripherici
  p. basilaris ossis occipitalis
  p. basilaris pontis
  p. basalis arteriae pulmonalis dextrae
  p. basalis arteriae pulmonalis sinistrae
  p. buccopharyngea musculi constrictoris pharyngis superioris
  p. canalis nervi optici
  p. cardiaca gastris
  p. cartilaginea septi nasi
  p. cartilaginea systematis skeletalis
  p. cartilaginea tubae auditivae

pars *(continued)*
  p. cartilaginea tubae auditoriae
  p. cavernosa arteriae carotidis internae
  p. centralis systematis nervosi
  p. centralis ventriculi lateralis
  p. ceratopharyngea musculi constrictoris pharyngis medii
  p. cerebralis arteriae carotidis internae
  p. cervicalis arteriae carotidis internae
  p. cervicalis arteriae vertebralis
  p. cervicalis ductus thoracici
  p. cervicalis medullae spinalis
  p. cervicalis oesophagi
  p. cervicalis tracheae
  p. chondropharyngea musculi constrictoris pharyngis medii
  p. ciliaris retinae
  p. clavicularis musculi pectoralis majoris
  p. coccygea medullae spinalis
  p. collis oesophagi
  p. compacta substantiae nigrae
  p. corneoscleralis reticuli trabecularis
  partes corporis humani
  p. costalis diaphragmatis
  p. cranialis partis parasympathici divisionis autonomici systematis nervosi
  p. cricopharyngea musculi constrictoris pharyngis inferioris
  p. cruciformis vaginae fibrosae digitorum manus

pars *(continued)*

p. cruciformis vaginae fibrosae digitorum pedis

p. cupularis recessus epitympanici

p. descendens aortae

p. descendens duodeni

p. dextra faciei diaphragmaticae hepatis

p. distalis adenohypophyseos

p. distalis lobi anterioris hypophyseos

p. dorsalis lobuli quadrangularis anterioris

p. duralis fili terminalis

p. flaccida membranae tympanicae

p. glossopharyngea musculi constrictoris pharyngis superioris

p. horizontalis arteriae cerebri mediae

p. horizontalis duodeni

p. inferior duodeni

p. inferior nervi vestibularis

p. inferior venae lingularis

p. infraclavicularis plexus brachialis

p. infralobaris rami posterior

p. insularis arteriae cerebri mediae

p. interarticularis

p. intercartilaginea rimae glottidis

p. intermedia adenohypophyseos

p. intermedia lobi anterioris hypophyseos

p. intermedia urethrae masculinae

p. intermembranacea rimae glottidis

p. intersegmentalis

p. intersegmentalis rami posterior

pars *(continued)*

p. intracanalicularis nervi optici

p. intracranialis arteriae vertebralis

p. intracranialis nervi optici

p. intralaminaris nervi optici intraocularis

p. intralobaris rami posterior

p. intraocularis nervi optici

p. intrasegmentalis

p. iridica retinae

p. lacrimalis musculi orbicularis oculi

p. laryngea pharyngis

p. lateralis arcus pedis longitudinalis

p. lateralis fornicis vaginae

p. lateralis musculorum intertransversariorum posteriorum cervicis

p. lateralis ossis occipitalis

p. lateralis ossis sacri

p. lateralis venae lobi medii

p. libera membri inferioris

p. libera membri superioris

p. lumbalis diaphragmatis

p. lumbalis medullae spinalis

p. magnocellularis nuclei rubri

p. medialis arcus pedis longitudinalis

p. medialis venae lobi medii

p. membranacea septi atriorum

p. membranacea septi interventricularis

p. membranacea septi nasi

p. membranacea urethrae masculinae

p. mobilis septi nasi

p. muscularis septi interventricularis

pars *(continued)*

    p. mylopharyngea musculi constrictoris pharyngis superioris

    p. nasalis ossis frontalis

    p. nasalis pharyngis

    p. nervosa neurohypophyseos

    p. obliqua musculi cricothyroidei

    p. occlusa arteriae umbilicalis

    p. olfactoria cavitatis nasi

    p. opercularis gyri frontalis inferioris

    p. optica retinae

    p. oralis pharyngis

    p. orbitalis glandulae lacrimalis

    p. orbitalis gyri frontalis inferioris

    p. orbitalis musculi orbicularis oculi

    p. orbitalis nervi optici

    p. orbitalis ossis frontalis

    p. ossea septi nasi

    p. ossea systematis skeletalis

    p. ossea tubae auditivae

    p. ossea tubae auditoriae

    p. palpebralis glandulae lacrimalis

    p. palpebralis musculi orbicularis oculi

    p. parasympathica divisionis autonomici systematis nervosi

    p. parvocellularis nuclei rubri

    p. patens arteriae umbilicalis

    p. pelvica partis parasympatheticae systematis nervosi autonomici

    p. pelvica ureteris

    p. peripherica systematis nervosi

pars *(continued)*

    p. petrosa arteriae carotidis internae

    p. petrosa ossis temporalis

    p. pialis fili terminalis

    p. postcommunicalis arteriae cerebri anterioris

    p. postcommunicalis arteriae cerebri posterioris

    p. posterior commissurae anterioris

    p. posterior commissurae rostralis

    p. posterior dorsi linguae

    p. posterior faciei diaphragmaticae hepatis

    p. posterior fornicis vaginae

    p. posterior lobuli quadrangularis anterioris

    p. posterior pedunculi cerebri

    p. postlaminaris nervi optici intraocularis

    p. postsulcalis dorsi linguae

    p. precommunicalis arteriae cerebri anterioris

    p. precommunicalis arteriae cerebri posterioris

    p. prelaminaris nervi optici intraocularis

    p. presulcalis dorsi linguae

    p. prevertebralis arteriae vertebralis

    p. profunda musculi masseteris

    p. profunda musculi sphincteris ani externus

    p. prostatica urethrae masculinae

    p. pterygopharyngea musculi constrictoris pharyngis superioris

    p. pylorica gastris

    p. pylorica ventriculi

    p. recta musculi cricothyroidei

pars *(continued)*
p. respiratoria cavitatis nasi
p. reticularis substantiae nigrae
p. retrolentiformis capsulae internae
p. sacralis medullae spinalis
p. sphenoidalis arteriae cerebri mediae
p. spinalis nervi accessorii
p. spongiosa urethrae masculinae
p. squamosa ossis temporalis
p. sternalis diaphragmatis
p. sternocostalis musculi pectoralis majoris
p. subcutanea musculi sphincteris ani externus
p. sublentiformis capsulae internae
p. superficialis musculi masseteris
p. superficialis musculi sphincteris ani externus
p. superior duodeni
p. superior faciei diaphragmaticae hepatis
p. superior nervi vestibularis
p. superior venae lingularis
p. supraclavicularis plexus brachialis
p. sympathica divisionis autonomici systematis nervosi
p. tensa membranae tympanicae
p. thoracica aortae
p. thoracica autonomica
p. thoracica ductus thoracici
p. thoracica medullae spinalis
p. thoracica oesophagi
p. thoracica tracheae

pars *(continued)*
p. thyroepiglottica musculi thyroarytenoidei
p. thyropharyngea musculi constrictoris pharyngis inferioris
p. tibiocalcanea ligamenti collateralis medialis
p. tibionavicularis ligamenti collateralis medialis
p. tibiotalaris anterior ligamenti collateralis medialis
p. tibiotalaris posterior ligamenti collateralis medialis
p. transversa musculi nasalis
p. transversa rami sinistri venae portae hepatis
p. transversaria arteriae vertebralis
p. triangularis gyri frontalis inferioris
p. tuberalis adenohypophyseos
p. tuberalis lobi anterioris hypophyseos
p. tympanica ossis temporalis
p. umbilicalis rami sinistri venae portae hepatis
p. uterina tubae uterinae
p. uvealis reticuli trabecularis
p. vagalis nervi accessorii
p. ventralis lobuli quadrangularis anterioris
p. vertebralis faciei costalis pulmonis

Parsidol

part
basilar p. of occipital bone
condylar p. of occipital bone
costal p. of diaphragm
exoccipital p. of occipital bone
jugular p. of occipital bone

part *(continued)*
  lateral p. of occipital bone
  lumbar p. of diaphragm
  nasal p. of frontal bone
  occipital p. of occipital
    bone
  pectineal p. of inguinal liga-
    ment
  squamous p. of frontal
    bone
  squamous p. of occipital
    bone
  squamous p. of temporal
    bone
  sternal p. of diaphragm
  sternocostal p. of dia-
    phragm
  tabular p. of occipital bone
  tendinous p. of epicranius
    muscle
  vertebral p. of diaphragm

partes (plural of pars)

passage of contrast material

particle
  alpha p.
  beta p.
  elementary p.
  high-velocity p's
  Zimmermann's elemen-
    tary p.

parumbilical

pastille

PAT
  paroxysmal auricular
    tachycardia

patch
  ash-leaf p.
  herald p.
  lance-ovate p.
  Peyer's p's
  salmon p.
  shagreen p.

patchy area of consolidation

patchy area of pneumonia

patella
  bipartite p.

patellectomy

patelliform

patency

path
  ionization p.

pathognomonic

pathologic

pathology
  p. report

pathological

pathway
  common p. of coagulation
  extrinsic p. of coagulation
  intrinsic p. of coagulation

pattern
  acinar p.
  bowel gas p.
  bronchovascular p.
  haustral p.
  intestinal gas p.
  lacy p.
  ladderlike p.
  mucosal p.
  pulmonary vascular p.
  reticulonodular p.
  rugal p.
  stromal p. of the breasts
  trabecular p.

patulin

patulous

paucity

Pautrier
  P's abscess
  P's microabscess

pavilion

Pavulon

P blood group

PCA
    porous-coated anatomic
        PCA prosthesis

peak
    Bragg p.
    kilovolts p.

PDA
    patent ductus arteriosus

pearl
    Ebstein's p.
    epidermic p's
    epithelial p's

Pearson's syndrome

pea-sized

peau
    p. de chagrin
    p. d'orange

Pecquet
    cistern of P.
    P's reservoir

pecten
    p. analis
    p. ossis pubis

pectinate

pectiniform

pectora (plural of pectus)

pectoral

pectoralis

pectus *pl.* pectora
    p. carinatum
    p. excavatum
    p. recurvatum (*same as*
        pectus excavatum)

pedes (plural of pes)

pedicellate, pedicellated

pedicellation

pedicle
    p's and pars

pedicled

pediculate

pediculation

pediculus *pl.* pediculi
    p. arcus vertebrae

peduncle
    cerebellar p.
    cerebral p.

peduncular

pedunculated

pedunculus *pl.* pedunculi
    pedunculi cerebellares
    p. cerebellaris inferior
    p. cerebellaris medius
    p. cerebellaris pontinus
    p. cerebellaris superior
    p. cerebralis
    p. cerebri
    p. flocculi

peel
    chemical p.
    pleural p.

peg
    rete p's

pelade

pelage

Pelger
    P's nuclear anomaly
    P.-Huët anomaly
    P.-Huët nuclear anomaly

peliosis

pellagrosis

Pellegrini-Stieda disease

peltate

Pelodera dermatitis

pelves (plural of pelvis)

pelvic
    p. brim
    p. films for IUD localization
    p. girdle

pelvic *(continued)*
    p. inflammatory disease
      (PID)
    p. inlet
    p. kidney
    p. measurements
    p. outlet

pelvicephalography

pelvimetry

pelviography

pelvioradiography

pelvioscopy

pelviradiography

pelvis *pl.* pelves
    android p.
    anthropoid p.
    bifid p.
    brim of the p.
    false p.
    gynecoid p.
    p. major
    maternal p.
    p. minor
    Otto p.
    p. renalis
    true p.

pelviscope

pelviscopy

pelviureteroradiography

pelvoscopy

pemphigoid
    benign mucosal p.
    benign mucous mem-
      brane p.
    bullous p.
    bullous p., localized
    cicatricial p.
    localized chronic p.

pemphigus
    benign familial p.
    Brazilian p.
    p. erythematosus

pemphigus *(continued)*
    p. foliaceus
    South American p.
    p. vegetans
    p. vegetans, benign
    p. vulgaris
    wildfire p.

penetrability

penetrometer

penicidin

penicilli

penicilliary

penicillus
    penicilli arteriae lienalis
    penicilli arteriae splenicae

penis

pennate

penniform

pentalogy of Fallot

pentamethylmelamine

pentetate

pentetic acid

pentetreotide

Penthrane

pentobarbital
    p. sodium

Pentothal

penumbra

Pepper
    P. syndrome
    P. tumor

peptide
    parathyroid hormone–
      like p.

percussion

percutaneous
    p. cholecystotomy tube in-
      sertion

perflubron

perfluorochemical

perforans

perforated hollow viscus

perforation
esophageal p.

perforator
incompetent p's

perfrigeration

perfusion
isolation-p.
myocardial p.

perfusionist

periacinal

periacinous

periadventitial

periampullary

periangiitis

periangioma

periapical

periaqueductal

periaxial

periaxillary

pericanalicular

pericapsular

pericardiopleural

pericardium
p. fibrosum
fibrous p.
p. serosum
serous p.

pericecal

pericentral

perichondrium

perichondroma

pericranial

pericranium

pericryptal

pericytoma

periderm

peridermal

periductal

periductile

peridurogram

peridurography

periencephalography

perifascicular

perifollicular

perifolliculitis
p. capitis abscedens et suffodiens
superficial pustular p.

perigemmal

periglandular

perihilar

periligamentous

perilobar

perilympha

perilymphangeal

perilymphatic

perimedullary

perimeter

perimetrium

perimyelography

perimysia

perimysium

perineal

perineum

perineurium

perinodal

period
    half-life p.

periodontal

periomphalic

perionychia

perionychium

perionyx

perioral

periorbita

periorbital

periosteal new bone formation

periosteum
    p. externum cranii

periostitis

peripherad

peripheral

peripheralis

peripheric

periphericus

peripherocentral

periphery

periporitis

perisinuous

perisplanchnic

perisplenic

perisplenitis
    p. cartilaginea

peristalsis
    hyperactive p.
    nonpropulsive p.

peristaltic

peristomal

perisyringitis

peritendinitis

perithelial

perithelioma

perithoracic

peritoneocentesis

peritoneography

peritoneopericardial

peritoneum
    abdominal p.
    p. parietale
    p. urogenitale
    p. viscerale

peritonitis

peritonsillar

periumbilical

periungual

perivasculitis

periventricular

perivisceral

PermCath (*not* PermaCath)

pernio

peroneal

peronealis

perpendicular

Persantine

persistence
    hereditary p. of fetal hemo-
      globin

perspiratio
    p. insensibilis

perspiration
    insensible p.
    sensible p.

pertechnetate

pes
  p. hippocampi
  p. planus

pessary

petechia
  calcaneal petechiae

petechiae

PET
  positron emission tomography
    PET scan

petechial

pethidine hydrochloride

petiolate, petiolated

petiole

petioled

petiolus
  p. epiglottidis

Petit's triangle

petroccipital

petro-occipital

Peutz-Jeghers syndrome

Peyer
  P's glands
  P's patches
  P's plaques

Peyronie's disease

phacoid

phagedena

phagedenic

phagocyte
  mononuclear p.

phagocytic

phagocytin

phalanx *pl.* phalanges
  phalanges digitorum manus

phalanx *(continued)*
  phalanges digitorum pedis
  p. distalis digitorum manus
  p. distalis digitorum pedis
  p. media digitorum manus
  p. media digitorum pedis
  p. proximalis digitorum manus
  p. proximalis digitorum pedis

Phalen's sign

phalloncus

phantom

pharcidous

pharmacoangiography

pharmacoradiography

pharyngeal

pharyngitid

pharynx

phase
  arterial p.
  expiratory p. of respiration
  growth p.
  growth p., radial
  growth p., vertical
  vascular p.
  wash-in p.
  wash-out p.

phenanthrene

phenomenon
  embolic p.
  Hamburger p.
  Herendeen p.
  Koebner's p.
  Lucio's p.
  Mach p.
  Meirowsky p.
  Raynaud's p.
  vacuum p.

phenopropazine hydrochloride

phenotype
  Bombay p.

phenotype *(continued)*
McLeod p.

phenylketonuria

pheochromoblastoma

pheochromocytoma

pheresis

Philadelphia (Ph¹) chromosome

philtrum

phlebectasia

phlebectasis

phlebitis

phlebogram
descending p.

phlebography
ascending p.
descending p.

phlebolith

phlebothrombosis

phlegmon

phlegmonous

phlycten

phlyctena

phlyctenar

phlyctenoid

phocomelia

phonation

phorbol
p. ester

phosphate
chromic p. P 32
chromic p. P 32
polyestradiol p.

phosphine

Phosphocol P 32

phosphorus
p. 32

phosphorus *(continued)*
p. 32

Phosphotec

photoaging

photochemotherapy

photocutaneous

photodermatitis

photodermatosis

photoerythema

photofluorogram

photofluorography

photofluoroscope

Photofrin

photon

photo-onycholysis

photopenia

photopenic

photopheresis

photoradiation

photoradiometer

photoscan

photoscanner

photoscope

photoscopy

photosensitive

photosensitivity

photosensitization

photosensitize

phototherapy
ultraviolet p.

phototimer

phototoxic

phototoxicity

phren

phrenic

phrenocolic

phrenogastric

phrenoglottic

phrenohepatic

phrenosplenic

phrynoderma

phthisis

phyllode

phyma *pl.* phymata

phymatorhusin

phymatorrhysin

physalides

physaliferous

physaliform

physaliphore

physaliphorous

physalis

physeal

physiologicoanatomical

physiologic for the patient's
    age

physique

physis

phytobezoar

phytophotodermatitis

pia mater
    p. m. cranialis
    p. m. encephali
    p. m. spinalis

piastrinemia

Piazza's fluid

PICC
    peripherally inserted cen-
       tral catheter

Picker (x-ray equipment)

picocurie

piebald

piebaldism

piedra
    black p.
    white p.

pigment
    blood p.
    hematogenous p.

pigmentation

pigmentophage

pila

pilae

pilar, pilary

pili (plural of pilus)

pilial

pillar
    p's of diaphragm
    tonsillar p.

pilocystic

piloerection

piloleiomyoma

pilomatricoma

pilomatrixoma

pilomotor

pilonidal

pilose

pilosebaceous

pilus *pl.* pili
    pili annulati
    pili canaliculi
    pili cuniculati

pilus *(continued)*
    pili incarnati
    pili incarnati recurvi
    pili multigemini
    pili torti
    pili trianguli et canaliculi

pimeloma

pimple

pin
    Hagie p.
    Smith-Petersen p.
    Steinmann p.

pinealoblastoma

pinealocytoma

pinealoma
    ectopic p.

pineoblastoma

pineocytoma

piniform

pinna of the ear

pinning
    hip p.

pion

piperocaine hydrochloride

PIPIDA scan

piroxantrone hydrochloride

pisiform

pisiformis

pit
    arm p.

pitchblende

Pitressin

pitting

pityriasis
    p. alba
    lichenoid p., acute
    lichenoid p., chronic
    p. lichenoides acuta

pityriasis *(continued)*
    p. lichenoides chronica
    p. lichenoides et variolifor-
      mis acuta
    p. maculata
    p. nigra
    p. rosea
    p. rotunda
    p. rubra
    p. rubra pilaris
    p. sicca
    p. simplex
    p. versicolor

pityroid

pixel

placenta
    p. previa (also placenta
      praevia)

placental

placentogram

placentography
    indirect p.

plafond
    tibial plafond

plain films (*not* plane films)

plana (plural of planum)

planchet

Planck's theory

plane
    Addison's p's
    Aeby's p.
    auriculoinfraorbital p.
    axial p.
    Baer's p.
    biparietal p.
    Blumenbach's p.
    Bolton-nasion p.
    Broadbent-Bolton p.
    coronal p's
    Daubenton's p.
    eye-ear p.
    facial p.
    fat p's

plane *(continued)*
    Frankfort horizontal p.
    frontal p's
    frontoparallel p.
    Hodge's p's
    horizontal p.
    interiliac p.
    interparietal p. of occipital
      bone
    interspinal p.
    interspinous p.
    intertubercular p.
    Ludwig's p.
    Meckel's p.
    median p.
    median-raphe p.
    median sagittal p.
    midclavicular p.
    midpelvic p.
    midsagittal p.
    Morton's p.
    nasion-postcondylare p.
    nuchal p.
    occipital p.
    orbital p.
    paramedian p's
    parasagittal p.
    pelvic p.
    pelvic p., narrow
    pelvic p., wide
    pelvic p. of outlet
    principal p.
    p's of reference
    sagittal p's
    semicircular p. of frontal
      bone
    semicircular p. of parietal
      bone
    semicircular p. of squama
      temporalis
    spinous p.
    sternoxiphoid p.
    subcostal p.
    supracrestal p.
    supracristal p.
    suprasternal p.
    temporal p.
    thoracic p.
    transpyloric p.

plane *(continued)*
    transtubercular p.
    transverse p's
    umbilical p.
    vertical p.

planigram

planigraphy

planimeter

planing

planithorax

planogram *(or* planigram)

planta

plantaris

planum *pl.* plana
    plana frontalia
    plana coronalia
    p. medianum
    plana horizontalia
    p. interspinale
    p. intertuberculare
    plana, lineae et regiones
    p. nuchale
    p. occipitale
    p. orbitale
    plana paramediana
    plana sagittalia
    p. sphenoidale
    p. subcostale
    p. supracristale
    p. temporale
    p. transpyloricum
    plana transversalia

plaque
    Hutchinson's p's
    Peyer's p's

plasma
    antihemophilic human p.
    blood p.
    citrated p.
    fresh frozen p.
    normal human p.
    oxalate p.
    pooled p.
    salt p.

plasma *(continued)*
    true p.

plasmacytoma
    multiple p. of bone

plasmacytosis

plasmapheresis

plasmatic

plasmic

plasmin

plasminogen

plasminogen activator

plasmocytoma

plasmoma

plate
    Casper p.
    p. of cranial bone, inner
    p. of cranial bone, outer
    cribriform p.
    growth p.
    nail p.
    quadrilateral p.

platelet
    blood p.

plateletpheresis

plateau
    tibial p.

Platinol

platybasia

platypelloid

platysma

platytrope

pleiades

pleomorphic

pleomorphism

plessigraph

plessimeter

plessimetric

plethora

plethysmograph
    digital p.
    finger p.

plethysmography
    impedance p.

pleura *pl.* pleurae
    parietal p.
    p. parietalis
    p. pulmonalis
    p. visceralis

pleural-based

pleurae (plural of pleura)

pleurisy

pleurocutaneous

pleuroesophageal

pleuroesophageus

pleurography

pleuroperitoneal

pleurovisceral

plexal

plexiform

pleximeter

pleximetric

pleximetry

plexogenic

plexometer

plexus
    p. aorticus
    p. aorticus abdominalis
    p. aorticus thoracicus
    p. autonomicus
    p. basilaris
    brachial p.
    p. brachialis
    p. cardiacus

plexus *(continued)*
- p. caroticus communis
- p. caroticus externus
- p. caroticus internus
- p. cavernosus
- p. cavernosus conchae
- celiac p.
- p. celiacus
- p. cervicalis
- choroid p.
- p. choroideus ventriculi lateralis
- p. choroideus ventriculi quarti
- p. choroideus ventriculi tertii
- p. coccygeus
- p. coeliacus
- p. deferentialis
- p. dentalis inferior
- p. dentalis superior
- p. entericus
- epigastric p.
- p. femoralis
- p. gastrici
- p. hepaticus
- p. hypogasticus
- p. hypogastricus inferior
- p. hypogastricus superior
- p. iliacus
- p. iliacus externus
- p. inguinalis
- p. intermesentericus
- p. intraparotideus
- p. jugularis
- p. lienalis
- p. lumbalis
- p. lumbosacralis
- lymphatic p.
- p. lymphaticus axillaris
- p. mesentericus inferior
- p. mesentericus superior
- p. myentericus
- p. nervorum spinalium
- p. oesophageus
- p. ovaricus
- p. pampiniformis

plexus *(continued)*
- p. pancreaticus
- Panizza's p's
- p. pelvicus
- p. periarterialis
- p. pharyngeus
- p. pharyngeus nervi vagi
- p. prostaticus
- p. pterygoideus
- p. pulmonalis
- Quénu's hemorrhoidal p.
- p. rectalis inferior
- p. rectalis medius
- p. rectalis superior
- p. renalis
- sacral lymphatic p.
- p. sacralis
- p. sacralis medius
- Sappey's subareolar p.
- p. splenicus
- p. subclavius
- p. submucosus
- p. subserosus
- p. suprarenalis
- p. testicularis
- p. tympanicus
- p. tympanicus [Jacobsoni]
- p. uretericus
- p. uterovaginalis
- p. vascularis
- p. vasculosus
- p. venosus
- p. venosus areolaris
- p. venosus canalis hypoglossi
- p. venosus caroticus internus
- p. venosus foraminis ovalis
- p. venosus prostaticus
- p. venosus rectalis
- p. venosus sacralis
- p. venosus suboccipitalis
- p. venosus uterinus
- p. venosus vaginalis
- p. venosus vertebralis externus anterior
- p. venosus vertebralis externus posterior

plexus *(continued)*
- p. venosus vertebralis internus anterior
- p. venosus vertebralis internus posterior
- p. venosus vesicalis
- p. vertebralis
- p. vesicalis
- p. visceralis

plica *pl.* plicae
- plicae alares
- p. aryepiglottica
- p. axillaris anterior
- p. axillaris posterior
- plicae caecales
- p. caecalis vascularis
- p. cecalis vascularis
- p. chordae tympani
- plicae ciliares
- plicae circulares
- p. duodenalis inferior
- p. duodenalis superior
- p. duodenojejunalis
- p. duodenomesocolica
- p. epigastrica
- p. fimbriata
- plicae gastricae
- p. gastropancreatica
- p. glossoepiglottica lateralis
- p. glossoepiglottica mediana
- p. hepatopancreatica
- p. hypogastrica
- p. ileocaecalis
- p. ileocecalis
- p. incudialis
- p. incudis
- p. interarytenoidea
- p. interureterica
- plicae iridis
- p. lacrimalis
- p. longitudinalis duodeni
- p. mallearis anterior membranae tympanicae
- p. mallearis anterior tunicae mucosae cavitatis tympanicae

plica *(continued)*
- p. mallearis posterior membranae tympanicae
- p. mallearis posterior tunicae mucosae cavitatis tympanicae
- plicae mucosae vesicae biliaris
- plicae mucosae vesicae felleae
- p. nervi laryngei superior
- plicae palmatae
- p. palpebronasalis
- p. paraduodenalis
- p. rectouterina
- p. salpingopalatina
- p. salpingopharyngea
- p. semilunaris faucium
- plicae semilunares coli
- p. semilunaris conjunctivae
- p. spiralis
- p. stapedialis
- p. sublingualis
- p. synovialis
- p. synovialis infrapatellaris
- plicae transversae recti
- plicae transversales recti
- plicae tubariae tubae uterinae
- p. triangularis
- plicae tubales tubae uterinae
- p. umbilicalis lateralis
- p. umbilicalis medialis
- p. umbilicalis mediana
- p. venae cavae sinistrae
- p. vesicalis transversa
- p. vestibularis
- plicae villosae gastris
- p. vocalis

plicae (plural of plica)

plicamycin

plicate

Plimmer's bodies

plot
- bull's-eye p.
- polar p.

plug

Plummer-Vinson syndrome

pluriglandular

pluriorificial

plurivisceral

PND
  paroxysmal nocturnal
    dyspnea

pneumarthrogram

pneumarthrography

pneumarthrosis

pneumatization

pneumatized

pneumatocele

pneumatosis
  p. coli
  p. intestinalis

pneumoalveolography

pneumoangiography

pneumoarthrography

pneumocardial

pneumococcal

pneumococcus

pneumoconiosis

Pneumocystis carinii pneumonia

pneumocystography

pneumocystotomography

pneumoderma

pneumoencephalogram

pneumoencephalography

pneumoencephalomyelogram

pneumoencephalomyelography

pneumofasciogram

pneumogastric

pneumogastrography

pneumogram

pneumography
  cerebral p.
  retroperitoneal p.

pneumogynogram

pneumohemothorax

pneumohydrothorax

pneumomediastinum

pneumomediastinogram

pneumomediastinography

pneumomyelography

pneumonectomy

pneumonia
  aspiration p.
  bacterial p.
  cryptococcal p.
  interstitial p.
  Klebsiella p.
  Pneumocystis carinii p.
  segmental p.
  unresolved p.
  varicella p.

pneumonitis
  traumatic p.
  viral p.

pneumonography

pneumoperitoneal

pneumoperitoneum

pneumopreperitoneum

pneumopyelography

pneumorachicentesis

pneumorachis

pneumoradiography

pneumoserosa

pneumosilicosis

pneumothorax
    apicolateral p.
    diagnostic p.
    spontaneous p.
    tension p.
    traumatic p.

pneumotomography

pneumoventriculography

pock

pocketing of barium

pockmark

poculum
    p. Diogenis

podophyllin

podophyllotoxin

podophyllum

poikilocarynosis

poikilocythemia

poikilocytosis

poikiloderma
    p. atrophicans vasculare
    p. of Civatte
    p. vasculare atrophicans

point
    Addison's p.
    p. Ba
    bleeding p.
    Broadbent registration p.
    Cannon's p.
    Desjardins' p.
    Hallé's p.
    Kienböck-Adamson p's
    Méglin's p.
    metopic p.
    nasal p.
    p. R
    p. SO

pointer
    metallic p.

Poirier's glands

poisoning
    carbon monoxide p.

poison ivy

poison oak

poison sumac

Polaroid films

pole

poli (plural of polus)

poliomyelitis

poliosis

polisography

pollex

polus *pl.* poli
    p. anterior bulbi oculi
    p. anterior lentis
    p. frontalis hemispherii cer-
        ebri
    p. occipitalis hemispherii
        cerebri
    p. posterior bulbi oculi
    p. posterior lentis
    p. temporalis hemispherii
        cerebri

poly

polyadenoma

polyadenomatosis

polyadenous

polyagglutination

polyangiitis

polyarteritis

polyarthritis

polychemotherapy

polychromasia

polychromatia

polychromatocytosis

polychromatophilia

polychromatophilic

polychromatosis

polychromemia

polychromophilia

polycythemia
    absolute p.
    appropriate p.
    benign p.
    compensatory p.
    hypertonic p.
    p. hypertonica
    inappropriate p.
    myelopathic p.
    primary p.
    relative p.
    p. rubra
    p. rubra vera
    relative p., chronic
    secondary p.
    splenomegalic p.
    spurious p.
    stress p.
    p. vera

polyembryoma

polyendocrinoma

polyestradiol phosphate

polyganglionic

polyglandular

polyhidrosis

polyhistiocytoma

polyhydramnios

polyidrosis

polymorph

polymorphocyte

polymorphonuclear

polyneuropathy
    carcinomatous p.
    paraneoplastic p.

polyoma

polyonychia

polyp
    adenomatous p.
    adenomatous p. of the colon
    adenomatous p. of the stomach
    cholesterol p.
    fibroepithelial p.
    gastric p.
    gelatinous p.
    pedunculated p.
    sessile p.

polypeptide
    parathyroid-like p.

polyphyletic

polyphyletism

polyphyletist

polyporous

polyposis
    p. coli
    familial p.
    familial adenomatous p.
    familial p. of the colon
    familial intestinal p.
    gastric p.
    intestinal p.
    multiple familial p.

polysplenia

polytomogram

polytomographic

polytomography

polytrichia

polytrichosis

polyunguia

polyvinyl
    p. alcohol

POMP
    prednisone, oncovin (vincristine), methotrexate, and 6-mercaptopurine

pompholyx

pons *pl.* pontes
    p. et cerebellum

ponticular

ponticulus

Pontocaine

pontocerebellum

pool
    storage p.

pooling of contrast material

poorly
    p. concentrated isotope
    p. defined
    p. marginated
    p. opacified
    p. visualized

poples

poradenia

poradenitis

poral

pore
    dilated p. of Winer
    sweat p.

porencephaly

porfimer sodium

porfiromycin

pori (plural of porus)

porocarcinoma
    eccrine p.

porokeratosis
    disseminated superficial
      actinic p.
    p. of Mibelli
    p. palmaris et plantaris dis-
      seminata

porokeratotic

poroma
    eccrine p.

porphyria

porta *pl.* portae
    p. hepatis
    p. lienis
    p. of spleen

portal

portio *pl.* portiones
    p. supravaginalis cervicis
    p. vaginalis cervicis

portion
    dependent p.
    prostatic p. of the urethra
    tufted p.

portiones (plural of portio)

portogram

portography
    portal p.
    splenic p.

portovenogram

portovenography

porus *pl.* pori
    p. acusticus
    p. acusticus externus
    p. acusticus internus
    p. gustatorius
    p. sudoriferus

position
    Albert's p.
    anatomical p.
    Caldwell's p.
    fetal p.
    Fowler's p.
    frog-leg p.
    Fuchs p.
    left-side-down p.
    lithotomy p.
    Mayer p.
    prone p.
    reclining p.
    recumbent p.
    right-side-down p.
    semiaxial p.
    semierect p.

position *(continued)*
    semisupine p.
    submentovertex p.
    supine p.
    Titterington's p.
    Trendelenburg p.
    verticosubmental p.
    Waters' p.
    Waters' p., reverse

positrocephalogram

positron

postalbumin

postbulbar

postcentral

postcondylare

postcranial

posteriad

posterior

posteroanterior

posteroexternal

posteroinferior

posterointernal

posterolateral

posteromedial

posteromedian

posteroparietal

posterosuperior

posterotemporal

postictal

posticus

postlingual

postmediastinal

postmediastinum

postmortem

postoperative

postsplenic

postural

posture

postsurgical

potassium
    p. 42

potential
    zeta p.

Pott's fracture

Potter
    P. Type IV kidney
    P.-Bucky diaphragm

pouch
    abdominovesical p.
    gastric p.
    Hartmann's p.
    Morison's p.
    perineal p., deep
    perineal p., superficial
    perineal p., subcutaneous
    suprapatellar p.

power
    carbon dioxide-combi-
      ning p.
    CO_2-combining p.

praeputium

pramoxine hydrochloride

preanesthetic

prebase

precancer

precancerous

precarcinomatous

precardium

precentral

precordia

precordial

precordium

precuneus

prednimustine

pregnancy
    ectopic p.
    intrauterine p. (IUP)
    tubal p.
    twin p.

preinvasive

preleukemia

preleukemic

prelimbic

premalignant

premaxilla

premedication

premonocyte

premyeloblast

premyelocyte

preneoplastic

preparation
    sterile p.

preperitoneal

prepuce

preputial

preputium
    p. clitoridis
    p. penis

presentation
    breech p.
    brow p.
    cephalic p.
    face p.
    footling breech p.
    frank breech p.
    shoulder p.

preseptal

prespondylolisthesis

pressure of injection

pressometer
    Jarcho p.

pressure
    blood p.
    diastolic blood p.
    systolic blood p.

presubiculum

presbyesophagus

pretarsal

prethrombotic

Price-Jones curve

prilocaine hydrochloride

Pringle's disease

Priscoline

proaccelerin

proactivator

probe
    localizing p.

procaine
    p. hydrochloride

procarbazine hydrochloride

procarcinogen

procedure
    Bankart p. for shoulder dis-
        location
    Billroth I p.
    Billroth II gastrectomy p.
    Caldwell-Luc p.
    cut-down p.
    fundoplication p.
    gastric pull-through p.
    Le Fort p.
    Nissen fundoplication p.
    pull-through p.
    Roux-en-Y p.
    TIPS (transverse intrahe-
        patic portocaval shunt) p.
    Whipple p.

procephalic

process
- acromion p.
- basilar p.
- coracoid p. of the clavicle
- coronoid p. of the ulna
- falciform p. of fascia lata
- falciform p. of pelvic fascia
- glenoid p.
- infectious p.
- infiltrative p.
- jugular p. of occipital bone, lateral
- jugular p. of occipital bone, middle
- lumbar transverse p.
- occipital p. of occipital bone
- odontoid p.
- olecranon p.
- paracondyloid p. of occipital bone
- paroccipital p. of occipital bone
- paramastoid p. of occipital bone
- pterygoid p.
- radial styloid p.
- spinous p.
- space-consuming p.
- space-occupying p.
- spinous p.
- styloid p.
- transverse p.
- ulnar styloid p.
- uncinate p.
- xiphoid p.

processus
- p. accessorius
- p. anterior mallei
- p. anterior mallei [Folii]
- p. articularis inferior vertebrae
- p. articularis superior ossis sacri
- p. articularis superior vertebrae

processus *(continued)*
- p. axillaris glandulae mammariae
- p. calcaneus ossis cuboidei
- p. caudatus hepatis
- p. ciliares
- p. clinoideus anterior
- p. clinoideus medius
- p. clinoideus posterior
- p. cochleariformis
- p. coracoideus scapulae
- p. coronoideus ulnae
- p. costalis vertebrae
- p. costiformis
- p. ethmoidalis conchae nasalis inferioris
- p. falciformis ligamenti sacrotuberalis
- p. frontalis maxillae
- p. frontalis ossis zygomatici
- p. frontosphenoidalis ossis zygomatici
- p. intrajugularis ossis occipitalis
- p. intrajugularis ossis temporalis
- p. jugularis ossis occipitalis
- p. lacrimalis conchae nasalis inferioris
- p. lateralis cartilaginis septi nasi
- p. lateralis glandulae mammariae
- p. lateralis mallei
- p. lateralis tali
- p. lateralis tuberis calcanei
- p. lenticularis incudis
- p. mammillaris
- p. mastoideus ossis temporalis
- p. maxillaris conchae nasalis inferioris
- p. medialis tuberis calcanei
- p. muscularis cartilaginis arytenoideae
- p. orbitalis ossis palatini

processus *(continued)*
  p. palatinus maxillae
  p. papillaris hepatis
  p. paramastoideus ossis occipitalis
  p. posterior cartilaginis septi nasi
  p. posterior tali
  p. pterygoideus ossis sphenoidalis
  p. pterygospinosus
  p. pterygospinosus [Civinini]
  p. pyramidalis ossis palatini
  p. sphenoidalis cartilaginis septi nasi
  p. sphenoidalis ossis palatini
  p. spinosus vertebrae
  p. styloideus ossis metacarpalis III
  p. styloideus ossis metacarpi III
  p. styloideus ossis temporalis
  p. styloideus radii
  p. styloideus ulnae
  p. supracondylaris humeri
  p. supracondyloideus humeri
  p. temporalis ossis zygomatici
  p. transversus vertebrae
  p. uncinatus ossis ethmoidalis
  p. uncinatus pancreatis
  p. vaginalis ossis sphenoidalis
  p. vocalis
  p. xiphoideus
  p. zygomaticus maxillae
  p. zygomaticus ossis frontalis
  p. zygomaticus ossis temporalis
procoagulant

proconvertin

proctitis

proctography

proctoscopy

procumbent

product
  contact activation p.
  decay p.
  fibrin degradation p's
  fibrin split p's
  fibrinogen degradation p's
  fission p.
  spallation p's

proerythroblast

proerythrocyte

profibrinolysin

Profichet's syndrome

profile
  biophysical p.

profondometer

profundus

proglossis

prognosis

progonoma
  melanotic p.

progranulocyte

ProHance

projection
  anteroposterior (AP) p.
  axial p.
  axillary p.
  brow-down p.
  brow-up p.
  Caldwell's p.
  carpal tunnel p.
  cross-table p.
  Didiée's p.
  dorsoplantar p.
  frog-leg p.

projection *(continued)*
    frontal p.
    half-axial p.
    Heinig's p.
    Hermodsson's p.
    Hughston's p.
    inferosuperior p.
    lateral p.
    Laurin's p.
    Merchant's p.
    mortise p.
    notch p.
    oblique p.
    open-mouth p.
    pillar p.
    posteroanterior (PA) p.
    radiographic p.
    Schüller's p.
    semiaxial p.
    Settegast's p.
    Stenvers p.
    stress p.
    Stryker's notch p.
    submentovertex p.
    sunrise p.
    swimmer's p.
    tangential p.
    Towne's p.
    tunnel p.
    verticosubmental p.
    Waters' p.
    West Point p.

Prokine

prolactinoma

prolapse
    p. of gastric mucosa
    uterine p.

Proleukin

proleukocyte

proliferation

promegakaryocyte

prominence

prominentia *pl.* prominentiae
    p. canalis facialis

prominentia *(continued)*
    p. canalis semicircularis
      lateralis
    p. laryngea
    p. mallearis membranae
      tympanicae
    p. mallearis membranae
      tympani
    p. malleolaris membranae
      tympani
    p. spiralis
    p. styloidea

prominentiae (plural of prominentia)

promonocyte

promontorium *pl.* promontoria
    p. ossis sacri
    p. tympani

promontory
    sacral p.

promoter

promotion

promyelocyte

pronate

pronation

prone

pronormoblast

propanidid

proparacaine hydrochloride

2-propenenitrile

properitoneal

proplasmin

propofol

proportion
    aneurysmal p's

propoxycaine hydrochloride

proptosis

propyliodone

prorsad

prorubricyte

prosection

prosector

prosencephalon

prostata

prostatography

prosthesis *pl.* prostheses
   Angelchik antireflux p.
   aortic valve p.
   Aufranc-Turner p.
   Austin Moore hip p.
   ball and socket p.
   Charnley-Mueller p.
   Christensen temporoman-
      dibular joint p.
   hip p.
   mammary p's
   mitral valve p.
   Moore p.
   Neer p.
   PCA (porous-coated ana-
      tomic) p.
   penile p.
   Swanson p.
   valve p.
   valvular p.

prosthetic

protein
   Bence Jones p.
   p. C
   parathyroid hormone–li-
      ke p.
   parathyroid hormone–rela-
      ted p.
   plasma p's
   p. S
   S-100 p.
   serum p's

proteinemia
   Bence Jones p.

proteinuria
   Bence Jones p.

prothrombin

prothrombinase

prothrombinogenic

prothrombinopenia

protoheme

protohemin

proton

proto-oncogene

protrusio acetabuli

protrusion
   disc p., disk p.

protuberance
   occipital p.
   occipital p., transverse
   occipital p., external
   occipital p., internal

protuberantia
   p. occipitalis externa
   p. occipitalis interna

prourokinase

Prower factor

proximad

proximal

proximalis

proximate

pruriginous

prurigo
   p. agria
   Besnier's p.
   p. of Besnier
   p. chronica multiformis
   p. estivalis
   p. ferox
   p. of Hebra
   melanotic p.
   p. mitis
   nodular p.

prurigo *(continued)*
    p. simplex
    summer p. of Hutchinson

pruritic

pruritogenic

pruritus
    p. ani
    p. hiemalis
    senile p.
    p. senilis
    aquagenic p.

psammocarcinoma

psammoma

psammomatous

pseudoacanthosis
    p. nigricans

pseudoagglutination

pseudoaneurysm

pseudoarthrosis

pseudoarticulation

pseudoatrophoderma colli

pseudobacillus

pseudochromidrosis

pseudocoarctation
    p. of the aorta

pseudocyst
    pterygomandibular p.

pseudodiverticulum

pseudoeosinophil

pseudofolliculitis

pseudofracture

pseudogout

pseudohemagglutination

pseudohemophilia

pseudoleukemia

pseudolymphoma
    Spiegler-Fendt p.

pseudomalignancy

pseudomelanoma

pseudomonilethrix

pseudo-obstruction

pseudoparalysis

pseudopelade

pseudopolycythemia

pseudopolyp

pseudorosette

pseudosarcoma

pseudosarcomatous

pseudotumor

pseudovacuole

psicofuranine

psoralen

psoas abscess
    psoas muscle
    psoas shadows
    psoas stripe

psoriasiform

psoriasis
    annular p.
    p. annularis
    p. annulata
    arthritic p.
    p. arthropathica
    p. arthopica
    Barber's p.
    circinate p.
    p. circinata
    discoid p.
    p. discoidea
    erythrodermic p.
    exfoliative p.
    p. figurata
    figurate p.
    flexural p.
    follicular p.
    p. guttata

psoriasis *(continued)*
    guttate p.
    p. gyrata
    gyrate p.
    inverse p.
    p. inveterata
    nummular p.
    p. nummularis
    p. ostracea
    ostraceous p.
    palmar p.
    p. of palms and soles
    pustular p., generalized
    pustular p., localized
    p. rupioides
    seborrheic p.
    volar p.
    von Zumbusch's p.
    p. vulgaris
    Zumbusch's p.

psoriatic

psychocutaneous

pterion

pterygoid

pterygomaxillary

ptosis

ptotic

ptyalography

puberty
    precocious p.

pubes

pubic

pubis

puboprostatic

puborectal

puborectalis

pubovesical

pudendum
    p. femininum

pulmo
    p. dexter
    p. sinister

pulmogram

Pulmolite

pulmonary consolidation

pulmonohepatic

pulmonoperitoneal

pulp
    red p.
    p. of spleen
    splenic p.
    white p.

pulpa
    p. lienalis
    p. splenica

pulpal

pulsate

pulsation
    myocardial p's

pulvinar
    p. thalami

pulvinate

pulse
    dorsalis pedis p.
    foot p's
    pedal p's
    p. generator
    thready p.

pulsus
    p. parvus et tardus

punched-out
    p.-o. areas
    p.-o. bony defects

puncta (plural of punctum)

punctate

punctograph

punctum *pl.* puncta
    p. lacrimale

puncture
lumbar p.
percutaneous p.

pupilla

Purinethol

puromycin

purpura
allergic p.
anaphylactoid p.
p. annularis telangiectodes
fibrinolytic p.
p. fibrinolytica
p. fulminans
p. hemorrhagica
Henoch's p.
Henoch-Schönlein p.
idiopathic p.
idiopathic thrombocyto-
penic p.
itching p.
Majocchi's p.
p. nervosa
p. of newborn
nonthrombocytopenic p.
palpable p.
psychogenic p.
p. rheumatica
Schönlein p.
Schönlein-Henoch p.
p. senilis
p. simplex
steroid p.
thrombocytopenic p.
thrombocytopenic p., idiopathic
thrombocytopenic p., sec-
ondary
thrombocytopenic p.,
thrombotic
thrombopenic p.
thrombocytopenic p., pri-
mary

purpuric

purulent

pus
frank p.

pustula

pustular

pustulation

pustule
multilocular p.
simple p.
spongiform p.
spongiform p. of Kogoj
unilocular p.

pustulosis
p. palmaris et plantaris
palmoplantar p.
p. vacciniformis acuta
p. varioliformis acuta

putamen

pyarthrosis

pyelectasis

pyelitis
p. cystica

pyelocaliectasis

pyelogram
dragon p.
excretory p.
intravenous p. (IVP)
retrograde p.

pyelograph

pyelography
air p.
antegrade p.
ascending p.
p. by elimination
excretion p.
intravenous p.
lateral p.
respiration p.
retrograde p.
wash-out p.

pyelonephritis

pyeloplasty

pyeloscopy

pyeloureterography

pygal

pyknocytosis

pyknotic

pyloroplasty

pylorospasm

pylorus *pl.* pylori

pyoderma
chancriform p.
p. chancriforme faciei
p. faciale
p. gangrenosum
malignant p.
p. vegetans

pyodermia

pyomyoma

pyopneumothorax

pyorrhea

pyosepsis

pyoureter

PYP
pyrophosphate
PYP myocardial scan

pyramid
petrous p's
renal p's

pyramidal

pyramidalis

pyramis *pl.* pyramides
p. bulbi
p. medullae oblongatae
pyramides renales
p. vermis
p. vestibuli
pyramides renales [Mal-
pighii]

pyrethrum

Pyribenzamine

pyroglobulinemia

Pyrolite

pyropoikilocytosis
hereditary p.

pyuria

Q

quadrant

quadrantal

quadrate

quadratus

quadriceps

quadrigeminal

quadrigeminus

quadrilocular

quadripartite

quadriplegia

quadriplegic

quadrisect

quadrisection

quadritubercular

quality

quantimeter

quantitative

quartisect

quenching

Quénu's hemorrhoidal plexus

Queyrat
    erythroplasia of Q.

Quincke's disease

quinolinic acid

quinquetubercular

Quotane

rachidial

rachitic

rad

radiability

radiable

radiad

radialis

radiate

radiatio *pl.* radiationes
    r. acustica
    r. corporis callosi
    r. optica
    r. thalami anterior
    r. thalami centralis
    r. thalami posterior
    r. thalami inferior

radiation
    α-r.
    alpha r.
    annihilation r.
    background r.
    β-r.
    beta r.
    braking r.
    Cerenkov r.
    corpuscular r's
    γ-r.
    gamma r.
    heterogeneous r.
    homogeneous r.
    interstitial r.
    ionizing r.
    monochromatic r.
    monoenergetic r.
    white r.

radices (plural of radix)

radiciform

radicle
    biliary r's
    intrahepatic r's

radicula

radicular

radiculography

radiculopathy

radii (plural of radius)

radioactive

radioactivity
    artificial r.
    induced r.

radioautogram

radioautograph

radioautography

radiobiological

radiobiologist

radiobiology

radiocalcium

radiocarbon

radiocarcinogenesis

radiocardiogram

radiocardiography

radiochemistry

radiochemotherapy

radiochroism

radiocolloid

radiocurable

radiode

radiodense

radiodensity

radiodermatitis

radiodiagnosis

radiodiagnostics

radioencephalogram

radioencephalography

radioepidermitis

radioepithelitis

radiogold

radiogram

radiograph
    conventional r's
    lateral skull r.
    maxillary sinus r.
    Waters' projection r.
    Waters' view r.

radiographic

radiographically

radiography
    body section r.
    digital r.
    double-contrast r.
    electron r.
    mucosal relief r.
    neutron r.
    serial r.
    spot-film r.

radioimmunity

radioimmunodetection

radioimmunoimaging

radioimmunoscintigraphy

radioiodine

radioiron

radioisotope
    carrier-free r.

radiolabel

radiolabeled

radiolesion

radiologic, radiological

radiologist

radiology
    interventional r.
    nuclear r.

radiolucency
    relative r.

radiolucent

radiomimetic

radiomuscular

radionecrosis

radionitrogen

radionuclide

radio-opacity

radiopacity

radiopaque

radioparency

radioparent

radiopharmaceutical

radiopharmacy

radiophosphorus

radiophotography

radiophylaxis

radiophysics

radiopotassium

radiopotentiation

radioprotectant

radioprotector

radioreaction

radioreceptor

radioresistance

radioresistant

radioscopy

radiosensibility

radiosensitive

radiosensitiveness

radiosensitivity

radiosensitizer

radiosodium

radiostereoscopy

radiostrontium

radiosulfur

radiosurgery
stereotactic r.
stereotaxic r.

radiotherapeutics

radiotherapist

radiotherapy
extended field r.
external beam r.
hemibody r.
high-voltage r.
hyperfractionated r.
interstitial r.
intracavitary r.
inverted Y field r.
involved field r.
mantle field r.
megavoltage r.
neoadjuvant r.
orthovoltage r.
preoperative r.
supervoltage r.

radiotomy

radiotracer

radiotransparency

radiotransparent

radiotropic

radioulnar

radium

radius *pl.* radii
r. fixus
radii lentis
radii medullares
r. and ulna

radix *pl.* radices
r. anterior nervi spinalis

radix *(continued)*
r. cranialis nervi accessorii
r. inferior ansae cervicalis
r. intermedia ganglii pterygopalatini
r. lateralis nervi mediani
r. lateralis tractus optici
r. linguae
r. medialis nervi mediani
r. medialis tractus optici
r. mesenterii
r. motoria nervi spinalis
r. motoria nervi trigemini
r. nasalis
r. nasi
r. nasociliaris ganglii ciliaris
r. oculomotoria ganglii ciliaris
r. parasympathica ganglii
ciliaris
r. parasympathica ganglii
otici
r. parasympathica ganglii
pterygopalatini
r. parasympathica ganglii
sublingualis
r. parasympathica ganglii
submandibularis
r. parasympathica gan-
gliorum pelvicorum
r. penis
r. pili
radices plexus brachialis
r. posterior nervi spinalis
r. pulmonis
r. sensoria ganglii ciliaris
r. sensoria ganglii otici
r. sensoria ganglii pterygopalatini
r. sensoria ganglii submandibularis
r. sensoria nervi spinalis
r. sensoria nervi trigemini
r. spinalis nervi accessorii
r. superior ansae cervicalis
r. sympathica ganglii ciliaris

radix *(continued)*
    r. sympathica ganglii ptery-
        gopalatini
    r. unguis

radon

RAI
        radioactive iodine
            RAI uptake

rale
        r's in the lungs

ramal

rami (plural of ramus)

ramification

ramify

Ramirez
        ashy dermatosis of R.

ramose

ramulus

ramus *pl.* rami
    r. accessorius arteriae men-
        ingeae mediae
    r. acetabularis arteriae cir-
        cumflexae femoris medi-
        alis
    r. acetabularis arteriae ob-
        turatoriae
    r. acromialis arteriae su-
        prascapularis
    r. acromialis arteriae thora-
        coacromialis
    rami alveolares superiores
        anteriores nervi maxillaris
    r. alveolaris superior med-
        ius nervi maxillaris
    rami alveolares superiores
        posteriores nervi maxil-
        laris
    r. anastomoticus arteriae
        lacrimalis cum arteria
        meningea media
    r. anastomoticus arteriae
        meningeae mediae cum
        arteria lacrimali

ramus *(continued)*
    r. anterior arteriae obtura-
        toriae
    r. anterior arteriae pancre-
        aticoduodenalis inferioris
    r. anterior arteriae recur-
        rentis ulnaris
    r. anterior arteriae renalis
    r. anterior ductus hepatici
        dextri
    r. anterior nervi auricularis
        magni
    rami anteriores nervorum
        cervicalium
    r. anterior nervi coccygei
    r. anterior nervi cutanei an-
        tebrachii medialis
    rami anteriores nervorum
        lumbalium
    r. anterior nervi obturatorii
    rami anteriores nervorum
        sacralium
    r. anterior nervi spinalis
    rami anteriores nervorum
        thoracicorum
    r. anterior sulci lateralis
        cerebri
    r. anterior venae pulmon-
        alis dextrae superioris
    r. anterior venae pulmon-
        alis sinistrae superioris
    r. apicalis arteriae pulmon-
        alis dextrae
    r. apicalis arteriae pulmon-
        alis sinistrae
    r. apicalis venae pulmon-
        alis dextrae superioris
    r. apicoposterior venae pul-
        monalis sinistrae superi-
        oris
    r. articularis
    rami articulares arteriae
        descendentis genicularis
    r. ascendens arteriae cir-
        cumflexae femoris latera-
        lis
    r. ascendens arteriae cir-
        cumflexae femoris medi-
        alis

ramus *(continued)*
- r. ascendens arteriae circumflexae ilium profundae
- r. ascendens arteriae segmentalis anterioris pulmonis dextri
- r. ascendens arteriae segmentalis anterioris pulmonis sinistri
- r. ascendens arteriae segmentalis posterioris pulmonis dextri
- r. ascendens arteriae segmentalis posterioris pulmonis sinistri
- r. ascendens rami superficialis arteriae transversae colli
- r. ascendens sulci lateralis cerebri
- r. atrialis anastomoticus rami circumflexi arteriae coronariae sinistrae
- rami atriales arteriae coronariae dextrae
- rami atriales rami circumflexi arteriae coronariae sinistrae
- r. atrialis intermedius arteriae coronariae dextrae
- r. atrialis intermedius rami circumflexi arteriae coronariae sinistri
- rami atrioventriculares rami circumflexi arteriae coronariae sinistrae
- rami auriculares anteriores arteriae temporalis superficialis
- r. auricularis arteriae auricularis posterioris
- r. auricularis arteriae occipitalis
- r. auricularis nervi vagi
- r. autonomicus
- r. basalis anterior venae basalis communis

ramus *(continued)*
- r. basalis tentorii arteriae carotidis internae
- rami bronchiales arteriae thoracicae internae
- rami bronchiales nervi vagi
- rami bronchiales partis thoracicae aortae
- rami buccales nervi facialis
- rami calcanei laterales nervi suralis
- rami calcanei mediales nervi tibialis
- rami calcanei ramorum malleolarium lateralium arteriae fibularis
- rami calcanei ramorum malleolarium lateralium arteriae peroneae
- rami calcanei arteriae tibialis posterioris
- r. calcarinus arteriae occipitalis medialis
- rami capsulae internae
- rami capsulares arteriae renalis
- rami cardiaci cervicales inferiores nervi vagi
- rami cardiaci cervicales superiores nervi vagi
- rami cardiaci thoracici
- rami cardiaci thoracici nervi vagi
- r. carpalis dorsalis arteriae radialis
- r. carpalis dorsalis arteriae ulnaris
- r. carpalis palmaris arteriae radialis
- r. carpalis palmaris arteriae ulnaris
- rami caudae nuclei caudati arteriae choroideae anterioris
- r. cervicalis nervi facialis
- r. chiasmaticus arteriae communicantis posterioris

ramus *(continued)*
rami choroidei posteriores
mediales arteriae cerebri
posterioris
rami choroidei posteriores
laterales arteriae cerebri
posterioris
rami choroidei ventriculi
lateralis
r. choroideus ventriculi
quarti arteriae inferioris
posterioris cerebelli
rami choroidei ventriculi
tertii
r. cingularis arteriae callosomarginalis
r. circumflexus arteriae coronariae sinistrae
r. circumflexus fibularis arteriae tibialis posterioris
r. circumflexus peronealis
arteriae tibialis poster-
ioris
r. clavicularis arteriae thoracoacromialis
rami clivales
r. cochlearis arteriae labyrinthinae
r. cochlearis arteriae vestibulocochlearis
rami coeliaci nervi vagi
r. colicus arteriae ileocolicae
r. collateralis arteriarum intercostalium posteriorum
r. colli nervi facialis
r. communicans albus
nervi spinalis
r. communicans arteriae fibularis
r. communicans arteriae
peroneae
r. communicans cochlearis
nervi vestibularis
r. communicans fibularis
nervi fibularis communis
r. communicans nervi glossopharyngei cum chorda
tympani

ramus *(continued)*
r. communicans nervi glossopharyngei cum nervo
auriculotemporali
r. communicans nervi glossopharyngei ramo menin-
geo nervi vagi
r. communicans griseus
nervi spinalis
rami communicantes nervi
auriculotemporalis cum
nervo faciali
r. communicans nervi facialis cum nervo glosso-
pharyngeo
r. communicans nervi glossopharyngei cum ramo
auriculari nervi vagi
r. communicans nervi intermedii cum nervo vago
r. communicans nervi intermedii cum plexu tympan-
ico
r. communicans nervi lacrimalis cum nervo zygoma-
tico
rami communicantes nervi
lingualis cum nervo hy-
poglosso
r. communicans nervi me-
diani cum nervo ulnari
r. communicans nervi nasociliaris cum ganglio ciliari
rami communicantes ner-
vorum spinalium
r. communicans nervi vagi
cum nervo glossopharyn-
geo
r. communicans peroneus
nervi peronei communis
r. communicans ulnaris
nervi radialis
r. coni arteriosi arteriae coronariae dextrae
r. coni arteriosi arteriae coronariae sinistrae
rami corporis amygdaloidei

ramus *(continued)*

    r. corporis callosi dorsalis arteriae occipitalis medialis

    rami corporis geniculati lateralis

    r. costalis lateralis arteriae thoracicae internae

    r. cricothyroideus arteriae thyroideae superioris

    r. cutaneus

    rami cutanei anteriores nervi femoralis

    r. cutaneus anterior nervi iliohypogastrici

    r. cutaneus anterior abdominalis nervi intercostalis

    r. cutaneus anterior pectoralis nervi intercostalis

    rami cutanei cruris mediales nervi sapheni

    r. cutaneus lateralis arteriarum intercostalium posteriorum

    r. cutaneus lateralis nervi iliohypogastrici

    r. cutaneus lateralis abdominalis nervi intercostalis

    r. cutaneus lateralis pectoralis nervi intercostalis

    r. cutaneus lateralis rami dorsalis arteriarum intercostalium posteriorum

    r. cutaneus medialis rami dorsalis arteriarum intercostalium posteriorum

    r. cutaneus nervi obturatorii

    r. cutaneus posterior rami posterioris nervi thoracici

    r. deltoideus arteriae profundae brachii

    r. deltoideus arteriae thoracoacromialis

    rami dentales arteriae alveolaris inferioris

ramus *(continued)*

    rami dentales arteriarum alveolarium superiorum anteriorum

    rami dentales arteriae alveolaris superioris posterioris

    rami dentales inferiores plexus dentalis inferioris

    rami dentales superiores plexus dentalis superioris

    r. descendens arteriae circumflexae femoris lateralis

    r. descendens arteriae occipitalis

    r. descendens arteriae segmentalis anterioris pulmonis dextri

    r. descendens arteriae segmentalis anterioris pulmonis sinistri

    r. descendens arteriae segmentalis posterioris pulmonis dextri

    r. descendens arteriae segmentalis posterioris pulmonis sinistri

    r. descendens rami superficialis arteriae transversae colli

    r. dexter arteriae hepaticae propriae

    r. dexter venae portae hepatis

    r. digastricus nervi facialis

    r. diploicus arteriae supraorbitalis

    r. dorsalis arteriarum intercostalium posteriorum

    rami dorsales arteriae intercostalis supremae

    r. dorsalis arteriarum lumbalium

    r. dorsalis arteriae subcostalis

    rami dorsales linguae arteriae lingualis

ramus *(continued)*
r. dorsalis nervi coccygei
rami dorsales nervorum lumbalium
rami dorsales nervorum sacralium
rami dorsales nervorum thoracicorum
r. dorsalis nervi ulnaris
r. dorsalis venae intercostalis posterioris
rami duodenales arteriae pancreaticoduodenalis superioris anterioris
rami duodenales arteriae pancreaticoduodenalis superioris posterioris
rami epididymales arteriae testicularis
r. externus nervi accessorii
r. externus nervi laryngei superioris
r. femoralis nervi genitofemoralis
r. frontalis anteromedialis arteriae callosomarginalis
r. frontalis arteriae meningeae mediae
r. frontalis arteriae temporalis superficialis
r. frontalis posteromedialis arteriae callosomarginalis
rami ganglionares nervi lingualis ad ganglion submandibulare
rami ganglionares nervi mandibularis ad ganglion oticum
rami ganglionares nervi maxillaris ad ganglion pterygopalatinum
rami ganglionares trigeminales
rami ganglionares trigemini
rami gastrici anteriores trunci vagalis anterioris
rami gastrici arteriae gastroomentalis dextrae

ramus *(continued)*
rami gastrici arteriae gastroomentalis sinistrae
rami gastrici posteriores trunci vagalis posterioris
r. genitalis nervi genitofemoralis
rami gingivales inferiores plexus dentalis inferioris
rami gingivales nervi mentalis
rami gingivales superiores plexus dentalis superioris
r. glandularis anterior arteriae thyroideae superioris
rami glandulares arteriae facialis
rami glandulares arteriae maxillaris externae
r. glandularis lateralis arteriae thyroideae superioris
r. glandularis posterior arteriae thyroideae superioris
rami globi pallidi
rami helicini arteriae uterinae
rami hepatici trunci vagalis anterioris
r. hypothalamicus arteriae communicantis posterioris
r. ilealis arteriae ileocolicae
r. iliacus arteriae iliolumbalis
inferior r.
r. inferior rami profundi arteriae gluteae superioris
r. inferior nervi oculomotorii
rami inferiores nervi transversi colli
r. inferior ossis pubis
r. infrahyoideus arteriae thyroideae superioris
r. infrapatellaris nervi sapheni

ramus *(continued)*
>rami inguinales arteriae pu-
dendae externae profun-
dae
>
>rami intercostales ante-
riores arteriae thoracicae
internae
>
>rami interganglionares
trunci sympathici
>
>r. internus nervi accessorii
>
>r. internus nervi laryngei
superioris
>
>r. interventricularis ante-
rior arteriae coronariae
sinistrae
>
>r. interventricularis poste-
rior arteriae coronariae
dextrae
>
>rami interventriculares sep-
tales arteriae coronariae
sinistrae
>
>rami interventriculares sep-
tales arteriae coronariae
dextrae
>
>ischiopubic r.
>
>r. ischiopubicus
>
>rami isthmi faucium nervi
lingualis
>
>rami intercostales arteriae
mammariae internae
>
>rami labiales anteriores ar-
teriae pudendae externae
profundae
>
>rami labiales nervi mentalis
>
>rami labiales posteriores
arteriae pudendae inter-
nae
>
>rami labiales superiores
nervi infraorbitalis
>
>rami laryngopharyngei gan-
glii cervicalis superioris
>
>r. lateralis ductus hepatici
sinistri
>
>r. lateralis interventricu-
laris anterioris arteriae
coronariae sinistrae
>
>r. lateralis nasi arteriae fa-
cialis

ramus *(continued)*
>r. lateralis nervi supraorbi-
talis
>
>r. lateralis rami posterioris
nervi cervicalis
>
>r. lateralis rami posterioris
nervi lumbalis
>
>r. lateralis rami posterioris
nervi sacralis
>
>r. lateralis rami posterioris
nervi thoracici
>
>rami lienales arteriae lien-
alis
>
>r. lingualis nervi facialis
>
>rami linguales nervi glosso-
pharyngei
>
>rami linguales nervi hypo-
glossi
>
>rami linguales nervi lin-
gualis
>
>r. lingularis venae pulmon-
alis sinistrae superioris
>
>rami lobi caudati partis
transversae venae portae
hepatis
>
>r. lobi medii venae pulmon-
alis dextrae superioris
>
>r. lumbalis arteriae iliolum-
balis
>
>rami malleolares laterales
arteriae fibularis
>
>rami malleolares laterales
arteriae peroneae
>
>rami malleolares mediales
arteriae tibiales poster-
ioris
>
>rami mammarii laterales ar-
teriae thoracicae lateralis
>
>rami mammarii laterales
rami cutanei lateralis arteriarum intercostalium
posteriorium
>
>rami mammarii laterales
rami cutanei lateralis pectoralis nervi intercostalis
>
>rami mammarii mediales
rami perforantium arte-
riae thoracicae internae

ramus *(continued)*

> rami mammarii mediales
> rami cutanei anterioris pectoralis nervi intercostalis
> mandibular r.
> r. marginalis dexter arteriae coronariae dextrae
> r. marginalis mandibularis nervi facialis
> r. marginalis sinister rami circumflexi arteriae coronariae sinistrae
> r. marginalis tentorii arteriae carotidis internae
> rami mastoidei arteriae auricularis posterioris
> r. mastoideus arteriae occipitalis
> rami mediales arteriarum centralium anterolateralium
> r. medialis ductus hepatici sinistri
> r. medialis nervi supraorbitalis
> r. medialis rami posterioris nervi cervicalis
> r. medialis rami posterioris nervi lumbalis
> r. medialis rami posterioris nervi sacralis
> r. medialis rami posterioris nervi thoracici
> rami mediastinales arteriae thoracicae internae
> rami mediastinales partis thoracicae aortae
> rami medullares laterales arteriae inferioris posterioris cerebelli
> rami medullares mediales arteriae inferioris posterioris cerebelli
> r. membranae tympani nervi auriculotemporalis
> r. meningeus anterior arteriae ethmoidalis anterioris

ramus *(continued)*

> r. meningeus arteriae carotidis internae
> r. meningeus arteriae occipitalis
> rami meningei arteriae vertebralis
> r. meningeus nervi maxillaris
> r. meningeus nervi mandibularis
> r. meningeus nervi spinalis
> r. meningeus nervi vagi
> r. meningeus recurrens arteriae lacrimalis
> r. meningeus recurrens nervi ophthalmici
> r. mentalis arteriae alveolaris inferioris
> rami mentales nervi mentalis
> r. muscularis
> rami musculares arteriae vertebralis
> rami musculares rami externi nervi accessorii
> rami musculares nervi axillaris
> rami musculares nervi femoralis
> rami musculares nervi fibularis profundi
> rami musculares nervi fibularis superficialis
> rami musculares nervorum intercostalium
> rami musculares nervi mediani
> rami musculares nervi musculocutanei
> rami musculares rami anterioris nervi obturatorii
> rami musculares nervi peronei profundi
> rami musculares nervi peronei superficialis
> rami musculares nervi radialis

ramus *(continued)*

rami musculares nervi tibialis

rami musculares nervi ulnaris

rami musculares rami posterioris nervi obturatorii

r. musculi stylopharyngei nervi glossopharyngei

r. mylohyoideus arteriae alveolaris inferioris

rami nasales anteriores laterales arteriae ethmoidalis anterioris

r. nasalis externus nervi ethmoidalis anterioris

rami nasales externi nervi infraorbitalis

rami nasales interni nervi ethmoidalis anterioris

rami nasales interni nervi infraorbitalis

rami nasales interni laterales nervi ethmoidalis anterioris

rami nasales interni mediales nervi ethmoidalis anterioris

rami nasales posteriores inferiores nervi palatini majoris

rami nasales posteriores superiores laterales nervi maxillaris

rami nasales posteriores superiores mediales nervi maxillaris

r. nervi oculomotorii arteriae communicantis posterioris

r. nodi atrioventricularis arteriae coronariae dextrae

r. nodi atrioventricularis rami circumflexi arteriae coronariae sinistrae

r. nodi sinuatrialis arteriae coronariae dextrae

ramus *(continued)*

r. nodi sinuatrialis rami circumflexi arteriae coronariae sinistrae

rami nuclei rubri

rami nucleorum hypothalamicorum

r. obturatorius rami pubici arteriae epigastricae inferioris

r. occipitalis arteriae auricularis posterioris

rami occipitales arteriae occipitalis

r. occipitalis nervi auricularis posterioris

r. occipitotemporalis arteriae occipitalis medialis

r. nervi oculomotorii ad ganglii ciliare

rami oesophageales arteriae gastricae sinistrae

rami oesophageales arteriae thyroideae inferioris

rami oesophageales gangliorum thoracicorum

rami oesophageales partis thoracicae aortae

rami oesophagei nervi laryngei recurrentis

rami omentales arteriae gastroomentalis dextrae

rami omentales arteriae gastroomentalis sinistrae

r. orbitalis arteriae meningeae mediae

rami orbitales ganglii pterygopalatini

rami orbitales nervi maxillaris

r. orbitofrontalis medialis arteriae cerebri anterioris

r. ossis ischii

r. ovaricus arteriae uterinae

r. palmaris nervi mediani

r. palmaris nervi ulnaris

r. palmaris profundus arteriae ulnaris

ramus *(continued)*

r. palmaris superficialis arteriae radialis

rami palpebrales inferiores nervi infraorbitalis

rami palpebrales nervi infratrochlearis

rami pancreatici arteriae lienalis

rami pancreatici arteriae pancreaticoduodenalis superioris anterioris

rami pancreatici arteriae pancreaticoduodenalis superioris posterioris

rami pancreatici arteriae splenicae

r. parietalis arteriae meningeae mediae

r. parietalis arteriae occipitalis medialis

r. parietalis arteriae temporalis superficialis

rami parietooccipitales arteriae cerebri anterioris

r. parietooccipitalis arteriae occipitalis medialis

r. parotideus arteriae auricularis posterioris

r. parotideus arteriae temporalis superficialis

rami parotidei nervi auriculotemporalis

rami parotidei venae facialis

rami pectorales arteriae thoracoacromialis

rami pedunculares arteriae cerebri posterioris

r. perforans arteriae fibularis

rami perforantes arcus palmaris profundus

rami perforantes arteriarum metatarsearum plantarium

rami perforantes arteriae thoracicae internae

ramus *(continued)*

r. pericardiacus nervi phrenici

rami pericardiaci partis thoracicae aortae

rami peridentales arteriae alveolaris inferioris

rami peridentales arteriae alveolaris superioris posterioris

rami perineales nervi cutanei femoris posterioris

r. petrosus arteriae meningeae mediae

r. petrosus superficialis arteriae meningeae mediae

rami pharyngeales arteriae pharyngeae ascendentis

rami pharyngeales arteriae thyroideae inferioris

r. pharyngeus arteriae canalis pterygoidei

rami pharyngei nervi glossopharyngei

rami pharyngei nervi laryngei recurrentis

r. pharyngeus nervi vagi

rami phrenicoabdominales nervi phrenici

r. posterior arteriae obturatoriae

r. posterior arteriae pancreaticoduodenalis inferioris

r. posterior arteriae recurrentis ulnaris

r. posterior arteriae renalis

r. posterior ductus hepatici dextri

r. posterior nervi auricularis magni

rami posteriores nervorum cervicalium

r. posterior nervi coccygei

r. posterior nervi cutanei antebrachii medialis

rami posteriores nervorum lumbalium

ramus *(continued)*
    r. posterior nervi obturatorii
    rami posteriores nervorum sacralium
    r. posterior nervi spinalis
    rami posteriores nervorum thoracicorum
    r. posterior sulci lateralis cerebri
    r. posterior venae pulmonalis dextrae superioris
    r. posterior ventriculi sinistri rami circumflexi arteriae coronariae sinistrae
    r. posterolateralis dexter arteriae coronariae dextrae
    r. profundus arteriae circumflexae femoris medialis
    r. profundus arteriae gluteae superioris
    r. profundus arteriae plantaris medialis
    r. profundus arteriae transversae cervicis
    r. profundus arteriae transversae colli
    r. profundus nervi plantaris lateralis
    r. profundus nervi radialis
    r. profundus nervi ulnaris
    rami prostatici arteriae vesicalis inferioris
    rami pterygoidei arteriae maxillaris
    rami pterygoidei arteriae maxillaris internae
    pubic r.
    r. pubicus arteriae epigastricae inferioris
    r. pubicus arteriae obturatoriae
    rami pulmonales plexus pulmonalis
    rami pulmonales thoracici gangliorum thoracicorum
    r. recurrens nervi spinalis

ramus *(continued)*
    r. renalis nervi splanchnici minoris
    rami renales nervi vagi
    rami sacrales laterales arteriae sacralis medianae
    r. saphenus arteriae descendentis genus
    rami scrotales anteriores arteriae pudendae externae profundae
    rami scrotales posteriores arteriae pudendae internae
    rami septales anteriores arteriae ethmoidalis anterioris
    rami septales posteriores arteriae sphenopalatinae
    r. septi nasi arteriae labialis superioris
    rami renales plexus coeliaci
    r. sinister arteriae hepaticae propriae
    r. sinister venae portae hepatis
    r. sinus carotici nervi glossopharyngei
    r. sinus cavernosi arteriae carotidis internae
    rami spinales arteriae cervicalis ascendentis
    rami spinales arteriarum intercostalium posteriorum
    rami spinales arteriae intercostalis supremae
    r. spinalis arteriarum lumbalium
    rami spinales arteriarum sacralium lateralium
    r. spinalis arteriae subcostalis
    rami spinales arteriae vertebralis
    r. spinalis rami dorsalis arteriarum intercostalium posteriorum

ramus *(continued)*
  r. spinalis arteriae iliolumbalis
  r. spinalis venae intercostalis
  r. spinalis venae intercostalis posterioris
  rami splenici arteriae splenicae
  r. stapedius arteriae auricularis posterioris
  rami sternales arteriae thoracicae internae
  rami sternocleidomastoidei arteriae occipitalis
  r. sternocleidomastoideus arteriae thyroideae superioris
  r. stylohyoideus nervi facialis
  rami subendocardiales
  rami subscapulares arteriae axillaris
  rami substantiae nigrae
  rami substantiae perforatae anterioris
  r. superficialis arteriae circumflexae femoris medialis
  r. superficialis arteriae gluteae superioris
  r. superficialis arteriae plantaris medialis
  r. superficialis arteriae transversae cervicis
  r. superficialis arteriae transversae colli
  r. superficialis nervi plantaris lateralis
  r. superficialis nervi radialis
  r. superficialis nervi ulnaris superior r.
  r. superior rami profundi arteriae gluteae superioris
  r. superior nervi oculomotorii

ramus *(continued)*
  rami superiores nervi transversi colli
  r. superior ossis pubis
  r. superior venae pulmonalis dextrae inferioris
  r. superior venae pulmonalis sinistrae inferioris
  r. suprahyoideus arteriae lingualis
  rami temporales anteriores arteriae occipitalis lateralis
  rami temporales intermedii mediales arteriae occipitalis lateralis
  rami temporales nervi facialis
  rami temporales posteriores arteriae occipitalis lateralis
  rami temporales superficiales nervi auriculotemporalis
  r. tentorii nervi ophthalmici
  rami thymici arteriae thoracicae internae
  r. thyrohyoideus ansae cervicalis
  r. tonsillae cerebelli arteriae inferioris posterioris cerebelli
  r. tonsillaris arteriae facialis
  r. tonsillaris arteriae maxillaris externi
  rami tonsillares nervi glossopharyngei
  rami tonsillares nervorum palatinorum minorum
  rami tracheales arteriae thoracicae internae
  rami tracheales arteriae thyroideae inferioris
  rami tracheales nervi laryngei recurrentis

ramus *(continued)*
> rami tracheales nervi recurrentis
> rami tractus optici
> r. transversus arteriae circumflexae femoris lateralis
> r. tubalis plexus tympanici
> rami tubarii arteriae ovaricae
> r. tubarius arteriae uterinae
> r. tubarius plexus tympanici
> rami tuberis cinerei
> rami ureterici arteriae ductus deferentis
> rami ureterici arteriae ovaricae
> rami ureterici arteriae renalis
> rami ureterici arteriae testicularis
> rami vaginales arteriae rectalis mediae
> rami vaginales arteriae uterinae
> rami ventrales nervorum cervicalium
> r. ventralis nervi coccygei
> rami ventrales nervorum thoracicorum
> rami vestibulares arteriae labyrinthinae
> rami zygomatici nervi facialis
> r. zygomaticofacialis nervi zygomatici
> r. zygomaticotemporalis nervi zygomatici

range of motion
> passive r. o. m.

ranine

Ranke's angle

raphae

raphe
> abdominal r.
> r. anococcygea

raphe *(continued)*
> anococcygeal r.
> median r.
> r. medullae oblongatae
> r. palati
> r. penis
> r. perinealis
> r. perinei
> r. pharyngis
> r. pontis
> r. pterygomandibularis
> r. scroti

Rappaport Classification

rarefaction

rash
> brown-tail r.
> butterfly r.
> drug r.
> papular r.

rate
> count r.
> erythrocyte sedimentation r.
> output exposure r.
> Westergren sedimentation r.

Rathke
> R's cleft cysts
> R's cysts
> R's pouch tumor
> R's tumor

ratio
> cardiothoracic r. (CTR)
> grid r.
> target-to-nontarget r.
> zeta sedimentation r.

ray
> α-r's
> alpha r's
> anode r's
> β-r's
> beta r's
> cathode r's
> central r.

ray *(continued)*
  characteristic r's
  characteristic fluorescent
    r's
  δ-r's
  delta r's
  direct r.
  fluorescent r's
  γ-r's
  gamma r's
  glass r's
  grenz r's
  hard r's
  indirect r's
  infra roentgen r's
  positive r's
  primary r's
  roentgen r's
  Sagnac r's
  scattered r's
  secondary r's
  soft r's
  x-r's

Raynaud's phenomenon

reaction
  allergic r.
  anaphylactic r.
  chromaffin r.
  erythrocyte sedimenta-
    tion r.
  id r.
  leukemic r.
  leukemoid r.
  periosteal r.
  peroxidase r.
  urticarial r.
  vagovagal r.
  vasovagal r.

reagent
  splenic r.

REAL Classification (of lymphomas)

real-time

recanalization

receptaculum *pl.* receptacula
  r. chyli

receptaculum *(continued)*
  r. ganglii petrosi
  r. Pecqueti

receptor
  estrogen r.

recess
  aorticomediastinal r.
  azygoesophageal r.
  azygomediastinal r.
  lateral reflex

recessus
  r. anterior membranae tym-
    panicae
  r. cochlearis vestibuli
  r. costodiaphragmaticus
    pleuralis
  r. costomediastinalis pleur-
    alis
  r. duodenalis inferior
  r. duodenalis superior
  r. duodenojejunalis
  r. ellipticus vestibuli
  r. epitympanicus
  r. hepatorenalis
  r. ileocaecalis inferior
  r. ileocaecalis superior
  r. inferior bursae omentalis
  r. infundibularis
  r. infundibuli
  r. intersigmoideus
  r. lateralis ventriculi quarti
  r. lienalis
  r. paraduodenalis
  r. pharyngeus
  r. pharyngeus [Rosenmül-
    leri]
  r. phrenicomediastinalis
    pleuralis
  r. pinealis
  r. piriformis
  r. pleurales
  r. posterior membranae
    tympanicae
  r. retrocaecalis
  r. retroduodenalis
  r. sacciformis articulationis
    radioulnaris distalis
  r. saccularis vestibuli

recessus *(continued)*
- r. sphenoethmoidalis
- r. sphericus vestibuli
- r. splenicus
- r. subhepatici
- r. subphrenici
- r. subpopliteus
- r. superior membranae tympanicae
- r. superior bursae omentalis
- r. suprapinealis
- r. supraopticus
- r. utriculi vestibularis
- r. utricularis vestibuli

Recklinghausen
- canals of R.
- R's tumor

reconstruction
- image r. from projections

rectischiac

rectococcygeal

rectococcygeus

rectocutaneous

rectouterine

rectum

rectus

recumbent

recurrent

reduction
- r. and application of plaster
- open r. and internal fixation (ORIF

redundancy

redundant

reduplication

Reed
- R. cells
- R.-Hodgkin disease
- R.-Sternberg cells

reflex
- pilomotor r.

reflux
- r. of barium
- esophageal r.
- r. esophagitis
- gastric r.
- gastroesophageal (GE) r.
- r. into the terminal ileum
- vesicoureteral r.

Regaud's tumor

regimen
- medical r.

regio *pl.* regiones
- regiones abdominales
- r. analis
- r. antebrachialis
- r. antebrachialis anterior
- r. antebrachii anterior
- r. antebrachii posterior
- r. auricularis
- r. axillaris
- r. brachialis
- r. brachialis anterior
- r. brachii anterior
- r. brachii posterior
- r. buccalis
- r. calcanea
- r. carpalis
- r. carpalis anterior
- r. carpalis posterior
- regiones capitis
- regiones cervicales
- r. cervicalis anterior
- r. cervicalis lateralis
- r. cervicalis posterior
- r. colli posterior
- r. coxae
- r. cruris
- r. cruris anterior
- r. cruris posterior
- r. cubitalis
- r. cubitalis anterior
- r. cubitalis posterior
- r. deltoidea

regio *(continued)*
regiones dorsales
r. dorsalis manus
r. dorsalis pedis
regiones dorsi
r. epigastrica
r. facialis
r. femoris
r. femoris anterior
r. femoris posterior
r. frontalis
r. genus
r. genus anterior
r. genus posterior
r. glutealis
r. hypochondriaca
r. hypogastrica
r. inframammaria
r. infraorbitalis
r. infrascapularis
r. infratemporalis
r. inguinalis
r. lateralis
r. lumbalis
r. lumbaris
r. mammaria
r. manus
r. mastoidea
regiones membri inferioris
regiones membri superioris
r. mentalis
r. metacarpalis
r. metatarsalis
r. nasalis
r. occipitalis
r. oralis
r. orbitalis
r. palmaris
r. parietalis
r. parotideomasseterica
r. pectoralis
regiones pectorales
r. pectoralis lateralis
r. pedis
r. perinealis
r. plantaris
regiones pleuropulmonales
r. presternalis

regio *(continued)*
r. pubica
r. retromalleolaris lateralis
r. retromalleolaris medialis
r. sacralis
r. scapularis
r. sternocleidomastoidea
r. surae
r. suralis
r. talocruralis anterior
r. talocruralis posterior
r. tarsalis
r. temporalis
regiones thoracicae ante-
riores et laterales
r. umbilicalis
r. urogenitalis
r. vertebralis
r. zygomatica

region
abdominal r's
anal r.
axillary r.
basilar r.
brachial r.
brachial r., anterior
brachial r., posterior
dorsal r's
epigastric r.
external r.
facial r.
frontal r.
genitourinary r.
gluteal r.
homogeneously staining r's
hypogastric r.
hypothenar r.
iliac r.
infraclavicular r.
inframammary r.
infrascapular r.
infratemporal r.
inguinal r.
intertrochanteric r.
lateral r.
leg r.
lumbar r.
mammary r.

region *(continued)*
    mastoid r.
    occipital r.
    occipitoparietal r.
    oral r.
    parietal r.
    pectoral r.
    pectoral r., lateral
    perineal r.
    pleuropulmonary r's
    precordial r.
    presternal r.
    pubic r.
    r's of back
    sacral r.
    scapular r.
    subauricular r.
    supraclavicular r.
    temporal r.
    umbilical r.
    urogenital r.
    vertebral r.

regional

regiones (plural of region)

regurgitation
    aortic r.

Reiter's syndrome

rem

remifentanil hydrochloride

ren *pl.* renes

renal
    r. and psoas shadows

reniform

renin
    renal vein r's
    renal vein r. assay

reninoma

Reno M drip

renocutaneous

renocystogram

renogastric

Renografin
    R.-60
    R.-76

renogram

renography

renointestinal

renovascular cause for hypertension

Renovist

reoxygenation

rep
    roentgen equivalent physical

replacement
    Marmor knee r.
    prosthetic hip r.
    prosthetic knee r.

replication

report
    pathology r.

reptilase

resection
    abdominoperineal r.
    gastric r.
    subtotal gastric r.
    transurethral r. (TUR)
    wedge r.

reserve
    alkali r.
    alkaline r.

reservoir
    Pecquet's r.

residual
    postvoid r.

resin
    podophyllum r.

resistance
    multidrug r.
    multiple drug r.
    pleiotropic drug r.

resonance
  nuclear magnetic r.

resorption
  bony r.
  periosteal r.
  subarticular bone r.

respiration
  stertorous r's

respirator

respiratory

response
  deconditioned exercise r.
  reticulocyte r.

rest
  aberrant r.
  embryonic r.
  epithelial r.
  fetal r.

resting left ventricular gated
  blood pool scan

restiform

restoration of the lumen

restoration of normal anatomic
  alignment

resuscitation

resupination

rete *pl.* retia
  r. acromiale
  r. arteriosum
  r. articulare cubiti
  r. articulare genus
  r. calcaneum
  r. carpale dorsale
  r. carpi dorsale
  r. lymphocapillare
  r. malleolare laterale
  r. malleolare mediale
  malpighian r.
  r. mirabile
  r. patellare
  r. testis
  r. testis [halleri]

rete *(continued)*
  r. vasculosum articulare
  r. venosum
  r. venosum dorsale manus
  r. venosum dorsale pedis
  r. venosum plantare

retention of urine in the bladder

retia (plural of rete)

retial

reticular

reticulated

reticulation

reticulocyte

reticulocytogenic

reticulocytopenia

reticulocytosis

reticuloendotheliosis
  leukemic r.

reticulohistiocytoma

reticulohistiocytosis
  multicentric r.

reticuloid
  actinic r.

reticulopenia

reticulosis
  familial hemophagocytic r.
  familial histiocytic r.
  histiocytic medullary r.
  lipomelanic r.
  malignant midline r.
  midline malignant r.
  pagetoid r.
  polymorphic r.

reticulum
  reticula lienis
  r. trabeculare

retiform

retina

retinaculum
r. caudale
retinacula cutis
r. flexorum manus
r. musculorum extensorum manus
r. musculorum extensorum inferius pedis
r. musculorum extensorum pedis inferius
r. musculorum extensorum pedis superius
r. musculorum extensorum superius pedis
r. musculorum fibularium inferius
r. musculorum fibularium superius
r. musculorum flexorum manus
r. musculorum flexorum pedis
r. musculorum peroneorum inferius
r. musculorum peroneorum superius
r. patellae laterale
r. patellae mediale
retinacula unguis

retinoblastoma
endophytic r.
r. endophytum
exophytic r.
r. exophytum

retinocytoma

retinoma

retraction
clot r.
mediastinal r.

retractor

retrad

retrocardiac

retrocaval

retrocrural

retrodisplacement

retrolisthesis

retroperitoneal

retroperitoneum

retropulsion

retrospectively

retrosternal

retrosymphysial

retroversion

Retzius space

reversal of the normal lordotic curvature

reverse 3 configuration of the duodenum

Revised European American Lymphoma Classification

Rh
R. antigen
R. blood group
R. factor

Rh_{null}

rhabdomyoblast

rhabdomyoblastic

rhabdomyoblastoma

rhabdomyochondroma

rhabdomyoma

rhabdomyomyxoma

rhabdomyosarcoma
alveolar r.
botryoid r.
embryonal r.
orbital r.
paratesticular r.
pleomorphic r.
r. of prostate

rhabdosarcoma

rhabdosphincter

rhagades

rhagadiform

rhaphe

rhenium
r. 186
r. 188

rheumatid

rhinion

rhinophyma

rhombencephalon

rhomboid
Michaelis' r.

Rhus

rhythm
sinus r.

rhythmeur

rhytid

rib
cervical r.
floating r.

Ribbert's theory

ribbon

Richard's screw

Richet's fascia

Richter
R.'s syndrome
R.-Monro line

rickets
oncogenous r.

rictal

rictus

ridge
alveolar r.
cerebral r's of cranial
bones
dermal r's
petrous r's

ridge *(continued)*
rete r's
semicircular r. of parietal
bone, inferior
semicircular r. of parietal
bone, superior
skin r's
sphenoid r.
superciliary r.
supraorbital r.
tentorial r.

Riedel's lobe

Rieder
R's cell
R's cell leukemia
R's lymphocyte

Riehl's melanosis

rim

rima *pl.* rimae
r. ani
r. clunium
r. glottidis
r. palpebrarum
r. pudendi
r. vestibuli

rimae (plural of rima)

rimal

ring
Albl's r.
annular r's
Cannon's r.
cardiac lymphatic r.
esophageal r.
hemosiderin r.
inguinal r.
pleural r's
Schatzki's r.

ringworm
r. of the beard
black-dot r.
r. of the body
r. of the face
r. of the foot
gray-patch r.
r. of the groin

ringworm *(continued)*
    r. of the hand
    honeycomb r.
    r. of the nails
    r. of the scalp
    Oriental r.
    Tokelau r.

Riolan
    R's bones
    R's nosegay
    R's ossicles

Ritter's disease

rivus
    r. lacrimalis

Robson's line

rocuronium bromide

rod
    Auer r's
    Harrington r.
    intramedullary r.
    medullary r.

roentgen

roentgenograph

roentgenographic
    r. findings

roentgenography

roentgenologist

roentgenology

roentgenoscope

roentgenoscopy

Roferon-A

Rokitansky-Aschoff sinuses

Rokus view

Rolando's line

roll

Rollet's stroma

Rommelaere's sign

roof
    acetabular r.
    r. of the antrum
    r. of the orbit
    orbital r.
    r. of skull

root
    anterior r. of zygomatic
        process of temporal bone
    aortic r.
    conjoined nerve r.
    r. of hair
    r. of nail
    nerve r.
    nerve r. sleeve
    posterior r. of zygomatic
        process of temporal bone

rootlet

rosacea
    granulomatous r.
    lupoid r.
    papular r.

Rosai-Dorfman disease

rose
    r. bengal sodium I 131

Rosenmüller
    R's fossa
    R's gland

Rosenthal syndrome

roseola
    syphilitic r.

Roser's line

rosette
    Flexner-Wintersteiner r.
    Homer Wright r.
    ependymal r.

rosin

rostra (plural of rostrum)

rostrad

rostral

rostralis

rostrally

rostrate

rostriform

rostrum *pl.* rostra
    r. corporis callosi
    r. sphenoidale

rot
    Barcoo r.

rotameter

rotate

rotation
    external r.
    internal r.
    internal and external r.
        views

rotexed

rotexion

Rothmann-Makai syndrome

rotoscoliosis

rouleau

Rous sarcoma

Roux-en-Y
    R.-en.-Y anastomosis
    R.-en.-Y procedure

row
    rudimentary r.

RS cells

RSDS
    reflex sympathetic dystro-
        phy syndrome

Rubex

rubidium
    r. 82
    r. chloride Rb 82

rubidomycin

rubriblast

rubricyte

rudimentary

rudimentum

rufous

ruga *pl.* rugae
    gastric rugae
    rugae vaginales
    rugae vesicae biliaris

"rugger jersey" appearance of
    the spine

rugose

rugosity

rugous

Rundles-Falls syndrome

rupia

rupial

rupioid

ruptured
    r. hollow viscus
    r. ulcer

Rush intramedullary nail

Russell
    R's viper venom
    R's viper venom time

rutherford

Rye Classification (of Hodgkin's
    disease)

SA, S-A
> sinoatrial
>> SA node

sac
> caudal s.
> pericardial s.
> serous s.
> thecal s.

saccate

sacci (plural of saccus)

sacciform

saccular

sacculated

sacculation

sacculus *pl.* sacculi
> s. laryngis

saccus *pl.* sacci
> s. conjunctivalis
> s. endolymphaticus
> s. lacrimalis
> s. profundus perinei
> s. subcutaneus perinei

sacrad

sacral

sacralization

sacroperineal

sacrouterine

sacrum

safrole

sagittal
> s. and coronal views
> s. magnetization transfer
> views
> s. plane
> s. suture

sagittalis

Sahli's method

St. Anthony's fire

Salem sump tube

saline
> D5 $\frac{1}{2}$ normal s.

salpingectomy

salpingion

salpingography

salpingo-oophorectomy

salpinx

Salter
> S. I fracture (*also* S. II frac-
> ture)
> S. III fracture
> S. IV fracture

samarium
> s. 153

sanguifacient

sanguiferous

sanguification

sanguineous

sanguinous

saphenography

saphenous

Sappey's subareolar plexus

sarcocarcinoma

sarcoenchondroma

sarcoid
> Boeck's s.
> Spiegler-Fendt s.

sarcoidosis
> Boeck's s.

sarcoma
> adipose s.
> alveolar soft part s.
> ameloblastic s.
> botryoid s.

sarcoma *(continued)*
    s. botryoides
    chloromatous s.
    chondroblastic s.
    clear cell s. of kidney
    embryonal s.
    endometrial stromal s.
    epithelioid s.
    Ewing's s.
    fascial s.
    fibroblastic s.
    giant cell s.
    granulocytic s.
    hemangioendothelial s.
    Hodgkin's s.
    idiopathic multiple pig-
        mented hemorrhagic s.
    immunoblastic s. of B cells
    immunoblastic s. of T cells
    Kaposi's s.
    Kupffer cell s.
    leukocytic s.
    lymphatic s.
    melanotic s.
    mixed cell s.
    multiple idiopathic hemor-
        rhagic s.
    multipotential primary s. of
        bone
    osteoblastic s.
    osteogenic s.
    parosteal s.
    polymorphous s.
    pseudo–Kaposi s.
    reticulum cell s.
    reticulum cell s. of the
        brain
    Rous s.
    soft tissue s.
    spindle cell s.
    stromal s.
    synovial s.
    telangiectatic s.

L-sarcolysin

sarcomagenic

sarcomata

sarcomatoid

sarcomatosis

sarcomatous

sargramostim

satumomab

saturation
    oxygen s.
    transferrin s.

saucer

Sauvage filamentous graft mate-
    rial

scabetic

scabies
    crusted s.
    Norwegian s.

scabietic

scala
    s. tympani
    s. vestibuli

scalariform

scald

scale
    gray s.

scaler

scalloping

scalp
    gyrate s.

scalpriform

scan
    A-s.
    B-s.
    Captopril renal s.
    CAT (computerized axial
        tomographic) s.
    CT computerized axial to-
        mographic) s.

scan *(continued)*
    diffusion s.
    gallium s.
    gastric emptying s.
    gated blood pool s.
    hepatobiliary s.
    left ventricular gated blood
      pool s.
    liver-spleen s.
    Meckel s.
    M-mode s.
    MUGA (multiple gated ac-
      quisition) s.
    perfusion lung s.
    PET (positron emission to-
      mography) s.
    PIPIDA s.
    PYP (pyrophosphate) my-
      ocardial s.
    resting left ventricular
      gated blood pool s.
    spiral CT s.
    three-phase bone s.
    ventilation lung s.
    ventilation-perfusion s.
    ventilation and perfusion
      lung s's
    V/Q s.
    whole-body bone s.

scanner
    EMI s.
    scintillation s.

scanning
    infarct avid s.
    MUGA (multiple gated ac-
      quisition) s.
    multiple gated acquisi-
      tion s.
    radioisotope s.
    sector s.
    thallium s.

scanogram

scanography

scapha

scaphion

scaphocephaly

scapholunate

scapula

scapus
    s. pili

scar
    hypertrophic s.

Scarpa
    S.'s fascia
    S.'s triangle

scarring
    pleural s.
    postinflammatory s.

scatter

scattered

scattering
    Compton s.
    Thomson s.

Schamberg
    S's dermatosis
    S's disease
    S's progressive pigmented
      purpuric dermatosis

Schatzki's ring

scheme
    decay s.

Scherer's secondary structures

Scheuermann's disease

Schilling's leukemia

schindylesis

schistocytosis

schistosomiasis
    cutaneous s.

schizocytosis

schizonychia

schizotrichia

Schmincke's tumor

Schmorl's nodule

Schoemaker's line

Schon dual line

Schönlein
  S. purpura
  S's disease
  S.-Henoch purpura
  S.-Henoch syndrome

Schüller's projection

Schultz
  S. syndrome
  S's angina

Schwachman's syndrome

Schwann cell tumor

schwannoglioma

schwannoma
  acoustic s.
  granular cell s.

Schweninger-Buzzi anetoderma

Scianna blood group

sciatic

sciatica

scintiangiography

scintigram

scintigraphic

scintigraphy
  antifibrin s.
  exercise thallium s.
  gated blood pool s.
  infarct avid s.
  technetium Tc 99m pyro-
    phosphate s.

scintillation

scintiphotograph

scintiphotography

scintirenography

scintiscan

scintiscanner

scirrhoid

scirrhoma

scirrhous

scirrhus

sclera

scleredema
  s. adultorum
  Buschke's s.

sclerema
  s. adultorum

sclerodactylia

sclerodactyly

scleroderma
  circumscribed s.
  diffuse s.
  generalized s.
  linear s.
  localized s.
  systemic s.

sclerodermatous

scleromyxedema

scleronychia

sclerosis
  diffuse systemic s.
  end plate s.
  gastric s.
  marginal s.
  multiple s.
  progressive systemic s.
  systemic s.
  variceal s.

scoliosis
  dextroconvex s.
  rotatory s.
  S-type s.

scoliotic

score
  Gleason s.

scorings

scout film

screen
    fluorescent s.
    intensifying s.

screening

screw
    Richard's s.
    interpedicular s's

scrobiculate

scrobiculus
    s. cordis

scrotum

scurvy

scutiform

scyphoid

seam

sebaceous

sebiferous

sebiparous

sebolith

seborrhea
    s. adiposa
    s. oleosa
    s. sicca

seborrheal

seborrheic

seborrhiasis

sebotropic

sebum
    cutaneous s.
    s. cutaneum

secretor

secretion
    retained s's

section
    caesarean s.

section *(continued)*
    coronal s.
    frontal s.
    frozen s.
    sagittal s.
    transverse s.

sedimentation
    erythrocyte s.

seed
    radiogold (198Au) s.
    radon s.

segment
    aganglionic s.
    axillary s. of the right up-
      per lobe
    cranial s's
    frontal s.
    lingular s.
    occipital s.
    parietal s.

segmentum *pl.* segmenta
    segmenta bronchopulmon-
      alia
    s. cardiacum
    segmenta cervicalia [1–8]
    segmenta coccygea [1–3]
    segmenta lumbalia [1–5]
    segmenta medullae spinalis
    segmenta renalia
    segmenta sacralia [1–5]
    segmenta thoracica [1–12]

seizure
    clonic-tonic s.
    grand mal s.
    petit mal s's
    tonic-clonic s.

Seldinger
    S. needle
    S. technique

selene
    s. unguium

selenium
    s. 75

selenomethylnorcholesterol

sella
    s. turcica

semiaxial

semicanal

semicanalis *pl.* semicanales
    s. musculi tensoris tympani
    s. tubae auditivae
    s. tubae auditoriae

seminoma
    anaplastic s.
    classical s.
    ovarian s.
    spermatocytic s.

semiopaque

semipronation

semiprone

semirecumbent

semisulcus

semisupination

semisupine

semustine (meCCNU)

Senear-Usher syndrome

senograph

senography

sensitization
    autoerythrocyte s.

Sensorcaine

Senter syndrome

separation
    meniscotibial s.
    acromioclavicular joint
        separation

sepsis

septa (plural of septum)

septal

septate

septation

septile

septomarginal

septula

septulum
    septula testis

septum *pl.* septa
    atrioventricular s. of heart
    s. atrioventriculare cordis
    s. canalis musculotubarii
    s. cavum interpositum
    s. cavum vergae
    cervical s., intermediate
    s. cervicale intermedium
    s. corporum cavernosorum
        clitoridis
    femoral s.
    s. femorale
    s. femorale [Cloqueti]
    s. glandis penis
    s. of glans penis
    hemal s.
    interatrial s. of heart
    s. interatriale cordis
    s. intermusculare brachii
        laterale
    s. intermusculare brachii
        mediale
    s. intermusculare cruris an-
        terius
    s. intermusculare cruris
        posterius
    s. intermusculare femoris
        laterale
    s. intermusculare femoris
        mediale
    interventricular s. of heart
    s. interventriculare cordis
    s. linguae
    s. linguale
    s. medianum posterius me-
        dullae spinalis
    mediastinal s.
    s. mediastinale
    nasal s.
    s. nasale

septum *(continued)*
- s. nasi
- s. nasi osseum
- neural s.
- orbital s.
- s. orbitale
- s. pellucidum
- s. penis
- rectovaginal s.
- s. rectovaginale
- rectovesical s.
- s. rectovesicale
- scrotal s.
- s. scrotale
- s. scroti
- s. sinuum frontalium
- s. sinuum sphenoidalium

sequela *pl.* sequelae

sequence
- adenoma-carcinoma s.
- pulse s.

sequential filming

sequestration

sequestrum *pl.* sequestra

sera (plural of serum)

seralbumin

serialograph

series
- abdominal s.
- basophil s.
- basophilic s.
- cardiac s.
- diagnostic skull s.
- eosinophil s.
- eosinophilic s.
- erythrocyte s.
- erythrocytic s.
- GB (gallbladder) s.
- GB-GI s.
- GI (gastrointestinal) s.
- granulocyte s.
- granulocytic s.
- leukocytic s.
- monocyte s.
- monocytic s.

series *(continued)*
- myelocytic s.
- myeloid s.
- neutrophil s.
- neutrophilic s.
- thrombocyte s.
- thrombocytic s.
- traumatic skull s.

serioscopy

seroalbuminous

seroma

serpiginous

serrated

serration

serratus

serrulate

Sertoli
- S. cell tumor
- S.-Leydig cell tumor

serum *pl.* sera
- blood s.
- blood grouping sera

sestamibi
- s. stress test

set
- introducer s.

Settegast's projection

sevoflurane

Sézary
- S. cell
- S. syndrome

SFA
- superficial femoral artery

shadow
- bat's wing s.
- cardiomediastinal s.
- cardiothymic s.
- concatenation of s's
- heart s.
- hilar s's

shadow *(continued)*
    overlying bowel s's
    psoas s's
    renal and psoas s's
    thymic s.

shadowing
    acoustical s.

shaft
    hair s.

shagreen

sheath
    bicipital tendon s.
    nerve root s.
    periarterial lymphatic s.
    periarterial lymphoid s.
    root s.
    rectus s.
    s. of rectus abdominis mus-
       cle
    tendon s.

shelf

Shenton
    S's arch
    S's line

shield
    lead s.

shift
    chloride s.
    s. to the left
    mediastinal s.
    midline s.
    s. of the midline structures
    s. to the right

shin

shotty *(not* shoddy) lymph
  nodes

shoulder
    frozen s.

shrapnel

shunt
    Cimino AV s.
    Cimino dialysis s.

shunt *(continued)*
    jejunoileal (JI) s.
    left-to-right s.
    LeVeen peritoneovenous s.
    s. to the lungs
    portal systemic s.
    portocaval s.
    right-to-left s.
    transjugular intrahepatic
       portosystemic s.
    s. tubing

shunting of tracer to the bone
  marrow

SI
    sacroiliac
          SI joints

sialadenitis

sialadenoma
    s. papilliferum

sialogram
    parotid gland s.
    submaxillary s.

sialography

sialoma

sialometaplasia

sialotomography

siboroxime

sickle cell
    s. c. anemia
    s. c. disease
    s. c. trait

sicklemia

sickling

sickness
    radiation s.
    x-ray s.

Sid blood group

side
    ipsilateral s.

sideroblast

siderocyte

siderophilin

siderosis

siderotic

SIDS
sudden infant death syndrome

Siemens

sievert

sigmoidoscopy

Sigmund's glands

sign
air-cushion s.
Ballance's s.
banana s.
Bergman's s.
bowler hat s.
broken straw s.
Carman's s.
Carman-Kirklin s.
Carman-Kirklin meniscus s.
Chilaiditi's s.
cobra head s.
coiled spring s.
Cole's s.
colon cutoff s.
crescent s.
Crowe's s.
Darier's s.
Dennie's s.
double bubble s.
E s.
Elliot's s.
fat pad s.
figure three s.
floating tooth s.
Gottron's s.
Granger's s.
halo s.
Haudek's s.
Hawkins s.
Hefke-Turner s.
Hitzelberger's s.

sign *(continued)*
Homans' s.
Horner's s.
Kantor's s.
Kehr's s.
Kernig's s.
Klemm's s.
Kussmaul's s.
lemon s.
Leser-Trélat s.
localizing s's
meniscus s.
Mercedes-Benz s.
Mexican hat s.
Murphy's s.
Mosler's s.
moulage s.
niche s.
Nikolsky's s.
obturator s.
patent bronchus s.
Phalen's s.
"railroad track" s.
reversed three s.
Rommelaere's s.
scimitar s.
silhouette s.
Spalding's s.
steeple s.
Stierlin's s.
string s.
string of beads s.
three s.
Troisier's s.
twin peak s.
Westermark's s.
Wimberger's s.
Wood's s.

silhouette
cardiac s.
cardiopericardial s.
cardiovascular s.
pericardial s.
s. sign

silhouetted-out

silhouetting

silicosis

Simmond's disease

Simmons catheter

sinal

sincipital

sinciput

sinister

sinistrad

sinistral

sinoaortic

Sinografin

sinography

sinopulmonary

sinuate

sinuous

sinus
    air s.
    anal s's
    s. anales
    s. aortae
    Aschoff-Rokitansky s's
    s. caroticus
    carotid s.
    s. cavernosus
    cavernous s.
    coccygeal s.
    s. coronarius
    coronary s.
    cortical s's
    s's of dura mater
    s. durae matris
    s. epididymidis
    s. of epididymis
    ethmoid s's
    Forssell's s.
    frontal s's
    s. frontalis
    s. intercavernosus anterior
    s. intercavernosus posterior
    intermediate s's
    lacteal s's

sinus *(continued)*
    s. lactiferi
    lactiferous s's
    s. lienalis
    lymph s's
    lymphatic s's
    marginal s's
    s. marginalis
    s. maxillaris
    s. maxillaris [Highmori]
    medullary s's
    oblique s. of pericardium
    s. obliquus pericardii
    occipital s.
    s. occipitalis
    paranasal s's
    s. paranasales
    s. petrosquamosus
    s. petrosus inferior
    s. petrosus superior
    pilonidal s.
    s. posterior cavitatis tympanicae
    prostatic s.
    s. prostaticus
    pyriform s's
    s. rectus
    renal s.
    renal s. lipomatosus
    s. renalis
    Rokitansky-Aschoff s's
    sacrococcygeal s.
    s. sagittalis inferior
    s. sagittalis superior
    sigmoid s.
    s. sigmoideus
    sphenoid s's
    s. sphenoidalis
    sphenoparietal s.
    s. sphenoparietalis
    s. of spleen
    splenic s.
    s. splenicus
    subcapsular s's
    tarsal s.
    s. tarsi
    s. tonsillaris
    s. transversus durae matris
    s. transversus pericardii

sinus *(continued)*
    s. trunci pulmonalis
    s. tympani
    s. unguis
    s. of venae cavae
    s. venarum cavarum
    s. venosus
    s. venosus sclerae
    s. ventriculi

sinusal

sinusitis
    antral s.

sinusoid

sinusoidal

siphon
    s. caroticum
    carotid s.

Sipple's syndrome

sissorexia

Sister Mary Joseph's nodule

site
    bleeding s.
    donor s.
    fracture s.

situs
    s. inversus
    s. solitus
    s. viscus inversus

Sitzmarks

size, position, and contour

Sjögren's syndrome

skeletography

skeletology

skeleton
    appendicular s.
    s. appendiculare
    axial s.
    s. axiale
    s. thoracis

skeletopia

skeletopy

skiagram

skiagraph

skiagraphy

skimming
    plasma s.

skin
    alligator s.
    collodion s.
    crocodile s.
    farmers' s.
    fish s.
    glossy s.
    lax s.
    loose s.
    marble s.
    piebald s.
    porcupine s.
    sailors' s.
    shagreen s.

Skinner's line

Skiodan

skull
    lacunar s.
    maplike s.
    West's lacuna s.
    West-Engstler's s.

sleep
    electric s.
    twilight s.

SLE
    systemic lupus erythemato-
      sus

slice

slipped capital femoral epiphy-
    sis

sludge in the gallbladder

sludging
    s. of blood

SMA
    superficial mesenteric ar-
      tery

small bowel
    s. b. follow-through exami-
        nation
    s. b. obstruction

smear
    Pap s.
    Papanicolaou s.
    Tzanck s.

smegma

smegmalith

smegmatic

Smith
    S.-Petersen nail
    S.-Petersen pin

smooth-bordered

Sneddon
    S's syndrome
    S.-Wilkinson disease

snuffbox

socia

socket

sodium
    s. 22
    s. 24
    s. acetate C 11
    s. chromate Cr 51
    s. diatrizoate
    s. iodide I 123
    s. iodide I 125
    s. ipodate
    s. pertechnetate Tc 99m
    s. phosphate P 32
    s. thiamylal

solenonychia

solution
    contrast s.
    diatrizoate sodium s.
    Drabkin's s.
    Fonio's s.
    Gowers' s.
    Hayem's s.
    hyperbaric s.

solution (continued)
    hypobaric s.
    indium In 111 chloride s.
    isobaric s.
    normobaric s.
    Toison's s.

soma

somal

somatic

somaticosplanchnic

somaticovisceral

somatogram

somatology

somatometry

somatostatinoma

somatotropinoma

sonarography

Sones
    S. coronary catheter
    S. technique

sonogram

sonographic

sonography

sonolucency

sonolucent

sore
    bed s.
    chrome s.
    desert s.
    pressure s.
    veldt s.

SOS catheter

souffle
    splenic s.

sound
    hypoactive bowel s's

space
    axillary s.

space *(continued)*
   ballooning of the disc s's
   Burns' s.
   cathodal dark s.
   Colles' s.
   s.-consuming process
   Crookes' s.
   disc s. narrowing
   disc s.–thecal sac interface
   extrapleural s.
   Henke's s.
   Holzknecht's s.
   iliocostal s.
   interpleural s.
   interradicular s.
   intervertebral disc s.
   joint s.
   joint s. narrowing
   Larrey's s's
   lymph s.
   mediastinal s.
   Mohrenheim's s.
   s.-occupying process
   osseous s.
   peridental s.
   perineal s., deep
   perineal s., superficial
   peritoneal s.
   phrenocostal s.
   pleural s.
   pneumatic s.
   predental s.
   preperitoneal s.
   prevertebral s.
   prevesical s.
   retrocardiac s.
   retroperitoneal s.
   retropubic s.
   retrosternal air s.
   Retzius s.
   semilunar s.
   subarachnoid s.
   subphrenic s.
   subumbilical s.
   suprapatellar s.
   suprasternal s.
   Traube's semilunar s.
   Virchow-Robin s's
   web s.

space *(continued)*
   Zang's s.

Spalding's sign

spallation

span

spasm

spatium *pl.* spatia
   spatia anguli iridis [Fon-
      tanae]
   spatia anguli iridocornealis
   s. epidurale
   s. episclerale
   s. extradurale
   s. extraperitoneale
   s. intercostale
   spatia interossea metacarpi
   spatia interossea metatarsi
   s. lateropharyngeum
   s. leptomeningeum
   s. perichoroideale
   s. perichoroideum
   s. peridurale
   s. perilymphaticum
   s. profundum perinei
   s. superficiale perinei
   s. peripharyngeum
   s. retroperitoneale
   s. retropharyngeum
   s. retropubicum
   s. subarachnoideum
   s. subdurale
   spatia zonularia

spatula

spatular

spatulate

specimen

SPECT
   single-photon emission
      computed tomography
         SPECT scan

spectrin

spectrum
   continuous x-ray s.

spectrum *(continued)*
    x-ray s.

spermatocytoma

spermocytoma

sphenoccipital

sphenofrontal

spheno-occipital

sphenoparietal

spherocytic

spherocytosis
    hereditary s.

sphincter
    s. of Oddi
    hypertensive lower esopha-
        geal s.
    pyloric s.

sphincteral

sphincteric

spica

spicular

spiculated

spicule
    bone s.

spiculum

spider
    arterial s.
    vascular s.

Spieghel's line

Spiegler
    S.-Fendt pseudolymphoma
    S.-Fendt sarcoid

spigelian line

Spigelius' line

spill
    ileal s.
    peritoneal s.

spill of contrast material

spin

spina *pl.* spinae
    s. bifida
    s. bifida occulta
    s. helicis
    s. iliaca anterior inferior
    s. iliaca anterior superior
    s. iliaca posterior inferior
    s. iliaca posterior superior
    s. ischiadica
    s. ischialis
    s. nasalis anterior maxillae
    s. nasalis ossis frontalis
    s. nasalis posterior ossis
        palatini
    s. ossis sphenoidalis
    spinae palatinae
    s. scapulae
    s. suprameatalis
    s. suprameatica
    s. trochlearis
    s. tympanica major
    s. tympanica minor

spinae (plural of spina)

spinalis

spine
    "bamboo s."
    cervical s.
    dorsal s.
    iliac s.
    ischial s.
    lumbosacral (LS) s.
    maternal s.
    nasal s.
    occipital s., external
    occipital s., internal
    thoracic s.
    tibial s.

spinocellular

spinocerebellum

spinogram

spinose

spinous

spintherometer

spintometer

spiradenoma
    eccrine s.

spiral
    Herxheimer's s's

spiroma

spirometry

Spitz nevus

splanchnapophyseal

splanchnapophysis

splanchnic

splanchnography

splanchnology

splanchnoskeleton

splanchnosomatic

splanchnotomy

splaying

spleen
    accessory s.
    enlarged s.
    flecked s. of Feitis
    floating s.
    Gandy-Gamna s.
    movable s.
    speckled s.
    wandering s.

splen
    s. accessorius

splenalgia

splenatrophy

splenauxe

splenculus

splenectasis

splenectopia

splenectopy

splenelcosis

spleneolus

splenic

splenitis
    spodogenous s.

splenium
    s. corporis callosi
    s. of the corpus callosum

splenoblast

splenocele

splenocolic

splenocyte

splenodynia

splenogenous

splenogram

splenography

splenology

splenolymphatic

splenoma

splenomalacia

splenomedullary

splenomegalia

splenomegaly
    congestive s.
    hemolytic s.
    infectious s.
    infective s.
    siderotic s.
    spodogenous s.

splenometry

splenomyelogenous

splenomyelomalacia

splenoncus

splenonephric

splenopancreatic

splenoparectasis

splenopathy

splenophrenic

splenoportography

splenoptosia

splenoptosis

splenorenal

splenorrhagia

splenosis

splenotoxin

splenulus

splenunculus

splint
Böhler's s.
Thomas s.

splinting

spondylitic

spondylitis
ankylosing s.

spondylodiscitis

spondylolisthesis

spondylolysis
reverse s.

spondylosis

sponge

spongioblastoma
s. multiforme
polar s.
s. polare
unipolar s.
s. unipolare

spongiocytoma

spongiosis

spongiotic

spot
ash-leaf s.
blue s.

spot *(continued)*
café au lait s's
Cayenne pepper s's
"cold" s.
De Morgan's s's
focal s.
Fordyce's s's
hot s.
lance-ovate s.
liver s.
mongolian s.
pelvic s's
sacral s.
shin s's
spongy s.

sprue
celiac s.

spur
heel s.
olecranon s.
plantar calcaneal s.

spurious finding

spurring
marginal s.
osteophytic s.

squama
s. of frontal bone
s. frontalis
mental s., external
occipital s.
occipital s., superior
s. occipitalis
perpendicular s.
temporal s.
s. of temporal bone
s. temporalis

squamate

squame

squamofrontal

squamomastoid

squamo-occipital

squamoparietal

squamopetrosal

squamosa

squamosal

squamosoparietal

squamotemporal

squamous

squamozygomatic

S-shaped

stability

stadium
    s. fluorescentiae

staff

stage
    eruptive s.

staging
    TNM s.

Stahr's gland

stain
    Gram's s.
    port-wine s.
    tumor s.

stalk
    pituitary s.

stannous
    s. pyrophosphate

stanolone

stapedectomy

stapes

Staphylococcus

staphylococcus

staphylococcal

staphyloderma

staphylokinase

staple
    four-pronged s.
    metallic s's
    two-pronged s.

star
    venus s.

stasis
    venous s.

state
    fasting s.
    hypercoagulable s.

static gray scale equipment (ultrasound)

station −

station +

statoconia

statoconium

stature

status
    s. asthmaticus
    s. epilepticus
    s. post

Stauffer syndrome

stay
    s. of white line

steal

stearaldehyde

steatocystoma
    s. multiplex

steatoma

steatomatosis

steatomery

Stein-Leventhal syndrome

Steinmann pin

steinstrasse

stellula

stem

stenosis *pl.* stenoses
    acquired spinal s.
    aortic s.

stenosis *(continued)*
    bronchial s.
    cicatricial s.
    foraminal s.
    hypertrophic pyloric s.
    idiopathic hypertrophic
      subaortic s. (IHSS)
    lateral recess s.
    meatal s.
    mitral s.
    pulmonary valvular s.
    pulmonic s.
    pyloric s.
    spinal s.

stenotic

Stensen's duct

stent
    biliary s.
    double-J ureteral s.
    ureteral s.

Stenvers
    S. views
    S. projection

stephanial

stephanion

Sterculia

sterculia

stereocinefluorography

stereofluoroscopy

stereogram

stereograph

stereoradiography

stereoradiometry

stereosalpingography

stereoskiagraphy

sterigmatocystin

sternad

Sternberg
    S's disease

Sternberg *(continued)*
    S's giant cells
    S.-Reed cells

sternogoniometer

sternohyoid

sternoid

sternopericardial

sternothyroid

sternotomy
    median s.

sternotracheal

sternum

Stevens-Johnson syndrome

Stewart-Treves syndrome

Stierlin's sign

stigma

stilbestrol

stippling
    epiphyseal s.

stomach
    cascade s.
    cup-and-spill s.
    fundus of the s.
    greater curvature of the s.
    J-shaped s.
    leather bottle s.
    lesser curvature of the s.
    sclerotic s.

stoma *pl.* stomas, stomata
    gastroenterostomy s.

stomal

stomatocytosis

stone
    common duct s.
    nonopaque s.
    skin s's
    ureteral s.

stool
    guaiac-negative s.

stool *(continued)*
  guaiac-positive s.
  Hemoccult-negative s.
  Hemoccult-positive s.
  impacted s.
  melenic s's
  tarry s's

storiform

strand
  Billroth's s's
  fibrotic s's

stranding

strand-like

strap

strata (plural of stratum)

stratification

stratified

stratiform

stratigraphy

stratum *pl.* strata
  s. basale epidermidis
  s. circulare tunicae muscularis coli
  s. circulare tunicae muscularis gastris
  s. circulare tunicae muscularis intestini tenuis
  s. circulare tunicae muscularis recti
  s. corneum epidermidis
  s. corneum unguis
  s. cylindricum epidermidis
  s. fibrosum capsulae articularis
  s. fibrosum vaginae tendinis
  ganglionic s. of retina
  s. ganglionicum retinae
  s. germinativum
  s. germinativum epidermidis [Malpighii]
  s. germinativum unguis
  s. granulosum cerebelli
  s. granulosum epidermidis

stratum *(continued)*
  s. granulosum ovarii
  s. griseum intermedium colliculi superioris
  s. griseum profundum colliculi superioris
  s. griseum superficiale colliculi superioris
  s. longitudinale tunicae muscularis coli
  s. longitudinale tunicae muscularis gastris
  s. longitudinale tunicae muscularis intestini tenuis
  s. longitudinale tunicae muscularis recti
  s. longitudinale tunicae muscularis ventriculi
  s. lucidum epidermidis
  s. malpighii
  s. medullare intermedium colliculi superioris
  s. medullare profundum colliculi superioris
  s. moleculare cerebelli
  s. nervosum retinae
  s. oriens hippocampi
  s. papillare corii
  s. papillare cutis
  s. papillare dermidis
  s. pigmentosum retinae
  s. purkinjense cerebelli
  s. pyramidale hippocampi
  s. radiatum hippocampi
  s. reticulare corii
  s. reticulare cutis
  s. reticulare dermidis
  s. spinosum epidermidis
  s. synoviale capsulae articularis
  s. synoviale vaginae tendinis
  s. zonale colliculi superioris

streak

stream
  blood s.

stream *(continued)*
    electron s.
    hair s's

strength
    magnetic field s.

streptococcal

Streptococcus

streptokinase

streptomycin

streptozocin

streptozotocin

stressing
    treadmill s.

stria *pl.* striae
    s. diagonalis
    s. diagonalis (Broca)
    s. laminae granularis externae
    s. laminae granularis internae
    s. laminae molecularis
    s. laminae pyramidalis internae
    s. longitudinalis lateralis corporis callosi
    s. longitudinalis medialis corporis callosi
    s. mallearis membranae tympanicae
    s. mallearis membranae tympani
    s. malleolaris membranae tympani
    s. medullaris thalami
    striae medullares ventriculi quarti
    striae olfactoriae
    s. olfactoria lateralis
    s. olfactoria medialis
    s. terminalis
    s. vascularis ductus cochlearis

striae (plural of stria)

striate

striated

striation

stricture
    esophageal s.

stridor

stridorous

stringy density

strip
    motor s.
    sensory s.

stripe
    psoas s.

stroma
    s. ganglii
    s. glandulae thyroideae
    s. iridis
    s. of iris
    s. ovarii
    s. of ovary
    Rollet's s.
    vitreous s.
    s. vitreum

stromatin

stromatolysis

strontium
    s. 85
    s. 87m
    s. 89
    s. 90
    s. chloride Sr 89

strontiuresis

strontiuretic

strophulus

structure
    echogenic s's
    glandular s's
    gyral s's
    invasion of adjacent s's
    mediastinal s's
    midline s's

structure *(continued)*
    osseous s's
    paired s's
    Scherer's secondary s's
    shift of the midline s's
    soft tissue s's
    vascular s's

struma
    s. ovarii

Stryker's notch projection

Stuart
    S. factor
    S.-Prower factor

study
    barium s.
    barium enema with air contrast s.
    baseline s.
    Doppler s's
    double contrast enema s.
    equilibrium s's
    flow s.
    leg length s.
    myelographic s.
    nerve conduction s.
    sputum s's

Sturge-Weber syndrome

Stypven time

sump
    van Sonnenberg s. *(pronounced* "von")

stump

styliform

styloid

subabdominal

subabdominoperitoneal

subacute

subanal

subapical

subarcuate

subareolar

subarticular

subatloidean

subatomic

subaxial

subaxillary

subbasal

subcapsular

subcarinal

subcartilaginous

subchondral

subclavian

subclavicular

subcostal

subcostalis

subcuticular

subcutis

subdeltoid

subdiaphragmatic

subdorsal

subendothelial

subependymoma

subepidermal, subepidermic

subepithelial

subfascial

subgaleal

subgemmal

subglottic

subhepatic

subhumeral

subiculum
    s. promontorii cavitatis tympanicae
    s. promontorii cavitatis tympani

subiliac

subjacent

Sublimaze

sublobe

sublobular

subluxation

submammary

submarginal

submedial

submedian

submentovertex

submucosa

submucosal

submucous

suboccipital

suboptimal

subpapillary

subpapular

subparietal

subpectoral

subpelviperitoneal

subpericardial

subperiosteal

subperitoneal

subperitoneoabdominal

subperitoneopelvic

subphrenic

subpleural

subpubic

subpulmonary

subpulmonic

subpyramidal

subrectal

subscapular

substance
   α-s.
   alpha s.
   blood group s's
   brain s.
   cortical s. of lymph node
   H s.
   medullary s. of lymph node
   metachromatic s.
   no-threshold s's
   onychogenic s.
   red s. of spleen
   reticular s.
   threshold s's
   thromboplastic s.
   zymoplastic s.

substantia
   s. alba
   s. alba medullae spinalis
   s. compacta ossium
   s. corticalis lymphoglandulae
   s. corticalis ossium
   s. gelatinosa cornu posterioris medullae spinalis
   s. gelatinosa centralis medullae spinalis
   s. grisea
   s. grisea centralis
   s. grisea medullae spinalis
   s. innominata
   s. intermedia centralis medullae spinalis
   s. intermedia lateralis medullae spinalis
   s. lentis
   s. medullaris lymphoglandulae
   s. muscularis prostatae
   s. nigra
   s. perforata anterior
   s. perforata interpeduncularis
   s. perforata posterior
   s. perforata rostralis

substantia *(continued)*
    s. propria corneae
    s. propria sclerae
    s. reticulofilamentosa
    s. spongiosa ossium
    s. trabecularis ossium
    s. visceralis secundaria medullae spinalis

substernal

substernomastoid

subsulcus

subtenial

subterminal

subthalamus

subtrapezial

subtrochanteric

subtrochlear

subtuberal

subumbilical

subungual

subvaginal

subzonal

succimer

succus

sudamen

sudaminal

sudation

Sudeck's atrophy

sudogram

sudomotor

sudoresis

sudoriferous

sudorific

sudoriparous

Sufenta

sufentanil citrate

sulcate

sulcation

sulci (plural of sulcus)

sulciform

sulculus

sulcus *pl.* sulci
    s. ampullaris
    ampullary s.
    s. anterolateralis medullae oblongatae
    s. anterolateralis medullae spinalis
    arterial sulci
    sulci arteriales
    s. arteriae meningeae mediae
    s. arteriae occipitalis
    s. arteriae subclaviae
    s. arteriae temporalis mediae
    s. arteriae vertebralis atlantis
    sulci arteriosi
    basilar s. of occipital bone
    basilar s. of pons
    s. basilaris pontis
    s. bicipitalis lateralis
    s. bicipitalis medialis
    s. bicipitalis radialis
    s. bicipitalis ulnaris
    bulbopontine s.
    s. bulbopontinus
    calcaneal s.
    s. calcanei
    calcarine s.
    s. calcarinus
    s. caroticus ossis sphenoidalis
    carotid s.
    carpal s.
    s. carpi
    s. centralis cerebri
    s. centralis insulae
    cerebral sulci
    sulci cerebri

sulcus *(continued)*
    sulci of cerebrum
    s. cinguli
    s. of cingulum
    circular s. of insula
    s. circularis insulae
    collateral s.
    s. collateralis
    s. coronarius cordis
    coronary s. of heart
    s. corporis callosi
    s. of corpus callosum
    s. costae
    costal s.
    costophrenic s.
    s. cruris helicis
    s. of crus of helix
    sulci cutis
    ethmoidal s. of nasal bone
    s. ethmoidalis ossis nasalis
    fimbriodentate s.
    s. fimbriodentatus
    s. frontalis inferior
    s. frontalis superior
    gluteal s.
    s. glutealis
    habenular s.
    s. habenularis
    s. hamuli pterygoidei
    hippocampal s.
    s. hippocampalis
    s. hippocampi
    hypothalamic s.
    s. hypothalamicus
    s. hypothalamicus [Monroi]
    s. for inferior petrosal sinus of occipital bone
    s. for inferior petrosal sinus of temporal bone
    infraorbital s. of maxilla
    s. infraorbitalis maxillae
    infrapalpebral s.
    s. infrapalpebralis
    sulci interlobares cerebri
    s. intermedius posterior medullae spinalis

sulcus *(continued)*
    intertubercular s. of humerus
    s. intertubercularis humeri
    s. interventricularis anterior
    s. interventricularis posterior
    intraparietal s.
    s. intraparietalis
    s. lacrimalis maxillae
    lacrimal s. of maxilla
    s. lacrimalis ossis lacrimalis
    lateral s. for lateral sinus of occipital bone
    lateral s. for lateral sinus of parietal bone
    lateral s. for sigmoidal part of lateral sinus
    s. lateralis cerebri
    s. lateralis mesencephali
    s. limitans fossae rhomboideae
    lunate s.
    s. lunatus
    s. malleolaris fibulae
    s. malleolaris tibiae
    s. matricis unguis
    s. of matrix of nail
    s. medianus linguae
    s. medianus posterior medullae oblongatae
    s. medianus posterior medullae spinalis
    s. medianus ventriculi quarti
    meningeal sulci
    mentolabial s.
    s. mentolabialis
    s. for middle temporal artery
    s. musculi subclavii
    nasolabial s.
    s. nasolabialis
    s. nervi oculomotorii
    s. nervi petrosi majoris

sulcus *(continued)*
- s. nervi petrosi minoris
- s. nervi radialis
- s. nervi spinalis
- s. nervi ulnaris
- obturator s. of pubis
- s. obturatorius ossis pubis
- s. for occipital artery
- s. occipitalis transversus
- occipitotemporal s.
- s. occipitotemporalis
- s. olfactorius lobi frontalis
- s. olfactorius nasi
- orbital sulci of frontal lobe
- sulci orbitales lobi frontalis
- palatinovaginal s.
- s. palatinovaginalis
- s. palatinus major maxillae
- s. palatinus major ossis palatini
- sulci palatini maxillae
- paracolic sulci
- sulci paracolici
- parietooccipital s.
- s. parietooccipitalis
- petrobasilar s.
- petrosal s. of occipital bone, inferior
- petrosal s. of temporal bone, inferior
- petrosal s. of temporal bone, posterior
- petrosal s. of temporal bone, superior
- s. petrosus inferior ossis occipitalis
- s. petrosus inferior ossis temporalis
- s. petrosus superior ossis temporalis
- s. popliteus femoris
- postcentral s.
- s. postcentralis
- s. posterior auriculae
- s. posterolateralis medullae oblongatae
- s. posterolateralis medullae spinalis

sulcus *(continued)*
- precentral s.
- s. precentralis
- prechiasmatic s.
- s. prechiasmaticus
- s. prechiasmatis
- s. promontorii cavitatis tympani
- s. pulmonalis
- pulmonary s.
- s. retroolivaris
- rhinal s.
- s. rhinalis
- sagittal s.
- s. sclerae
- scleral s.
- sclerocorneal s.
- sigmoid s.
- s. of sigmoid sinus
- s. for sigmoid sinus of occipital bone
- s. for sigmoid sinus of parietal bone
- s. for sigmoid sinus of temporal bone
- s. sigmoideus ossis temporalis
- s. sinus petrosi inferioris ossis occipitalis
- s. sinus petrosi inferioris ossis temporalis
- s. sinus petrosi superioris
- s. sinus sagittalis superioris
- s. sinus sigmoidei
- s. sinus sigmoidei ossis occipitalis
- s. sinus sigmoidei ossis parietalis
- s. sinus sigmoidei ossis temporalis
- s. sinus transversi
- sulci of skin
- s. spiralis externus
- s. spiralis internus
- subparietal s.
- s. subparietalis

sulcus *(continued)*
  superior s.
  s. for superior petrosal sinus
  supra-acetabular s.
  s. supraacetabularis
  supraorbital s.
  suprapalpebral s.
  s. suprapalpebralis
  s. tali
  s. of talus
  s. temporalis inferior
  s. temporalis superior
  s. temporalis transversus
  s. tendinis musculi fibularis longi
  s. tendinis musculi flexoris hallucis longi calcanei
  s. tendinis musculi flexoris hallucis longi tali
  s. tendinis musculi peronei longi
  s. tendinum musculorum fibularium calcanei
  s. tendinum musculorum peroneorum calcanei
  s. terminalis atrii dextri
  s. terminalis cordis
  s. terminalis linguae
  transverse s. of occipital bone
  transverse s. of parietal bone
  s. for transverse sinus
  transverse s. of temporal bone
  s. transversus ossis occipitalis
  s. transversus ossis parietalis
  s. tubae auditivae
  s. tubae auditoriae
  s. tympanicus ossis temporalis
  sulci for veins
  s. for vena cava
  s. venae cavae
  s. venae subclaviae
  sulci venosi

sulcus *(continued)*
  venous sulci
  s. vomeris
  vomerovaginal s.
  s. vomerovaginalis

sulfhemoglobinemia

sulfur
  s. 35

Sulzberger-Garbe syndrome

summit

sunburn

supercentral

supercilia

supercilium

superficial

superficialis

superficies

superimposed

superior

superjacent

supermedial

superoccipital

superolateral

superomedial

supersoft

supersonic

supersphenoid

superstructure

supervascularization

supervoltage

supinate

supination

supine

suppression
  bone marrow s.

suppurative

supra-anal

supra-axillary

supracarinal

supraceliac

supraclavicular

supraclavicularis

supraclinoid

supracondylar

supracranial

supradiaphragmatic

suprahepatic

suprahilar

suprainguinal

supraintestinal

supralumbar

supramarginal

suprameatal

supraoccipital

supraorbital

suprapatellar

suprapelvic

suprapubic

suprarenal

suprasellar

supraseptal

supraspinal

supraspinous

suprasternal

supratentorial

suprathoracic

supratrochlear

supraumbilical

supravaginal

supravalvar

supravesical

supraxiphoid

suprazygomatic

sura

sural

suramin sodium

surface
    anterior s.
    articular s.
    cerebral s. of parietal bone
    diaphragmatic s.
    distal s.
    dorsal s.
    external s. of cranial base
    inferior s.
    lateral s.
    medial s.
    palmar s.
    posterior s.
    proximal s.
    proximate s.
    superior s.
    temporal s. of frontal bone
    ventral s.

surgery
    gastric bypass s.
    Mohs' s.

Surital

surveillance
    immune s.
    immunological s.

survey
    long bone s.
    metabolic bone s.
    metastatic bone s.
    traumatic bone s.

suspension
    barium s.

suspension *(continued)*
   propyliodone s., sterile
   propyliodone injectable
      oil s.

suspensorius

suspensory

sustentacular

sustentaculum
   s. tali
   s. of talus

Sutton's nevus

sutura *pl.* suturae
   s. coronalis
   suturae craniales
   suturae cranii
   s. dentata
   s. ethmoidolacrimalis
   s. ethmoidomaxillaris
   s. frontalis
   s. frontalis metopica
   s. frontalis persistens
   s. frontoethmoidalis
   s. frontolacrimalis
   s. frontomaxillaris
   s. frontonasalis
   s. frontozygomatica
   s. harmonia
   s. infraorbitalis
   s. intermaxillaris
   s. internasalis
   s. lacrimoconchalis
   s. lacrimomaxillaris
   s. lambdoidea
   s. limbosa
   s. nasomaxillaris
   s. occipitomastoidea
   s. palatina mediana
   s. palatina transversa
   s. palatoethmoidalis
   s. palatomaxillaris
   s. parietomastoidea
   s. plana
   s. sagittalis
   s. serrata
   s. sphenoethmoidalis
   s. sphenofrontalis

sutura *(continued)*
   s. sphenomaxillaris
   s. sphenoparietalis
   s. sphenosquamosa
   s. sphenovomeralis
   s. sphenovomeriana
   s. sphenozygomatica
   s. squamomastoidea
   s. squamosa
   s. squamosa cranii
   s. squamosomastoidea
   s. temporozygomatica
   s. vera
   s. zygomaticomaxillaris

suturae (plural of sutura)

sutural

suture
   arcuate s.
   basilar s.
   biparietal s.
   bony s.
   bregmatomastoid s.
   coronal s.
   cranial s's
   dentate s.
   ethmoidomaxillary s.
   false s.
   flat s.
   frontal s.
   frontoethmoidal s.
   frontoparietal s.
   frontozygomatic s.
   interparietal s.
   jugal s.
   lambdoid s.
   limbous s.
   longitudinal s.
   mammillary s.
   mastoid s.
   metallic s's
   metopic s.
   occipital s.
   occipitomastoid s.
   occipitoparietal s.
   occipitosphenoidal s.
   palatine s.
   parietal s.

suture *(continued)*
    parietomastoid s.
    parietooccipital s.
    petrobasilar s.
    persistent metopic s.
    petrosphenobasilar s.
    petrosphenooccipital s. of
      Gruber
    petrosquamous s.
    rhabdoid s.
    sagittal s.
    serrated s.
    skin s's
    s's of skull
    sphenooccipital s.
    sphenoparietal s.
    sphenopetrosal s.
    sphenosquamous s.
    sphenotemporal s.
    squamomastoid s.
    squamosal s.
    squamosomastoid s.
    squamosoparietal s.
    squamososphenoid s.
    squamous s.
    squamous s. of cranium
    sternal s's
    temporal s.
    temporozygomatic s.
    true s.
    wire s's
    zygomaticofrontal s.

swallow
    barium s.
    video barium s.

Swan-Ganz catheter

Swanson prosthesis

sweat
    bloody s.
    blue s.
    fetid s.
    green s.
    phosphorescent s.

sweating

sweep
    duodenal s.

swelling

sycosiform

sycosis
    s. barbae
    lupoid s.
    s. nuchae
    s. vulgaris

sym-dichloromethyl ether

Symington's body

Symmers's disease

symmetrical

symmetry
    bilateral s.
    inverse s.

sympathicoblastoma

sympathicogonioma

sympathoblastoma

sympathogonioma

symphysis *pl.* symphyses
    s. intervertebralis
    s. of the mandible
    s. manubriosternalis
    s. pubica
    s. pubis

symptom
    crossbar s. of Fraenkel
    objective s's

symptomatology

synapsis

synarthrosis

syncelom

synchondrosis *pl.* synchon-
    droses
    synchondroses craniales
    synchondroses cranii
    intraoccipital s., anterior

synchondrosis *(continued)*
    intraoccipital s., posterior
    s. intraoccipitalis anterior
    s. intraoccipitalis posterior
    s. manubriosternalis
    s. petrooccipitalis
    s's of skull
    s. sphenoethmoidalis
    spheno-occipital s.
    s. sphenooccipitalis
    s. sphenopetrosa
    s. sternalis
    s. sternocostalis costae primae
    s. xiphisternalis

synchrotron

synclitic

syncliticism

synclitism

syncope
    near s.

Syncurine

syncytioma
    s. malignum

syndesmography

syndesmophyte

syndesmosis
    s. radioulnaris
    s. tibiofibularis
    s. tympanostapedialis

syndrome
    acquired autoimmune deficiency s. (AIDS)
    acute chest s.
    acute radiation s.
    adult respiratory distress s. (ARDS)
    Alezzandrini's s.
    anorexia-cachexia s.
    argentaffinoma s.
    Arnold-Chiari s.
    autoerythrocyte sensitization s.

syndrome *(continued)*
    BADS s.
    Bäfverstedt's s.
    Bart's s.
    basal cell nevus s.
    Bazex's s.
    Bernard-Soulier s.
    Blackfan-Diamond s.
    blind loop s.
    Boerhaave's s.
    Brown-Séquard s.
    Brunsting's s.
    Budd-Chiari s.
    Buschke-Ollendorff s.
    Caffey's s.
    Canada-Cronkhite s.
    capillary leak s.
    carcinoid s.
    Carney's s.
    carpal tunnel s. (CTS)
    Chilaiditi s.
    CHILD s.
    Courvoisier-Terrier s.
    CREST s. (calcinosis, Raynaud's phenomenon, esophageal dysmotility, sclerodactyly, and telangiectasia)
    Cronkhite-Canada s.
    Crow-Fukase s.
    CRST s.
    Dandy-Walker s.
    defibrination s.
    Degos' s.
    Di Guglielmo's s.
    Diamond-Blackfan s.
    diarrheogenic s.
    disseminated intravascular coagulation s.
    Down s.
    Dresbach's s.
    dumping s.
    dysplastic nevus s.
    Eaton-Lambert s.
    ectrodactyly-ectodermal dysplasia-clefting s.
    EEC s.
    empty sella s.

syndrome *(continued)*

erythrocyte autosensitization s.

Evans's s.

Faber's s.

Fanconi's s.

Favre-Racouchot s.

Felty's s.

Feuerstein-Mims s.

Forsius-Eriksson s.

Gardner-Diamond s.

Gasser's s.

Gianotti-Crosti s.

giant platelet s.

glioma-polyposis s.

Goodpasture's s.

Gorlin's s.

Gorlin-Goltz s.

Gougerot-Blum s.

Gougerot-Carteaud s.

Graham Little s.

gray platelet s.

Guillain-Barré s.

Hamman-Rich s.

hand-foot-and-mouth s.

Hare's s.

Hayem-Widal s.

hemangioma-thrombocytopenia s.

hemolytic uremic s.

hemophagocytic s.

Henoch-Schönlein s.

hereditary flat adenoma s.

Hermansky-Pudlak s.

Howel-Evans' s.

Hutchison s.

hypereosinophilic s.

hyperviscosity s.

Imerslund s.

Imerslund-Graesbeck s.

inferior s. of red nucleus

inhibitory s.

irritable bowel s.

Jadassohn-Lewandowsky s.

Kartagener's s.

Kasabach-Merritt s.

Kast's s.

syndrome *(continued)*

keratitis-ichthyosis-deafness s.

KID s.

Kimmelstiel-Wilson s.

King s.

Klinefelter's s.

Klippel-Feil s.

Kostmann's s.

Lambert-Eaton s.

Lambert-Eaton myasthenic s.

lazy leukocyte s.

Li-Fraumeni s.

linear sebaceous nevus s.

Loeffler's s.

Löfgren's s.

Lyell's s.

lymphoproliferative s's

lymphoreticular s's

Maffucci's s.

malabsorption s.

Mallory-Weiss s.

Marchiafava-Micheli s.

Marcus Gunn s.

Marfan's s.

McLeod s.

meconium aspiration s. (MES)

Meigs' s.

Meigs-Salmon s.

Mendelson's s.

Meniere's s.

Mickulicz' s.

Mikity-Wilson s.

Mikulicz s.

Milkman's s.

Minkowski-Chauffard s.

Minot-von Willebrand s.

Mosse's s.

mucosal neuroma s.

Muir-Torre s.

myasthenic s.

myelodysplastic s.

myelofibrosis-osteosclerosis s.

myeloproliferative s's

nephrotic s.

syndrome *(continued)*
- Netherton's s.
- nevoid basal cell carcinoma s.
- nevoid basalioma s.
- nonstaphylococcal scalded skin s.
- Omenn's s.
- opsoclonus-myoclonus s.
- painful bruising s.
- Pancoast's s.
- pancreatic cholera s.
- pancytopenia-dysmelia s.
- paraneoplastic s.
- Pearson's s.
- PEP s.
- Pepper s.
- Peutz-Jeghers s.
- Plummer-Vinson s.
- POEMS s.
- postirradiation s.
- postpolio s.
- Profichet's s.
- prune belly s.
- pulmonary acid aspiration s.
- reflex sympathetic dystrophy s. (RSDS)
- Reiter's s.
- Rh-null s.
- Richter's s.
- Rosenthal s.
- Rothmann-Makai s.
- Rundles-Falls s.
- Schönlein-Henoch s.
- Schultz s.
- Schwachman's s.
- Senear-Usher s.
- Senter s.
- Sézary s.
- sinus tarsi s.
- subclavian steal s.
- sudden infant death s. (SIDS)
- Sipple's s.
- Sjögren's s.
- Sneddon's s.
- spun glass hair s.

syndrome *(continued)*
- staphylococcal scalded skin s.
- Stauffer s.
- Stein-Leventhal s.
- Stevens-Johnson s.
- Stewart-Treves s.
- Sturge-Weber s.
- Sulzberger-Garbe s.
- superior sulcus tumor s.
- sweat retention s.
- Sweet's s.
- Taussig-Bing s.
- Tietze's s.
- Torre's s.
- Touraine-Solente-Golé s.
- Treacher Collins s.
- Trousseau's s.
- tumor lysis s.
- Turcot's s.
- uncombable hair s.
- unilateral nevoid telangiectasia s.
- Unna-Thost s.
- Verner-Morrison s.
- Vohwinkel's s.
- WAGR s.
- WDHA s.
- WDHH s.
- Weber-Christian s.
- Weber-Cockayne s.
- Wells' s.
- Wermer's s.
- "wet lung" s.
- Widal s.
- Willebrand's s.
- Wilson-Mikity s.
- Woringer-Kolopp s.
- yellow nail s.
- Zinsser-Cole-Engman s.

synechia *pl.* synechiae

synophridia

synophrys

synosteosis

synostosis

synovectomy
- radiation s.

synovectomy *(continued)*
  radioisotope s.

synovia

synovialoma

synovitis
  pigmented villonodular s.
  (PVNS)

synovioma
  benign s.
  malignant s.

synoviorthesis

synoviosarcoma

synovitis
  villonodular s.

syntopy

syntropic

syntropy

syphilid
  annular s.
  corymbose s.
  follicular s.
  lenticular s.
  macular s.
  maculopapular s.
  palmar s.
  papular s.
  plantar s.

syphilis

syphilitic

syphilide

syringadenoma
  s. papilliferum

syringoacanthoma

syringoadenoma

syringocarcinoma

syringocystadenoma
  s. papilliferum

syringocystoma

syringoma
  chondroid s.

syringomyelia

syrinx

syssarcosic

syssarcosis

syssarcotic

system
  AJCC s.
  Ancure Endograft S.
  BAK interbody fusion s.
  blood group s.
  Breast Imaging Reporting
    and Data S. (BIRADS)
  central nervous s. (CNS)
  dermal s.
  dermoid s.
  duplicate collecting s.
  glandular s.
  hematopoietic s.
  keratinizing s.
  lymphatic s.
  lymphoid s.
  malpighian s.
  melanocyte s.
  muscular s.
  nervous s.
  parasympathetic nervous s.
  pelvocaliceal s.
  pelvocalyceal s.
  pigmentary s.
  pyelocaliceal s.
  pyelocalyceal s.
  retroendothelial s.
  UICC s.
  vertebrobasilar s.

systema
  s. cardiovasculare
  s. conducens cordis
  s. digestorium
  s. lymphaticum
  s. lymphoideum
  s. musculare
  s. nervosum
  s. nervosum centrale

systema *(continued)*
    s. nervosum periphericum
    s. respiratorium
    s. skeletale
    s. urogenitale
    s. vasorum

systematic

systemoid

T1
T1-weighted images

T2
T2 images

T-1824

TA

table
external t. of calvaria
inner t. of frontal bone
inner t. of skull
internal t. of calvaria
outer t. of frontal bone
outer t. of skull
vitreous t.

tabula
t. externa ossis cranii
t. interna ossis cranii
t. vitrea

TACE

tache
t's bleuâtres
t's laiteuses

tachycardia
paroxysmal auricular t.
(PAT)
paroxysmal supraventricu-
lar t.
supraventricular t.

tachypnea
transient t. of the newborn

TAD
6-thioguanine, ara-C (cytarabine), and daunomycin

TAD wire

taenia *pl.* taeniae
t. choroidea
taeniae coli
t. fornicis
t. libera
t. mesocolica
t. omentalis

taenia *(continued)*
t. thalami
t. ventriculi quarti

taeniae (plural of tenia)

taenial

taeniola

tag
auricular t's
cutaneous t.
radioactive t.
skin t.

Tagamet

tagging
isotope t.

tail
t. of the breast
t. of the pancreas
t. of Spence
t. of the spleen

take-off

talc on the skin

tali (plural of talus)

talon
t. noir

talus *pl.* tali

tamoxifen citrate

tamponade
ferromagnetic t.

T antigen

tapetal

tapetum
t. corporis callosi

tapiroid

tar
coal t.

target

Tarlov's cyst

tarsometatarsal

tarsophalangeal

tarsotarsal

tarsotibial

tarsus *pl.* tarsi
    t. inferior palpebrae
    t. osseus
    t. superior palpebrae

tattooing

Taussig-Bing syndrome

taxane

Taxol

Taxotere

Tay-Sachs disease

TB
    tuberculosis

TE
    tracheoesophageal
        TE fistula

tear
    bucket-handle t.
    intimal t.
    Mallory-Weiss t.
    meniscal t.
    rotator cuff t.

teboroxime

Techneplex

TechneScan
    T. Gluceptate
    T. HDP
    T. HIDA
    T. MAA
    T. MAG3
    T. MDP
    T. PYP
    T. Sulfur Colloid

technetium
    t. 99m
    t. Tc 99m aggregated albumin

technetium *(continued)*
    t. Tc 99m albumin microspheres
    t. Tc 99m DISIDA
    t. Tc 99m DTPA
    t. Tc 99m HDP
    t. Tc 99m HSA
    t.-labeled red blood cells
    t. Tc 99m MAA
    t. Tc 99m MDP
    t. 99m pertechnetate
    t. Tc 99m pyrophosphate
    t. Tc 99m sestamibi
    t. Tc 99m sulfur colloid

technical
    t. difficulties
    t. factors

technique
    Amplatz t.
    Braasch bulb t.
    isolation-perfusion t.
    "kissing balloon" t.
    Judkins t.
    Mohs' t.
    needle-through-needle t.
    scintillation counting t.
    Seldinger t.
    Sones t.

tectorial

tectum
    t. mesencephali
    t. mesencephalicum

tegafur

tegmen *pl.* tegmina
    t. tympani
    t. ventriculi quarti

tegmental

tegmentum *pl.* tegmenta
    t. mesencephali
    t. pontis

Teichmann's crystals

tela *pl.* telae
    t. choroidea ventriculi quarti

tela *(continued)*
    t. choroidea ventriculi tertii
    t. subcutanea
    t. submucosa
    t. submucosa bronchiorum
    t. submucosa gastris
    t. submucosa intestini tenuis
    t. submucosa oesophagi
    t. submucosa pharyngis
    t. submucosa vesicae urinariae
    t. subserosa
    t. subserosa gastris
    t. subserosa hepatis
    t. subserosa intestini tenuis
    t. subserosa peritonei
    t. subserosa tubae uterinae
    t. subserosa uteri
    t. subserosa vesicae biliaris
    t. subserosa vesicae felleae
    t. subserosa vesicae urinariae

telae (plural of tela)

telangiectasia
    t. lymphatica
    t. macularis eruptiva perstans
    spider t.
    unilateral nevoid t.

telangiectasis

telar

telecord

telecurietherapy

telefluoroscopy

telencephalon

Telepaque

teleradiogram

teleradiography

teleradium

teleroentgentherapy

teletherapy

telogen

telognosis

temple

tempora

temporal

temporalis

temporoauricular

temporofrontal

temporo-occipital

temporoparietal

temporoparietalis

Tenckhoff peritoneal catheter

tenaculum

tendinitis

tendo *pl.* tendines
    t. calcaneus
    t. conjunctivus
    t. cordiformis
    t. cricooesophageus
    t. infundibuli

tendon
    biceps t.
    central t. of diaphragm
    cordiform t. of diaphragm
    flexor carpi radialis t.
    flexor pollicis longus t.
    infrapatellar t.
    infraspinatus t.
    intermediate t. of diaphragm
    t. sheath
    trefoil t.

tenia *pl.* teniae

tenial

teniposide

tenosynovitis
    nodular t.

Tensilon

tentorial

tentorium *pl.* tentoria
    ,t. cerebelli
    t. of cerebellum

teratoblastoma

teratocarcinogenesis

teratocarcinoma

teratoma *pl.* teratomas, teratomata
    benign cystic t.
    cystic t.
    immature t.
    malignant t.
    mature t.
    solid t.

teratomata (plural of teratoma)

teratomatous

teres

tergal

terminad

terminal

terminatio *pl.* terminationes

termination

terminationes (plural of terminatio)

terminology
    International Anatomical T.

tessellated

test
    acid elution t.
    acidified serum t.
    alkali denaturation t.
    Ames t.
    Apt t.
    aspirin tolerance t.
    autohemolysis t.
    Beta HCG t.

test *(continued)*
    bleeding time t.
    D-dimer t.
    Duke's t.
    euglobulin lysis t.
    Graham's t.
    Ham's t.
    hemadsorption t.
    histamine t.
    isopropanol precipitation t.
    Ivy's t.
    Kleihauer t.
    Kleihauer-Betke t.
    Linsman's water t.
    liver function t.
    osmotic fragility t.
    partial thromboplastin ti-
     me t.
    porphobilinogen t.
    prothrombin t.
    prothrombin t., one-stage
    prothrombin t., two-stage
    prothrombin consump-
     tion t.
    prothrombin time t.
    prothrombin time t., one-
     stage
    prothrombin time t., two-
     stage
    prothrombin-proconver-
     tin t.
    Quick's t.
    Russell's viper venom t.
    Schilling t.
    sestamibi stress t.
    sickling t.
    smear t.
    Stypven time t.
    sucrose hemolysis t.
    thallium stress t.
    thallium treadmill t.
    thromboplastin genera-
     tion t.
    Watson-Schwartz t.
    Whitaker t.

testes

testiculoma
    t. ovarii

testis

test meal
    motor t. m.

testicular

testis *pl.* testes

testolactone

testosterone
    t. propionate

tetiothalein sodium

tetrabromophthalein sodium

tetracaine
    t. hydrochloride

2,3,7,8-tetrachlorodibenzo-*p*-di-
    oxin

tetradecanoyl phorbol acetate

tetragonum
    t. lumbale

tetraiodophenolphthalein

tetraiodophthalein sodium

tetralogy
    t. of Fallot

tetrofosmin

tetter

6-TG (6-thioguanine)

thalamic hemorrhage

thalamus *pl.* thalami

thalassanemia

thalassemia
    α-t.
    β-t.
    δ-t.
    δβ-t.
    hemoglobin C–t.
    hemoglobin E–t.
    hemoglobin S–t.
    t. intermedia
    t. major

thalassemia *(continued)*
    t. minor
    sickle cell–t.

thallium
    t. 201
    t. stress test
    t. treadmill test

theca *pl.* thecae

thecal

thecoma

Theile's muscle

thelium

thenad

thenar

theory
    Cohnheim's t.
    dualistic t.
    hit t.
    monophyletic t.
    Planck's t.
    polyphyletic t.
    quantum t.
    Ribbert's t.
    single hit t.
    target t.
    trialistic t.
    undulatory t.
    unitarian t.
    wave t.

theque

therapy
    adjuvant t.
    anticoagulant t.
    antiplatelet t.
    beam t.
    Chaoul t.
    combined modality t.
    crossfire radiation t.
    deep roentgen-ray t.
    external beam t.
    fibrinolytic t.

therapy *(continued)*
    first line t.
    grid t.
    heparin t.
    high-voltage roentgen t.
    hormone t.
    I-131 t.
    induction t.
    light t.
    multimodality t.
    neoadjuvant t.
    photodynamic t.
    plasma t.
    preoperative t.
    presurgical t.
    PUVA t.
    radiation t.
    radium t.
    rotation t.
    steroid t.
    thrombolytic t.
    t-PA or tPA (tissue plasmin-
      ogen activator) t.
    ulcer t.
    virus-directed enzyme/
      prodrug t.

thermion

thermionics

thermocoagulation

thermogram

thermograph
    continuous scan t.

thermographic

thermography

thermomastography

thermoplacentography

thermoradiotherapy

thesaurosis

thickening
    mucosal t.
    peribronchial t.
    pericardial t.

thickening *(continued)*
    periosteal t.
    pleural t.
    skin t.

thigh

thinning

thiocarbamide

thioguanine

thiopental sodium

thiopentone

thiotepa

thiourea

Thoma
    T.-Zeiss counting cell
    T.-Zeiss counting chamber

thoracal

thoracentesis

thoraces (plural of thorax)

thoracic

thoracicoabdominal

thoracicohumeral

thoracoabdominal

thoracoacromial

thoracoplasty

thorax *pl.* thoraces
    bony t.

thorium
    t. dioxide
    sodium t. tartrate

Thorotrast

threaded screw

thread-like

threshold
    erythema t.

thrix

thrombapheresis

thrombase

thrombasthenia
   Glanzmann's t.

thrombi (plural of thrombus)

thrombin

thrombinogen

thromboasthenia

thromboclasis

thromboclastic

thrombocytapheresis

thrombocyte

thrombocythemia
   essential t.
   hemorrhagic t.
   idiopathic t.
   primary t.

thrombocytic

thrombocytocrit

thrombocytolysis

thrombocytopathia

thrombocytopathic

thrombocytopathy
   constitutional t.

thrombocytopenia
   immune t.
   neonatal t.
   neonatal alloimmune t.

thrombocytopoiesis

thrombocytopoietic

thrombocytosis
   primary t.
   reactive t.
   secondary t.

thromboelastogram

thromboelastograph

thromboelastography

thromboembolic

thromboembolus *pl.* thromboemboli

thrombogenesis

thrombogenic

α-thromboglobulin

thrombokinase

thrombokinesis

thrombokinetics

thrombolymphangitis

thrombolysis

thrombolytic

thrombomodulin

thrombon

thrombopathy

thrombopenia

thrombophlebitis

thromboplastic

thromboplastid

thromboplastin
   tissue t.

thromboplastinogen

thrombopoiesis

thrombopoietic

thrombopoietin

thrombosis
   coronary t.
   deep vein t.
   deep venous t. (DVT)
   mural t.

thrombospondin

thrombosthenin

thromboxane

thrombus *pl.* thrombi

thumb

thumbprinting

thymelcosis

thymic
    t. shadow

thymicolymphatic

thymion

thymitis

thymokesis

thymokinetic

thymolysis

thymolytic

thymoma

thymopathic

thymopathy

thymoprivic

thymoprivous

thymotoxic

thymotoxin

thymotrophic

thymus
    accessory t.
    t. persistens hyperplastica
    persistent t.

thyrohyoid

thyroiditis

thyromegaly

thyrotoxicosis

thyrotropinoma

TIA
    transient ischemic attack

tibia
    Blount's t. vara
    tibia and fibula

tibialis

tibiofemoral

tibiofibular

tibionavicular

tibiotalar

tic douloureux

Tietze's syndrome

time
    activated partial thrombo-
        plastin t.
    bleeding t.
    clot retraction t.
    clotting t.
    coagulation t.
    dead t.
    longitudinal relaxation t.
    motility t.
    one-stage prothrombin t.
    partial thromboplastin t.
    prothrombin t.
    recalcification t.
    relaxation t.
    reptilase t.
    Russell's viper venom t.
    spin-lattice relaxation t.
    spin-spin relaxation t.
    Stypven t.
    thermal relaxation t.
    thrombin t.
    thrombin clotting t.
    transit t.
    transverse relaxation t.
    T1 relaxation t.
    T2 relaxation t.

tinea
    t. amiantacea
    asbestos-like t.
    t. axillaris
    t. barbae
    t. capitis
    t. ciliorum
    t. circinata
    t. circinata tropical
    t. corporis

tinea *(continued)*
    t. cruris
    t. faciei
    t. favosa
    t. flava
    t. glabrosa
    t. imbricata
    t. manus
    t. manuum
    t. nigra
    t. pedis
    t. profunda
    t. sycosis
    t. tonsurans
    t. unguium
    t. versicolor

tinnitus

tip
    t. of the Dobbhoff tube
    t. of the endotracheal tube
    t. of the feeding tube
    mercury t. of the Dobbhoff
        tube

TIPS
    transverse intrahepatic
        portocaval shunt
            TIPS procedure

tissue
    adenoid t.
    adipose t.
    fibrofatty breast t.
    glandular t.
    granulation t.
    gut-associated lymphoid t.
    hematopoietic t.
    heterotopic t.
    lymphadenoid t.
    lymphatic t.
    lymphoid t.
    mucosa-associated lym-
        phoid t.
    paratracheal t. stripe
    prevertebral soft t's
    retropharyngeal soft t's
    soft t's
    soft t. swelling
    splenic t.

tissue *(continued)*
    subcutaneous t.
    subcutaneous fatty t.

Titterington's position

TMJ
    temporomandibular joint

toadskin

toe
    tennis t.

toenail
    ingrowing t.
    ingrown t.

Toison
    T's fluid
    T's solution

tolazoline hydrochloride

tolonium chloride

toluidine
    t. blue O
    o-t.

tomogram

tomograph

tomography
    computed t. (CT)
    computerized axial t. (CAT)
    electron beam computed t.
    high-resolution computed t.
    hypocycloidal t.
    linear t.
    positron emission t. (PET)
    single-photon emission
        computed t. (SPECT)
    spiral computed t.
    trispiral t.
    ultrasonic t.

tongs
    Crutchfield t.

tongue

tonsil
    adenoid t.
    buried t.

tonsil *(continued)*
    eustachian t.
    faucial t.
    Gerlach's t.
    intestinal t.
    lingual t.
    Luschka's t.
    pharyngeal t.
    submerged t.
    third t.
    t. of torus tubarius
    tubal t.

tonsilla *pl.* tonsillae
    t. adenoidea
    t. cerebelli
    t. intestinalis
    t. lingualis
    t. palatina
    t. pharyngea
    t. pharyngealis
    t. tubaria

tonsillar

topholipoma

tooth
    loose teeth

tophus *pl.* tophi

top normal

topogram

topographic

topographical

topography

topology

toponym

toponymy

topotecan hydrochloride

Torcon blue catheter

torcular

toremifene citrate

tori (plural of torus)

toric

torose

torous

torpedo
    Gelfoam t's

Torre's syndrome

torsion

torso

torticollis

tortuosity

tortuous

torulus *pl.* toruli
    toruli tactiles

torus *pl.* tori
    t. frontalis
    t. levatorius
    t. mandibularis
    t. occipitalis
    t. palatinus
    t. tubarius

Touraine-Solente-Golé syndrome

tourniquet
    scalp t.

Towne
    T's projection
    T's view

toxanemia

toxemia

toxemic

toxicemia

Toxicodendron

toxicohemia

toxicosis
    hemorrhagic capillary t.

toxoplasmosis

t-plasminogen activator (t-PA, tPA)

t-PA, tPA
  tissue plasminogen activator
    t-PA therapy

TPN
  total parenteral nutrition

trabecula *pl.* trabeculae
  trabeculae arachnoideae
  trabeculae carneae cordis
  trabeculae corporum cavernosorum penis
  trabeculae corporis spongiosi penis
  trabeculae lienis
  trabeculae nodi lymphatici
  trabeculae nodi lymphoidei
  t. septomarginalis
  trabeculae splenicae

trabeculae (plural of trabecula)

trabecular

trabecularism

trabeculate

trabeculation

tracer
  radioactive t.

trachea

tracheae

tracheobronchitis

tracheoesophageal (TE)

tracheopharyngeal

tracheostenosis

trachyonychia

track
  ionization t.
  metallic t. of bullet

Tracrium

tract
  aerodigestive t., upper
  biliary t.

tract *(continued)*
  bronchial t.
  fistulous t.
  gastrointestinal t.
  pulmonary outflow t.
  sinus t.
  urinary t.

traction

tractus
  t. anterolaterales
  t. bulboreticulospinalis
  t. centralis thymi
  t. corticopontinus
  t. corticospinalis anterior
  t. corticospinalis lateralis
  t. frontopontinus
  t. habenulointerpeduncularis
  t. hypothalamohypophysialis
  t. iliopubicus
  t. iliotibialis
  t. interstitiospinalis
  t. mesencephalicus nervi trigeminalis
  t. mesencephalicus nervi trigemini
  t. olfactorius
  t. olivocerebellaris
  t. olivocochlearis
  t. opticus
  t. paraventriculohypophysialis
  t. pontoreticulospinalis
  t. posterolateralis
  t. pyramidalis
  t. reticulospinalis anterior
  t. reticulospinalis ventralis
  t. rubrobulbaris
  t. rubrospinalis
  t. solitarius medullae oblongatae
  t. spinalis nervi trigeminalis
  t. spinalis nervi trigemini
  t. spinocerebellaris anterior
  t. spinocerebellaris posterior

tractus *(continued)*
    t. spinocervicalis
    t. spinoolivaris
    t. spinoreticularis
    t. spinotectalis
    t. spinothalamicus anterior
    t. spinothalamicus lateralis
    t. spiralis foraminosus
    t. supraopticohypophysi-
        alis
    t. tectobulbaris
    t. tectospinalis
    t. tegmentalis centralis
    t. trigeminothalamicus
    t. vestibulospinalis lateralis
    t. vestibulospinalis medi-
        alis

tragomaschalia

tragus *pl.* tragi

trait
    sickle cell t.
    hemoglobin C t.

tramline effect in the liver

transabdominal

transaxial

transbronchial

transcoelomic

transcrural

transducer
    ultrasound t.

transepidermal

transfer
    linear energy t.

transferrin

transfixed

transformation

transfusion
    autologous t.
    direct t.
    exchange t.

transfusion *(continued)*
    exsanguination t.
    immediate t.
    indirect t.
    mediate t.
    replacement t.
    substitution t.

transglutaminase

transhiatal

transiliac

transischiac

transition
    isobaric t.

translateral

transmigration

transmutation

transpiration

transplantation
    bone marrow t.

transposition of great vessels

transsegmental

transseptal

transversalis

transverse
    t. abdominal

transversus
    t. abdominis
    t. nuchae

trapezial

trapeziform

trapezium

Traube's semilunar space

trauma

Treacher Collins syndrome

treatment
    conservative t.
    eventration t.

treatment *(continued)*
    Goeckerman t.
    light t.
    light t.
    slush t.

tree
    biliary t.
    bronchial t.
    tracheobronchial t.

Treitz
    T's fascia
    ligament of T.

Trendelenburg position

tretinoin

triad
    Carney's t.
    Kartagener's t.
    Whipple's t.

trialism

triangle
    anal t.
    t. of auscultation
    auscultatory t.
    axillary t.
    brachial t.
    Bryant's t.
    cardiohepatic t.
    cephalic t.
    Codman's t.
    crural t.
    Elant's t.
    femoral t.
    Henke's t.
    Hesselbach's t.
    iliofemoral t.
    infraclavicular t.
    inguinal t.
    Labbé's t.
    Langenbeck's t.
    lumbar t.
    lumbar t., inferior
    lumbar t., superior
    lumbocostoabdominal t.
    Macewen's t.
    Minor's t.
    Mohrenheim's t.

triangle *(continued)*
    Petit's t.
    pubourethral t.
    Scarpa's t.
    sternocostal t.
    subinguinal t.
    suboccipital t.
    suprameatal t.
    sylvian t.
    umbilicomammillary t.

triangularis

triazene

triceps

trichiasis

trichilemmoma

trichoadenoma

trichobezoar

trichoclasia

trichoclasis

trichodiscoma

trichoepithelioma
    desmoplastic t.
    t. papillosum multiplex

trichofolliculoma

trichographism

trichohyalin

tricholemmoma

tricholeukocyte

trichology

trichomycosis
    t. axillaris
    t. nodosa
    t. nodularis

trichonodosis

trichopathic

trichopathy

trichophytic

trichophytid

trichophytosis

trichoptilosis

trichorrhexis
t. nodosa

trichoschisis

trichoscopy

trichosiderin

trichosis

trichostasis spinulosa

trichothiodystrophy

tricornute

tridermal

tridermoma

triethylenethiophosphoramide

trifurcation

trigona (plural of trigonum)

trigonal

trigone
t. of the bladder
t. of the fourth ventricle
Henke's t.
iliopectineal t.

trigonum *pl.* trigona
t. auscultationis
t. caroticum
t. cervicale anterius
t. cervicale posterius
t. clavipectorale
t. collaterale ventriculi lateralis
t. colli anterius
t. colli laterale
t. coracoacromiale
t. deltoideopectorale
t. deltopectorale
t. femorale
t. femoris
t. fibrosum dextrum cordis
t. fibrosum sinistrum cordis

trigonum *(continued)*
t. habenulae
t. habenulare
t. hypoglossale
t. inguinale
t. lemnisci lateralis
t. lumbale inferius
t. lumbale superius
t. lumbare
t. lumbare [Petiti]
t. lumbocostale
t. musculare
t. nervi hypoglossi
t. nervi vagi
t. olfactorium
t. omoclaviculare
t. omotracheale
t. sternocostale
t. submandibulare
t. submentale
t. vagale
t. vesicae
t. vesicae [Lieutaudi]

triiodoethionic acid

trilobate

trilobed

trilocular

TR images

trimester

trimethylene

trimetrexate

tripartite

triptorelin

triquetral

triquetrum

triradial

triradiate

triradiation

tris

tris(2,3-dibromopropyl) phosphate

trisegmentectomy
    right t.

trisplanchnic

trisulcate

tritium

trizonal

TRND
    transient respiratory distress of the newborn

trochanter
    greater t.
    lesser t.
    t. major
    t. minor
    t. tertius

trochlea
    t. fibularis calcanei
    t. humeri
    t. muscularis
    t. musculi obliqui superioris bulbi
    t. musculi obliqui superioris oculi
    peroneal t. of calcaneus
    t. peronealis calcanei
    t. phalangis manus
    t. phalangis pedis
    t. tali

trochlear

trochleariform

trochlearis

trochoid

Troisier
    T's ganglion
    T's node
    T's sign

trombiculiasis

trombiculidiasis

trombidiiasis

trombidiosis

Tronothane

trough

Trousseau's syndrome

Tru-Cut needle

truncal

truncation

truncus *pl.* trunci
    t. brachiocephalicus
    t. bronchomediastinalis
    t. coeliacus
    t. corporis callosi
    t. costocervicalis
    t. encephali
    t. encephalicus
    t. inferior plexus brachialis
    trunci intestinales
    t. jugularis
    t. linguofacialis
    t. lumbalis
    t. lumbaris
    t. lumbosacralis
    trunci lymphatici
    t. medius plexus brachialis
    t. nervi accessorii
    t. nervi spinalis
    trunci plexus brachialis
    t. pulmonalis
    t. subclavius
    t. superior plexus brachialis
    t. sympatheticus
    t. sympathicus
    t. thyrocervicalis
    t. vagalis anterior
    t. vagalis posterior

trunk
    bronchomediastinal t.
    intestinal t's
    jugular t.
    lumbar t.
    lymphatic t's
    subclavian t.

trypanid

trypanosomid

T-shaped

T-tube cholangiogram

tuba *pl.* tubae
    t. auditiva
    t. auditoria
    t. uterina

tubal

tube
    Cantor t.
    Celestin's t.
    Chaoul t.
    chest t.
    Coolidge t.
    Dennis t.
    Dobbhoff t.
    endotracheal t.
    eustachian t.
    feeding t.
    gastrostomy t.
    Herring t.
    hot-cathode t.
    Levine t.
    mediastinal drainage t.
    metallic distal end of t.
    Miller-Abbott t.
    Minnesota t.
    nasogastric (NG) t.
    Olshevsky t.
    photomultiplier t.
    Salem sump t.
    suction t.
    thoracostomy t.
    tracheostomy t.
    U-t.
    Westergren t.
    Wintrobe hematocrit t.
    x-ray t.
    Y-t.

tuber *pl.* tubera
    t. calcanei
    t. cinereum
    t. frontale
    t. ischiadicum
    t. ischiale
    t. maxillae
    t. maxillare

tuber *(continued)*
    maxillary t.
    t. omentale hepatis
    t. omentale corporis pancreatis
    t. parietale
    t. vermis
    t. zygomaticum

tubera (plural of tuber)

tubercle
    anatomical t.
    articular t. of temporal bone
    Farre's t's
    jugular t. of occipital bone
    postglenoid t.
    t. of root of zygoma
    tibial t.
    zygomatic t.
    t. of zygomatic arch

tubercula

tuberculate

tuberculated

tuberculid
    micronodular t.
    papulonecrotic t.
    rosacea-like t.

tuberculoderma

tuberculosis (TB)
    t. cutis
    t. cutis indurativa
    t. cutis lichenoides
    t. cutis miliaris disseminata
    t. indurativa
    t. lichenoides
    t. miliaris disseminata (miliary tuberculosis)
    papulonecrotic t.
    pulmonary t.
    t. of skin
    t. verrucosa cutis
    warty t.

tuberculum *pl.* tubercula
    t. adductorium femoris
    t. anterius atlantis

tuberculum *(continued)*
  t. anterius thalami
  t. anterius vertebrae cervi-
    calis
  t. articulare ossis temporalis
  t. auriculae
  t. auriculare
  t. calcanei
  t. conoideum
  t. corniculatum
  t. corniculatum [Santorini]
  t. costae
  t. cuneatum
  t. cuneiforme
  t. cuneiforme [Wrisbergi]
  t. dorsale radii
  t. epiglotticum
  t. gracile
  t. iliacum
  t. infraglenoidale
  t. intercondylare laterale
  t. intercondylare mediale
  t. intervenosum
  t. jugulare ossis occipitalis
  t. labii superioris
  t. laterale processus pos-
    terioris tali
  t. majus humeri
  t. marginale ossis zygoma-
    tici
  t. mediale processus pos-
    terioris tali
  t. minus humeri
  t. musculi scaleni anterioris
  t. obturatorium anterius
  t. obturatorium posterius
  t. ossis scaphoidei
  t. ossis trapezii
  t. pharyngeum
  t. posterius atlantis
  t. posterius vertebrae cer-
    vicalis
  t. pubicum ossis pubis
  t. quadratum femoris
  t. sellae turcicae
  t. supraglenoidale
  t. supratragicum
  t. thyroideum inferius

tuberculum *(continued)*
  t. thyroideum superius
  t. trigeminale

tuberositas *pl.* tuberositates
  t. deltoidea humeri
  t. glutea femoris
  t. iliaca
  t. ligamenti coracoclavicu-
    laris
  t. musculi serrati anterioris
  t. ossis cuboidei
  t. ossis metatarsalis primi
  t. ossis metatarsalis quinti
  t. ossis navicularis
  t. ossis sacri
  t. phalangis distalis manus
  t. phalangis distalis pedis
  t. pronatoria
  t. radii
  t. tibiae
  t. ulnae

tuberositates (plural of tuberositas)

tuberosity
  bicipital t.
  iliac t.
  ischial t.
  malar t.
  pyramidal t. of palatine
    bone
  radial t.
  tibial t.

tubi (plural of tubus)

tubing
  dialysis t.
  polyethylene t.
  Silastic t.
  ventriculoperitoneal (VP)
    shunt t.

tubular

tubule
  discharging t's

tubuli (plural of tubulus)

tubuloacinar

tubulosaccular

tubulous

tubulus *pl.* tubuli
    tubuli seminiferi contorti
    tubuli seminiferi recti

tubus *pl.* tubi

tuft
    hair t's
    ungual t.

tumefaction

tumeur
    t. perlée

tumor
    Abrikosov's (Abrikos-
      soff's) t.
    acinar cell t.
    acinic cell t.
    adenoid t.
    adenomatoid t.
    adenomatoid odontogen-
      ic t.
    adipose t.
    adrenal t.
    adrenal rest t.
    aldosterone-producing t.
    aldosterone-secreting t.
    alveolar cell t.
    ameloblastic adenoma-
      toid t.
    aniline t.
    Askin's t.
    benign t.
    benign epithelial odonto-
      genic t.
    Brenner t.
    bronchial carcinoid t.
    Brooke's t.
    brown t.
    Burkitt's t.
    Buschke-Löwenstein t.
    calcifying epithelial odonto-
      genic t.
    carcinoid t.

tumor *(continued)*
    carcinoid t. of bronchus
    carcinoma ex mixed t.
    carotid body t.
    cartilaginous t.
    cellular t.
    chromaffin cell t.
    clear cell odontogenic t.
    Codman's t.
    collision t.
    colloid t.
    connective-tissue t.
    corticotrope t.
    corticotroph t.
    craniopharyngeal duct t.
    cystic t.
    dermal analogue t.
    dermal duct t.
    dermoid t.
    desmoid t.
    diarrheogenic t.
    dumbbell t.
    eighth nerve t.
    embryonal t.
    embryoplastic t.
    endodermal sinus t.
    epidermoid t.
    Ewing's t.
    fatty t.
    feminizing t.
    fibrocellular t.
    fibrohistiocytic t.
    fibroid t.
    fibroplastic t.
    t. of follicular infundibulum
    functional t.
    functioning t.
    gelatinous t.
    germ cell t.
    giant cell t.
    giant cell t. of bone
    giant cell t. of tendon
      sheath
    glomus t.
    glomus jugulare t.
    glomus tympanicum t.
    glomus vagale t.
    gonadal stromal t.

tumor *(continued)*
 granular cell t.
 granulosa t.
 granulosa cell t.
 granulosa-theca cell t.
 Grawitz's t.
 heterologous t.
 heterotypic t.
 histioid t.
 homoiotypic t.
 homologous t.
 hourglass t.
 Hürthle cell t.
 innocent t.
 interstitial cell t.
 intracranial t.
 intramural t.
 islet cell t.
 ivory-like t.
 juxtaglomerular t.
 juxtaglomerular cell t.
 Klatskin's t.
 Koenen's t.
 Krukenberg's t.
 Leydig cell t.
 Lindau's t.
 lipoid cell t. of ovary
 luteinized granulosa-theca cell t.
 malignant t.
 margaroid t.
 melanotic neuroectodermal t.
 Merkel cell t.
 mesodermal mixed t.
 mixed t.
 mixed t., benign
 mixed t., malignant
 mixed t. of skin
 mucoepidermoid t.
 mucous t.
 müllerian mixed t.
 muscular t.
 Nélaton's t.
 nerve sheath t.
 neuroectodermal t. of infancy

tumor *(continued)*
 neuroendocrine t.
 neuroendocrine cell t.
 neuroepithelial t.
 nonfunctional t.
 nonfunctioning t.
 t. of Oddi
 odontogenic t.
 organoid t.
 oxyphil cell t.
 Pancoast's t.
 papillary t.
 papillary cystic t. of pancreas
 pearl t.
 pearly t.
 Pepper t.
 peripheral neuroectodermal t.
 phyllodes t.
 Pindborg t.
 pineal t.
 plasma cell t.
 potato t.
 premalignant fibroepithelial t.
 primary t.
 primitive neuroectodermal t.
 primitive neuroepithelial t.
 prolactin-secreting t.
 proliferating trichilemmal t.
 pulmonary sulcus t.
 Rathke's t.
 Rathke's pouch t.
 Recklinghausen's t.
 Regaud's t.
 retinal anlage t.
 rhabdoid t. of the kidney
 sand t.
 Schmincke's t.
 scrotal t.
 Schwann cell t.
 serous borderline t.
 Sertoli cell t.
 Sertoli-Leydig cell t.
 sex cord–stromal t's

tumor *(continued)*
 sheath t.
 solid-cystic t. of pancreas
 solid pseudopapillary t. of pancreas
 solitary fibrous t.
 squamous odontogenic t.
 stromal t's
 superior sulcus t.
 teratoid t.
 testicular t.
 theca cell t.
 thyrotrope t.
 thyrotroph t.
 tomato t.
 tridermic t.
 turban t.
 vascular t.
 villous t.
 virilizing t.
 Warthin's t.
 Wilms' t.
 yolk sac t.

tumoraffin

tumoricidal

tumorigenesis

tumorigenic

tumorlet

tumorous

tungiasis

tunic

tunica *pl.* tunicae
 t. adventitia
 t. adventitia ductus deferentis
 t. adventitia glandulae seminalis
 t. adventitia glandulae vesiculosae
 t. adventitia oesophagi
 t. adventitia ureteris

tunica *(continued)*
 t. adventitia vesiculae seminalis
 t. albuginea
 t. albuginea corporum cavernosorum
 t. albuginea corporis spongiosi
 t. albuginea ovarii
 t. albuginea testis
 t. conjunctiva
 t. conjunctiva bulbaris
 t. conjunctiva bulbi
 t. conjunctiva palpebrarum
 t. conjunctiva palpebralis
 t. dartos
 t. externa vasorum
 t. fibrosa
 t. fibrosa bulbi
 t. fibrosa hepatis
 t. fibrosa lienis
 t. fibrosa splenis
 t. interna bulbi
 t. intima vasorum
 t. media vasorum
 t. mucosa
 t. mucosa bronchiorum
 t. mucosa cavitatis tympanicae
 t. mucosa ductus deferentis
 t. mucosa glandulae seminalis
 t. mucosa glandulae vesiculosae
 t. mucosa intestini crassi
 t. mucosa intestini tenuis
 t. mucosa laryngis
 t. mucosa linguae
 t. mucosa nasi
 t. mucosa oesophagi
 t. mucosa oris
 t. mucosa pharyngis
 t. mucosa tracheae
 t. mucosa tubae auditivae
 t. mucosa tubae auditoriae
 t. mucosa tubae uterinae
 t. mucosa ureteris

tunica *(continued)*
   t. mucosa urethrae femini-
      nae
   t. mucosa urethrae mulie-
      bris
   t. mucosa uteri
   t. mucosa vaginae
   t. mucosa ventriculi
   t. mucosa vesicae biliaris
   t. mucosa vesicae felleae
   t. mucosa vesicae urinariae
   t. mucosa vesiculae semin-
      alis
   t. muscularis
   t. muscularis coli
   t. muscularis ductus defer-
      entis
   t. muscularis gastris
   t. muscularis glandulae
      seminalis
   t. muscularis glandulae ves-
      iculosae
   t. muscularis intestini ten-
      uis
   t. muscularis oesophagi
   t. muscularis pharyngis
   t. muscularis recti
   t. muscularis tubae uteri-
      nae
   t. muscularis ureteris
   t. muscularis urethrae femi-
      ninae
   t. muscularis urethrae mu-
      liebris
   t. muscularis uteri
   t. muscularis vaginae
   t. muscularis vesicae bil-
      iaris
   t. muscularis vesicae fel-
      leae
   t. muscularis vesicae uri-
      nariae
   t. muscularis vesiculae
      seminalis
   t. propria
   t. propria corii
   t. serosa
   t. serosa gastris

tunica *(continued)*
   t. serosa hepatis
   t. serosa intestini crassi
   t. serosa intestini tenuis
   t. serosa lienis
   t. serosa peritonei
   t. serosa splenis
   t. serosa tubae uterinae
   t. serosa uteri
   t. serosa ventriculi
   t. serosa vesicae biliaris
   t. serosa vesicae felleae
   t. serosa vesicae urinariae
   t. spongiosa urethrae femi-
      ninae
   t. spongiosa vaginae
   t. vaginalis testis
   t. vasculosa
   t. vasculosa bulbi

tunicary

tunicate

TUR
   transurethral resection

tunnel

turban
   ice t.

turbinate
   nasal t's

turnover
   erythrocyte iron t.
   plasma iron t.
   red blood cell iron t.

tutamen

twig

tyloma

tylosis
   t. palmaris et plantaris

tylotic

tympanoplasty

tympanosquamosal

typing
  t. of blood

type
  blood t.

tyropanoate sodium

Tzanck smear

ulcer
    amebic u.
    burrowing phagedenic u.
    Buruli u.
    chrome u.
    collar-button u's
    Curling's u.
    decubital u.
    decubitus u.
    diphtheritic u.
    duodenal u.
    healed gastric u.
    healing u.
    Jacob's u.
    lupoid u.
    Marjolin's u.
    Meleney's u.
    Meleney's chronic under-
       mining u.
    u. niche
    penetrating u.
    penetrating u. of foot
    perambulating u.
    perforated u.
    phagedenic u.
    plantar u.
    prepyloric u.
    pressure u.
    rodent u.
    ruptured u.
    sloughing u.
    tanner's u.
    u. therapy
    undermining burrowing u.
    varicose u.

ulceration
    marginal u.
    mucosal u.

ulcus
    u. ambulans
    u. interdigitale

ulerythema
    u. ophryogenes

ulna

ulnaris

Ultane

Ultiva

ultrasonic

ultrasonics

ultrasonogram

ultrasonographic

ultrasonography
    Doppler u.
    duplex u.
    Doppler u., continuous
       wave
    Doppler u., pulsed wave
    endorectal u.
    endoscopic u.
    gray-scale u.
    intravascular u.
    real-time u.

ultrasonometry

ultrasound
    graded-compression u.
    gray-scale u.

UltraTag RBC

ultraviolet
    u. A
    u. B
    u. C

Ultravist

umbauzonen

umbilical

umbilicate

umbilicated

umbilication

umbilicus

umbo *pl.* umbones
    u. membranae tympani
    u. membranae tympanicae

umbonate

umbones (plural of umbo)

umbra

umbrella-shaped

unci (plural of uncus)

unciform

uncoiling of the aorta

unco-ossified

uncovertebral

uncus *pl.* unci
    u. corporis vertebrae cervi-
       calis

undifferentiated

undifferentiation

ungual

unguis *pl.* ungues
    u. incarnatus

uniaxial

unibasal

unicameral

unicentral

unicentric

unicornous

uniglandular

unilateral

unilobar

unilocular

union
    fibrous u.
    osseous u.
    non-bony u. (frequently
       dictated for "bony nonun-
       ion")

uniseptate

unit
    Behnken's u.

unit *(continued)*
    Bethesda u.
    burst-forming u.–erythroid
    C-arm fluoroscopic u.
    colony-forming u.
    colony-forming u.–culture
    colony-forming u.–ery-
       throid
    colony-forming u.–granulo-
       cyte-macrophage
    colony-forming u.–spleen
    Hampson u.
    Hounsfield u.
    Kienböck u.
    pilosebaceous u.
    pressor u.
    x-ray u.

Unna
    U's boot
    U's nevus
    U's paste boot
    U.-Thost disease
    U.-Thost syndrome

unsharpness

unstriated

u-plasminogen activator

UPJ
    ureteropelvic junction

upright compression spot films

upsiloid

uptake
    heterogeneous u.
    increased isotope u.
    isotope u.
    RAI (radioactive iodine) u.
    thyroid u.

urceiform

urceolate

ureter
    bifid u.

ureterectasis

ureterocele

ureterogram

ureterography

ureterolithiasis

ureteropyelography

urethra
  u. feminina
  u. masculina

urethral

urethrocystogram

urethrocystography

urethrography

urhidrosis
  u. crystallina

uric acid level

urinate

urine

urinidrosis

urinogenital

urinosexual

uroanthelone

uroenterone

urogenital

Urografin

urogram
  excretory u.

urography
  ascending u.
  cystoscopic u.
  descending u.
  excretion u.
  excretory u.
  intravenous u.
  oral u.
  retrograde u.

urokinase

uropathy
  obstructive u.

uropod

uroradiology

urticant

urticaria
  acute u.
  aquagenic u.
  u. bullosa
  bullous u.
  cholinergic u.
  chronic u.
  cold u.
  colonic u.
  contact u.
  giant u.
  heat u.
  light u.
  u. medicamentosa
  u. multiformis endemica
  papular u.
  u. pigmentosa
  pressure u.
  solar u.
  u. solaris

urticarial

urticariogenic

urticarious

urticate

urtication

uteri (plural of uterus)

uterography

uterosacral

uterosalpingography

uterotubography

uterus *pl.* uteri
  anteflexed u.
  anteverted u.
  bicornuate u.
  fibroid u.
  fundus of the u.
  gravid u.

uterus *(continued)*
   retroflexed u.
   retroverted u.

UTI
   urinary tract infection

utilization
   red cell u.

utricular

utriculi

utriculus
   u. prostaticus

utriform

U-tube

uviform

UVJ
   ureterovesical junction

uvula
   u. palatina
   u. vermis
   u. vesicae

VAC
  vincristine, dactinomycin,
  and cyclophosphamide

vaccine
  BCG v.

vagina *pl.* vaginae
  v. bulbi
  v. carotica fasciae cervi-
    calis
  v. communis musculorum
    flexorum
  v. communis tendinum
    musculorum fibularium
  v. communis tendinum
    musculorum peroneorum
  v. externa nervi optici
  v. fibrosa
  vaginae fibrosae digitorum
    manus
  vaginae fibrosae digitorum
    pedis
  v. interna nervi optici
  v. musculi recti abdominis
  v. plantaris tendinis mus-
    culi fibularis longi
  v. plantaris tendinis mus-
    culi peronei longi
  v. processus styloidei
  v. synovialis
  vaginae synoviales digito-
    rum manus
  vaginae synoviales digito-
    rum pedis
  v. synovialis intertubercu-
    laris
  v. synovialis tendinis
  v. tendinis
  vaginae tendinum digito-
    rum pedis
  v. tendinum musculorum
    abductoris longi et exten-
    soris pollicis brevis
  v. tendinum musculorum
    extensorum carpi radi-
    alium
  v. tendinis musculi exten-
    soris carpi ulnaris

vagina *(continued)*
  v. tendinum musculorum
    extensoris digitorum et
    extensoris indicis
  v. tendinis musculi exten-
    soris digiti minmimi
  vaginae tendinum musculi
    extensoris digitorum longi
    pedis
  v. tendinis musculi exten-
    soris hallucis longi
  v. tendinis musculi exten-
    soris pollicis longi
  v. tendinis musculi flexoris
    carpi radialis
  vaginae tendinum musculi
    flexoris digitorum longi
    pedis
  v. tendinis musculi flexoris
    hallucis longi
  v. tendinis musculi flexoris
    pollicis longi
  v. tendinis musculi obliqui
    superioris
  v. tendinis musculi tibialis
    anterioris
  v. tendinis musculi tibialis
    posterioris

vaginae (plural of vagina)

vaginal

vaginate

vaginogram

vaginography

vagotomy
  medical v.

vallate

vallecula *pl.* valleculae
  v. cerebelli
  v. epiglottica
  v. for petrosal ganglion
  v. unguis

vallecular

vallum
  v. unguis

Valsalva maneuver

valva *pl.* valvae
  v. aortae
  v. atrioventricularis dextra
  v. atrioventricularis sinistra
  v. mitralis
  v. tricuspidalis
  v. trunci pulmonalis

valval

valvar

valvate

valve
  aortic v.
  v. of Heister
  ileocecal v.
  incompetent v.
  lymphatic v.
  prolapsed mitral v.
  prosthetic v.

valved

valviform

valvula *pl.* valvulae
  valvulae anales
  valvulae conniventes
  v. coronaria dextra valvae
    aortae
  v. coronaria sinistra valvae
    aortae
  v. non coronaria valvae
    aortae
  v. foraminis ovalis
  v. fossae navicularis
  v. lymphaticum
  v. semilunaris anterior val-
    vae trunci pulmonalis
  v. semilunaris dextra val-
    vae aortae
  v. semilunaris dextra val-
    vae trunci pulmonalis
  v. semilunaris posterior
    valvae aortae

valvula *(continued)*
  v. semilunaris sinistra val-
    vae aortae
  v. semilunaris sinistra val-
    vae trunci pulmonalis
  v. sinus coronarii
  v. venae cavae inferioris
  v. venosa

valvulae (plural of valvula)

valvular

valvule

VAMP
  vincristine, methotrexate,
    6-mercaptopurine, and
    prednisone

Van Hoorne's canal

vanillism

van Sonnenberg sump *(pro-
  nounced* "von")

Vaquez
  V's disease
  V.-Osler disease

variant
  normal v.

variation
  developmental v.

varication

variceal

varices (plural of varix)

variciform

varicocele

varicography

varicoid

varicose

varicosity

varix *pl.* varices
  esophageal varices
  lymph v.

varix *(continued)*
    v. lymphaticus

vas *pl.* vasa
    vasa afferentia
    vasa afferentia lymphoglan-
        dulae
    vasa afferentia nodi lym-
        phatici
    v. anastomoticum
    v. capillare
    v. collaterale
    v. deferens
    vasa efferentia
    vasa efferentia lymphoglan-
        dulae
    vasa efferentia nodi lym-
        phatici
    vasa lymphatica
    v. lymphaticum profundum
    v. lymphaticum superficiale
    v. lymphocapillare
    vasa nervorum
    v. prominens ductus coch-
        learis
    vasa recta renis
    vasa sanguinea auris inter-
        nae
    vasa sanguinea retinae
    v. sinusoideum
    v. spirale
    vasa vasorum

vasa (plural of vas)

vasal

Vascoray

vascular

vascularity
    increased v.

vascularization

vasculature

vasodilation

vasculitis
    hypocomplementemic v.
    urticarial v.

vasculolymphatic

vasculum

vasiform

vasoepididymography

vasography

vasospasm

Vater's fold

vault
    cranial v.

vecuronium bromide

vegetation
    dendritic v.

veil

vein
    antecubital v.
    azygos v.
    azygous v.
    basilic v.
    cephalic v.
    deep v. thrombosis
    draining v.
    inferior mesenteric v.
    innominate v.
    jugular v.
    peroneal v.
    petrosal v.
    portal v.
    renal v.
    saphenous v.
    scalp v.
    subclavian v.
    varicose v's
    v. of Galen
    vermian v's

Vel blood group

velamen

velamenta

velamentous

velamentum

velar

Velban

veliform

vellus

velum *pl.* vela
  v. medullare inferius
  v. medullare posterius
  v. medullare rostralis
  v. medullare superius
  v. palatinum

vena *pl.* venae
  v. anastomotica inferior
  v. anastomotica superior
  v. angularis
  venae anteriores cerebri
  v. anterior lobi superioris
    pulmonis dextri
  v. anterior lobi superioris
    pulmonis sinistri
  v. anterior septi pellucidi
  v. apicalis lobi superioris
    pulmonis dextri
  v. apicoposterior lobi supe-
    rioris pulmonis sinistri
  v. appendicularis
  v. aqueductus cochleae
  v. aqueductus vestibuli
  venae arciformes renis
  venae arcuatae renis
  venae articulares
  venae atriales dextrae
  venae atriales sinistrae
  venae atrioventriculares
    cordis
  venae auriculares ante-
    riores
  v. auricularis posterior
  v. axillaris
  v. azygos
  v. basalis
  v. basalis anterior
  v. basalis communis
  v. basalis inferior

vena *(continued)*
  v. basalis superior
  v. basilica
  venae basivertebrales
  venae brachiales
  v. brachiocephalica
  venae bronchiales
  v. bulbi penis
  v. bulbi vestibuli
  v. canalis pterygoidei
  v. cardiaca magna
  v. cardiaca media
  venae cardiacae minimae
  v. cardiaca parva
  v. cava inferior
  v. cava superior
  venae cavernosae penis
  v. centralis glandulae su-
    prarenalis
  venae centrales hepatis
  v. centralis retinae
  v. cephalica
  v. cephalica accessoria
  venae cerebelli
  v. cervicalis profunda
  v. choroidea inferior
  v. choroidea superior
  venae ciliares
  venae circumflexae femoris
    laterales
  venae circumflexae femoris
    mediales
  v. circumflexa ilium pro-
    funda
  v. circumflexa ilium superfi-
    cialis
  v. circumflexa superficialis
    ilium
  v. colica dextra
  v. colica intermedia
  v. colica media
  v. colica sinistra
  venae columnae vertebralis
  v. comitans
  v. comitans nervi hypo-
    glossi
  venae conjunctivales
  venae cordis
  v. cordis magna

vena *(continued)*
  v. cordis media
  venae cordis minimae
  v. cordis parva
  v. cutanea
  v. cystica
  venae digitales dorsales pedis
  venae digitales palmares
  venae digitales plantares
  venae diploicae
  v. diploica frontalis
  v. diploica occipitalis
  v. diploica temporalis anterior
  v. diploica temporalis posterior
  venae directae laterales
  v. dorsalis corporis callosi
  venae dorsales linguae
  v. dorsalis profunda clitoridis
  v. dorsalis profunda penis
  venae dorsales superficiales clitoridis
  venae dorsales superficiales penis
  v. emissaria
  v. emissaria condylaris
  v. emissaria condyloidea
  v. emissaria mastoidea
  v. emissaria occipitalis
  v. emissaria parietalis
  venae encephali
  v. epigastrica inferior
  v. epigastrica superficialis
  venae epigastricae superiores
  venae episclerales
  venae ethmoidales
  v. facialis
  v. femoralis
  venae fibulares
  venae frontales
  venae gastricae breves
  v. gastrica dextra
  v. gastrica sinistra
  v. gastroepiploica dextra
  v. gastroepiploica sinistra

vena *(continued)*
  v. gastroomentalis dextra
  v. gastroomentalis sinistra
  venae geniculares
  venae genus
  venae gluteae inferiores
  venae gluteae superiores
  v. gyri olfactorii
  v. hemiazygos
  v. hemiazygos accessoria
  venae hepaticae
  venae hepaticae dextrae
  venae hepaticae intermediae
  venae hepaticae sinistrae
  venae ileales
  v. ileocolica
  v. iliaca communis
  v. iliaca externa
  v. iliaca interna
  v. iliolumbalis
  inferior v. cava
  venae inferiores cerebri
  venae inferiores cerebelli
  v. inferior vermis
  venae insulares
  venae intercapitulares manus
  venae intercapitulares pedis
  venae intercostales anteriores
  venae intercostales posteriores
  v. intercostalis superior dextra
  v. intercostalis superior sinistra
  v. intercostalis suprema
  venae interlobares renis
  venae interlobulares hepatis
  venae interlobulares renis
  v. mediana antebrachii
  v. mediana cubiti
  venae internae cerebri
  venae interosseae anteriores

vena *(continued)*
  venae interosseae poster-
    iores
  v. interventricularis ante-
    rior
  v. interventricularis poste-
    rior
  v. intervertebralis
  venae jejunales
  v. jugularis anterior
  v. jugularis externa
  v. jugularis interna
  venae labiales anteriores
  venae labiales inferiores
  venae labiales posteriores
  v. labialis superior
  venae labyrinthinae
  venae labyrinthi
  v. lacrimalis
  v. laryngea inferior
  v. laryngea superior
  v. lateralis ventriculi latera-
    lis
  v. lingularis
  v. lingualis
  v. lobi medii pulmonis dex-
    tri
  venae lumbales
  v. lumbalis ascendens
  v. magna cerebri
  v. marginalis dextra
  v. marginalis lateralis
  v. marginalis medialis
  venae maxillares
  v. media profunda cerebri
  v. media superficialis cere-
    bri
  v. medialis ventriculi later-
    alis
  venae mediastinales
  venae medullae oblongatae
  venae membri inferioris
  venae membri superioris
  venae meningeae
  venae meningeae mediae
  v. mesenterica inferior
  v. mesenterica superior
  venae metacarpales dor-
    sales

vena *(continued)*
  venae metacarpales palma-
    res
  venae metatarsales dor-
    sales
  venae metatarsales planta-
    res
  venae musculophrenicae
  venae nasales externae
  v. nasofrontalis
  venae nuclei caudati
  v. obliqua atrii sinistri
  venae obturatoriae
  venae occipitales
  v. occipitalis
  venae oesophageales
  v. ophthalmica inferior
  v. ophthalmica superior
  venae orbitae
  v. ovarica dextra
  v. ovarica sinistra
  v. palatina externa
  venae palpebrales
  venae palpebrales infe-
    riores
  venae palpebrales supe-
    riores
  venae pancreaticae
  venae pancreaticoduodena-
    les
  venae paraumbilicales
  venae parietales
  venae parotideae
  venae pectorales
  venae pedunculares
  venae perforantes
  venae pericardiacophreni-
    cae
  venae pericardiacae
  venae peroneae
  v. petrosa
  venae pharyngeae
  venae pharyngeales
  venae phrenicae inferiores
  venae phrenicae superiores
  venae pontis
  v. pontomesencephalica
    anterior
  v. poplitea

vena *(continued)*
    v. portae hepatis
    v. portalis hepatis
    venae portales hypophysiales
    venae portales hypophysiales
    v. posterior corporis callosi
    v. posterior lobi superioris pulmonis dextri
    v. posterior septi pellucidi
    v. precentralis cerebelli
    venae prefrontales
    v. prepylorica
    v. profunda
    venae profundae cerebri
    venae profundae clitoridis
    v. profunda facialis
    v. profunda faciei
    v. profunda femoris
    v. profunda linguae
    venae profundae membri inferioris
    venae profundae membri superioris
    venae profundae penis
    venae pudendae externae
    v. pudenda interna
    venae pulmonales
    v. pulmonalis dextra inferior
    v. pulmonalis dextra superior
    v. pulmonalis sinistra inferior
    v. pulmonalis sinistra superior
    venae radiales
    v. recessus lateralis ventriculi quarti
    venae rectales inferiores
    venae rectales mediae
    v. rectalis superior
    venae renis
    venae renales
    v. retromandibularis
    venae sacrales laterales
    v. sacralis mediana

vena *(continued)*
    v. saphena accessoria
    v. saphena magna
    v. saphena parva
    v. scapularis dorsalis
    venae sclerales
    venae scrotales anteriores
    venae scrotales posteriores
    venae sigmoideae
    venae spinales anteriores
    venae spinales posteriores
    v. splenica
    venae stellatae renis
    v. sternocleidomastoidea
    v. stylomastoidea
    v. subclavia
    v. subcostalis
    venae subcutaneae abdominis
    v. sublingualis
    v. submentalis
    v. superficialis
    venae superficiales cerebri
    venae superficiales membri inferioris
    venae superficiales membri superioris
    venae superiores cerebelli
    venae superiores cerebri
    v. superior lobi inferioris pulmonis dextri
    v. superior lobi inferioris pulmonis sinistri
    v. superior vermis
    v. supraorbitalis
    v. suprarenalis dextra
    v. suprarenalis sinistra
    v. suprascapularis
    venae supratrochleares
    venae surales
    v. temporalis media
    venae temporales profundae
    venae temporales superficiales
    v. terminalis
    v. testicularis dextra
    v. testicularis sinistra

vena *(continued)*
    venae thalamostriatae inferiores
    v. thalamostriata superior
    venae thoracicae internae
    v. thoracica lateralis
    v. thoracoacromialis
    venae thoracoepigastricae
    venae thymicae
    v. thyroidea inferioris
    venae thyroideae mediae
    v. thyroidea superior
    venae tibiales anteriores
    venae tibiales posteriores
    venae tracheales
    venae transversae cervicis
    venae transversae colli
    v. transversa facialis
    v. transversa faciei
    venae trunci encephalici
    venae tympanicae
    venae ulnares
    v. umbilicalis
    v. uncalis
    venae uterinae
    venae ventriculares cordis
    v. ventricularis inferior
    venae ventriculi dextri anteriores
    v. ventriculi sinistri posterior
    v. vertebralis
    v. vertebralis accessoria
    v. vertebralis anterior
    venae vesicales
    venae vestibulares
    venae vorticosae

venacavogram
    inferior v.

venacavography

venae (plural of vena)

venepuncture

venesection

venogram

venography
    intraosseous v.

venography *(continued)*
    portal v.
    splenic v.

venom
    Russell's viper v.

vent

venter
    v. anterior musculi digastrici
    v. frontalis musculi occipitofrontalis
    v. inferior musculi omohyoidei
    v. occipitalis musculi occipitofrontalis
    v. posterior musculi digastrici
    v. superior musculi omohyoidei

ventilation
    high-frequency v.
    v. and perfusion lung scans

ventilator

ventrad

ventral

ventralis

ventralward

ventricle
    fourth v.
    lateral v.
    third v.

ventricose

ventricular

ventricular system and brain substance

ventriculi (plural of ventriculus)

ventriculogram

ventriculography
    first pass v.
    gated blood pool v.

ventriculography *(continued)*
   left v.
   radionuclide v.

ventriculus *pl.* ventriculi
   v. cordis dexter/sinister
   v. dexter cordis
   v. laryngis
   v. laryngis [Morgagnii]
   v. lateralis cerebri
   v. quartus cerebri
   v. sinister cordis
   v. terminalis medullae spinalis
   v. tertius cerebri

ventricumbent

ventriduct

ventriduction

ventriflexion

ventrimesal

ventrimeson

ventrodorsad

ventrodorsal

ventroinguinal

ventrolateral

ventromedian

ventroposterior

ventrose

venula *pl.* venulae
   v. macularis inferior
   v. macularis media
   v. macularis superior
   v. nasalis retinae inferior
   v. nasalis retinae superior
   venulae rectae renis
   v. temporalis retinae inferior
   v. temporalis retinae superior

venulae (plural of venula)

venulitis
   cutaneous necrotizing v.

VePesid

Vercyte

verge

vermetoid

vermicular

vermiform

vermis
   v. cerebelli

vermography

Verner-Morrison syndrome

Verneuil's neuroma

verruca *pl.* verrucae
   v. acuminata
   v. digitata
   v. filiformis
   v. necrogenica
   v. plana
   v. plana juvenilis
   v. plantaris
   v. seborrheica
   v. vulgaris

verrucae (plural of verruca)

verruciform

verrucose

verrucosis

verrucous

verruga

version

vertebra *pl.* vertebrae
   block vertebrae
   cervical v.
   vertebrae cervicales
   vertebrae coccygeae
   coccygeal v.
   cranial v.
   fishtail v.
   four lumbar vertebrae
   fused vertebrae
   "ivory" v.

vertebra *(continued)*
    vertebrae lumbales
    lumbar v.
    non–rib-bearing v.
    v. prominens
    rib-bearing v.
    sacral v.
    vertebrae sacrales
    vertebrae thoracales
    thoracic v.
    vertebrae thoracicae
    transitional v.

vertebrectomy

vertebromammary

vertex
    v. of bony cranium
    v. corneae
    v. cranii
    v. cranii ossei

vertical

verticalis

verticillate

verticomental

vertigraphy

Vesalius
    foramen of V.
    foramen Vesalii

vesica *pl.* vesicae
    v. biliaris
    v. fellea
    v. urinaria

vesical

vesicant

vesication

vesicatory

vesicle
    seminal v's

vesicocavernous

vesicorectal

vesicosigmoid

vesicospinal

vesicoumbilical

vesicula *pl.* vesiculae

vesicular

vesiculated

vesiculation

vesiculiform

vesiculogram

vesiculography

vesiculopapular

vesiculopustular

vessel
    absorbent v.
    afferent v's of lymph node
    brachiocephalic v's
    chyliferous v.
    efferent v's of lymph node
    great v's
    lacteal v.
    lenticulostiate v's
    lymphatic v's
    lymphatic v., deep
    lymphatic v., superficial
    lymphocapillary v.
    native v.
    Windkessel v's

vestibula (plural of vestibulum)

vestibular

vestibule

vestibulocerebellum

vestibulogenic

vestibulum *pl.* vestibula
    v. auris
    v. bursae omentalis
    v. laryngis
    v. nasale
    v. nasi
    v. vaginae

vestige
     coccygeal v.

vestigia (plural of vestigium)

vestigial

vestigium *pl.* vestigia
     v. processus vaginalis

vibex *pl.* vibices

viable

vibrissae

video barium swallow

videodensitometry

videofluorography

videofluoroscopy

videognosis

view
     air contrast v's of the stom-
          ach
     Alexander v.
     anteroposterior (AP) v.
     apical lordotic v.
     Broden v.
     bull's eye v's
     Caldwell v.
     Carter-Rowe v.
     Chamberlain-Towne v.
     Cleopatra v.
     closed-mouth v.
     cone-down (or coned-
          down) v.
     coronal reconstruction v's
     cross-table lateral v.
     craniocaudad v.
     decubitus v.
     dens v. of the cervical
          spine
     Eklund v.
     expiratory v.
     fast spin echo (FSE) v's
     Fleckinger v. (*same as*
          swimmer's view)
     flexion and extension v's
     frog-leg v. of the hips

view *(continued)*
     frontal v.
     full column v's
     Hampton v.
     Hughston v. of the knee
     infrapatellar v.
     inspiration and expiration
          v's (*not* inspiration-expira-
          tion)
     inspiratory v.
     internal and external rota-
          tion v's
     internal rotation v.
     internal and external rota-
          tion v's
     Judet v.
     lateral decubitus v.
     lateral flexion and exten-
          sion v's
     Law's v.
     left anterior oblique v.
     lordotic v.
     Mayer v.
     mediolateral v.
     mortise v.
     navicular v.
     oblique v.
     odontoid v.
     open-mouth odontoid v.
     orthogonal v's
     Panorex v's
     plumbline v's
     portable v.
     posteroanterior (PA) v.
     reconstruction v's
     recumbent v.
     Rokus v.
     sagittal and coronal v's
     sagittal magnetization
          transfer v's
     Stenver's v's
     semiupright v.
     stereoscopic v's
     stress v's
     submaxillary v.
     submentovertex v.
     subtalar v.
     sunrise v.
     supine v. Towne's v.

view *(continued)*
    swimmer's v.
    tangential v.
    transthoracic v.
    tunnel v.
    ulnar deviation v.
    upright v.

villi (plural of villus)

villiferous

villoma

villose

villosity

villous

villus *pl.* villi
    villi intestinales
    villi synoviales

vinblastine sulfate

vincristine sulfate

vinculum *pl.* vincula
    v. breve digitorum manus
    v. longum digitorum manus
    vincula tendinum digito-
        rum manus
    vincula tendinum digito-
        rum pedis

vindesine sulfate

vinorelbine ditartrate

vinorelbine tartrate

vinyl
    v. chloride
    v. cyanide

violaceous

violet
    gentian v.

VIPoma

Virchow
    V's gland
    V's law
    V's node

Virchow *(continued)*
    V.-Robin spaces

viscera (plural of viscera)

viscerad

visceral

viscerocranium
    cartilaginous v.
    membranous v.

viscerography

visceromegaly

visceroparietal

visceroperitoneal

visceropleural

viscerosomatic

viscous

viscus *pl.* viscera

Visipaque

visualization
    double contrast v.
    fractional v.
    limited v.

visualize

vitiligines

vitiliginous

vitiligo

VM-26 (teniposide)

Vohwinkel's syndrome

void

Voigt's line

vola

volaris

volume
    blood v.
    mean corpuscular v.
    mean platelet v.

volume *(continued)*
    packed-cell v. (PCV)
    v. of packed red cells
      (VPRC)
    plasma v.
    red cell v.

volute

volvulus
    cecal v.

vomer

vomerobasilar

vomited

vomiting

v-*onc*

von Hippel
    von H's disease
    von H.-Lindau disease

von Recklinghausen's disease

von Willebrand
    von W's disease
    von W's factor

vortex *pl.* vortices
    v. coccygeus
    v. cordis
    vortices pilorum

vortices (plural of vortex)

voxel

VP-16 (etoposide)

VP
    ventriculoperitoneal
      VP shunt tubing

vulvitis
    atrophic v.
    leukoplakic v.
    pseudoleukoplakic v.

Waters' view

waist

wall
>   bowel w.
>   chest w.
>   nail w.

warfarin

wart
>   acuminate w.
>   anatomical w.
>   common w.
>   digitate w.
>   filiform w.
>   flat w.
>   fugitive w.
>   genital w.
>   juvenile w.
>   moist w.
>   mosaic w.
>   necrogenic w.
>   pitch w's
>   plane w.
>   plantar w.
>   pointed w.
>   postmortem w.
>   prosector's w.
>   seborrheic w.
>   seed w.
>   soot w.
>   telangiectatic w.
>   tuberculous w.
>   venereal w.

wave
>   sound w's

Warthin's tumor

water
>   heavy w.
>   w. O 15

Waters
>   W's position
>   W's position, reverse
>   W's projection
>   W's projection radiograph

Waters *(continued)*
>   W's view
>   W's view radiograph

watershed

wavelength
>   effective w.
>   equivalent w.
>   minimum w.

wax
>   sticky w.

web
>   esophageal w.

Weber
>   W.-Christian disease
>   W.-Christian panniculitis
>   W.-Christian syndrome
>   W.-Cockayne syndrome

wedge
>   step w.

wedged

wedge-shaped

wedging

weep

Wegener's granulomatosis

Welcker's angle

Wells' syndrome

welt

Werlhof's disease

Wermer's syndrome

Werner Schultz disease

West
>   W's lacuna skull
>   W.-Engstler's skull

Westergren
>   W. method
>   W. tube

Westermark's sign

West Point projection

"wet reading"

Wharton's duct

wheal

Whipple
W. disease
W. procedure
W's triad

whitehead

whitlow
herpetic w.
melanotic w.
thecal w.

whorl

Wickersheimer's fluid

Widal syndrome

widening
mediastinal w.

width
window w.

Willebrand's syndrome

Willis
circle of W.

Wilms' tumor

Wilson-Mikity syndrome

Wimberger's sign

windburn

window
aortic w.
aorticopulmonary w. (*not* aortopulmonary)
bone w.
coronal meniscal w's

wing
w. of the ilium

wing *(continued)*
w. of the scapula

Winkler's disease

Wintrobe
W. hematocrit tube
W. method

wire
Kirschner w's (also K wires)
Lunderquist w.
safety J w.
TAD w.

witkop

Wolfe's classification of breast carcinoma

Wölfler's glands

Wood
W's filter
W's lamp
W's light
W's sign

Woringer-Kolopp disease

Woringer-Kolopp syndrome

Working Formulation

Working Formulation of National Cancer Institute

Working Formulation of Non-Hodgkin's Lymphomas for Clinical Usage

worm

wound
gunshot w. (GSW

Wright blood group

wrist

wryneck

xanthelasmatosis

xanthism

xanthochromia
  x. striata palmaris

xanthoderma

xanthoerythrodermia
  x. perstans

xanthogranuloma
  juvenile x.

xanthoma
  diabetic x.
  x. diabeticorum
  disseminated x.
  x. disseminatum
  eruptive x.
  x. eruptivum
  fibrous x.
  x. multiplex
  planar x.
  plane x.
  x. planum
  x. striatum palmare
  tuberoeruptive x.
  x. tuberosum
  x. tuberosum multiplex
  tuberous x.
  verruciform x.

xanthomatosis
  biliary hypercholesterol-
    emic x.

xanthomatous

xanthosarcoma

xenon
  x. Xe 127
  x. Xe 133

xenylamine

xerocytosis
  hereditary x.

xeroderma
  x. pigmentosum

xerodermatic

xerodermia

xerodermoid
  pigmented x.

xerography

xeromammography

xeroradiography

xerosis
  x. cutis
  x. generalisata

xerotomography

Xg blood group

x-ray

Xylocaine

xyphoid

yellow
    butter y.
    methyl y.

yoke

ypsiliform

ypsiloid

Y-shaped

Yt blood group

yttrium
   y. 90

Y-tube

Y view

Zamia

zamia

Zanosar

Zang's space

Zappert's chamber

Zemuron

zetacrit

Zetafuge

zeugopodium

Zimmermann's elementary particle

Zinecard

Z-line

Zinn
    cap of Z.

Zinsser-Cole-Engman syndrome

zoacanthosis

Zoladex

zona *pl.* zonae
    z. incerta
    z. orbicularis articulationis
        coxae
    z. vasculosa

zonae (plural of zona)

zonal

zonary

zone
    abdominal z's
    border z.
    epigastric z.
    grenz z.
    hypogastric z.
    keratogenous z.
    Looser's transformation z's
    lung z.
    marginal z.
    transition z.
    transitional z.
    umbau z's
    vascular z.

zonifugal

zonipetal

zonoskeleton

zonula
    z. ciliaris
    z. ciliaris [Zinnii]

zonulae

Zoon's erythroplasia

zonular

zootomist

zygal

zygapophysis
    z. inferior
    z. superior

zygoma *pl.* zygomas, zygomata

zygopodium

Drugs Used in Radiology & Oncology

Below are the names of generic and ℞ brand name drugs used in radiology and oncology, as shown in the *Saunders Pharmaceutical Xref Book*. The drugs are categorized by their "indications"—also called "designated use," "approved use," or "therapeutic action"—which group together drugs used for a similar purpose. The indications shown below are broad categories of therapeutic action. Individual drugs may be placed in subcategories or have specifically targeted diseases beyond the scope of this listing. For complete information about the drugs listed below, including each drug's availability, specific indications, forms of administration, and dosages, please consult the current edition of *Saunders Pharmaceutical Word Book*.

Antineoplastics
[*see also: Immunostimulants; Immunosuppressants*]
Antineoplastics, Alkylating
Alkeran
BiCNU
busulfan
Busulfex
carboplatin
carmustine
CeeNu
chlorambucil
cisplatin
cyclophosphamide
Cytoxan
Dacplat
Eloxatin
Emcyt
estramustine phosphate sodium
Foloxatine
Gliadel
Ifex
ifosfamide
IntraDose
Leukeran
lomustine
mechlorethamine HCl
melphalan (MPL)
Mustargen
Myleran
Neosar
oxaliplatin

Antineoplastics, Alkylating (cont.)
Paraplatin
Platinol
Platinol-AQ
streptozocin
Temodar
temozolomide
Thioplex
thiotepa
Transplatin
Triapine
Zanosar
Antineoplastics, Angiogenesis Inhibitors
AE-941
BeneFin
Neovastat
squalamine
SU-5416
Vitaxin
Antineoplastics, Antibiotics
Adriamycin PFS
Adriamycin RDF
Blenoxane
bleomycin sulfate
Cerubidine
Cosmegen
dactinomycin
DaunoXome
daunorubicin citrate, liposomal
daunorubicin HCl
Doxil

Antineoplastics, Antibiotics (cont.)
  doxorubicin HCl
  epirubicin HCl
  Evacet
  Idamycin
  Idamycin PFS
  idarubicin HCl
  Lysodren
  Mithracin
  mitomycin
  mitotane
  mitoxantrone HCl
  Mutamycin
  Nipent
  Novantrone
  pentostatin
  Pharmorubicin PFS; Pharmorubicin
    RDF ⊕
  plicamycin
  Rubex
  valrubicin
  Valstar

Antineoplastics, Antimetabolites
  Abitrexate
  Adrucil
  capecitabine
  cladribine
  cytarabine
  cytarabine, liposomal
  Cytosar-U
  DepoCyt
  Efudex
  floxuridine
  Fluoroplex
  fluorouracil (5-FU)
  Folex PFS
  FUDR
  gemcitabine
  Gemzar
  Hydrea
  hydroxyurea
  Leustatin
  mercaptopurine (6-MP)
  methotrexate (MTX)
  methotrexate sodium
  Methotrexate LPF Sodium
  Purinethol
  raltitrexed
  Rheumatrex
  Tarabine PFS

Antineoplastics, Antimetabolites (cont.)
  tegafur
  thioguanine (6-TG)
  Tomudex
  UFT
  Xeloda

Antineoplastics, Hormones
  Andro L.A. 200
  Android-10; Android-25
  Andropository-200
  Aquest
  buserelin acetate
  chlorotrianisene
  Deladiol-40
  Delatestryl
  Delestrogen
  depAndro 100; depAndro 200
  Depo-Provera
  Depo-Testosterone
  Depotest 100; Depotest 200
  diethylstilbestrol (DES)
  diethylstilbestrol diphosphate
  Dioval XX; Dioval 40
  Durabolin
  Duragen-20; Duragen-40
  Duratest 100; Duratest 200
  Durathate-200
  DUROS
  Estinyl
  Estra-L 20
  Estra-L 40
  Estrace
  estradiol
  estradiol valerate
  Estratab
  Estrogenic Substance Aqueous
  estrogens, conjugated
  estrogens, esterified
  estrone
  Estrone 5
  Estrone Aqueous
  ethinyl estradiol
  Everone 200
  fluoxymesterone
  goserelin acetate
  Gynogen L.A. 20
  Gynogen L.A. 40
  Halotestin
  Histerone 100

Antineoplastics, Hormones (cont.)
Hybolin Improved
Kestrone 5
leuprolide acetate
Lupron Depot
Lupron Depot–3 month; Lupron
    Depot–4 month
Lupron; Lupron Pediatric
medroxyprogesterone acetate
Megace
megestrol acetate
Menest
methyltestosterone
nandrolone phenpropionate
Oreton Methyl
PEG-camptothecin
Premarin
ProMaxx-100
Prothecan
Stilphostrol
Suprefact ⓒ
Suprefact; Suprefact Depot ⓒ
Tace
Tesamone
Teslac
Testandro
testolactone
testosterone
testosterone cypionate
testosterone enanthate
Testosterone Aqueous
Testred
Theelin Aqueous
Valergen 10
Valergen 20; Valergen 40
Virilon
Wehgen
Zoladex

Antineoplastics, Hormone Antagonists
aminoglutethimide
Anandron ⓒ
anastrozole
Arimidex
bicalutamide
Casodex
cyproterone acetate
Cytadren
Euflex ⓒ
Eulexin

Antineoplastics, Hormone Antagonists (cont.)
Fareston
Femara
flutamide
letrozole
MGI-114
Modrastane
Nilandron
nilutamide
Nolvadex
Novo-Cyproterone ⓒ
tamoxifen citrate
toremifene citrate
trilostane

Antineoplastics, Plant Alkaloids and Other Natural Products
Alkaban-AQ
Camptosar
docetaxel
Eldisine
Etopophos
etoposide
etoposide phosphate
irinotecan HCl
Navelbine
Oncovin
paclitaxel
Paxene
Taxol
Taxotere
teniposide
Toposar
Velban
VePesid
vinblastine sulfate
Vincasar PFS
vincristine sulfate
vindesine sulfate
vinorelbine tartrate
Vumon

Antineoplastics, Protective and Rescue Agents
amifostine
dexrazoxane
Ethyol
Isovorin
L-leucovorin
leucovorin calcium
mesna

Antineoplastics, Protective and Rescue Agents (cont.)

Mesnex
pilocarpine HCl
Salagen
sucralfate
Wellcovorin
Zinecard

Antineoplastics, Therapeutic Vaccines (Theraccines)

AdjuVax-100a
Avicine
BrevaRex
Gastrimmune
GVAX
M-Vax
Melacine
melanoma vaccine
monoclonal antibody B43.13
O-Vax
OncoVax-CL
OncoVax-P
OvaRex
TA-HPV
Theratope-STn
vaccinia virus vaccine for human papillomavirus (HPV), recombinant

Antineoplastics, Unclassified and Adjuncts

AdjuVax-100a
allopurinol sodium
Allovectin-7
altretamine
amsacrine
Amsidyl
Armour Thyroid
asparaginase (L-asparaginase)
Atragen
Avicidin
bexarotene
Bexxar
biricodar dicitrate
blood mononuclear cells, allogenic peripheral
Bondronat
Bonefos
Bonviva
Broxine
broxuridine

Antineoplastics, Unclassified and Adjuncts (cont.)

C-225
CEA-Cide
Ceprate SC
chromic phosphate P 32
coumarin
CYT-103-Y-90
CytoImplant
dacarbazine
Decapeptyl
denileukin diftitox
disaccharide tripeptide glycerol dipalmitoyl
disodium clodronate tetrahydrate
DTIC-Dome
edrecolomab
Elspar
EpiLeukin
Ergamisol
Erwinase
erwinia L-asparaginase
Fludara
fludarabine phosphate
Herceptin
Hexalen
Hycamtin
ibandronate sodium
ImmTher
ImmuRAIT-LL2
Imuvert
Incel
iodine I 131 Lym-1 MAb
iodine I 131 murine MAb IgG_2a to B cell
iodine I 131 murine MAb to alpha-fetoprotein (AFP)
iodine I 131 murine MAb to human chorionic gonadotropin (hCG)
iodine I 131 radiolabeled B1 MAb
iodine I 131 tositumomab
Iodotope
Leucotropin
Leuvectin
levamisole HCl
Lu-Tex
lutetium texaphyrin
LymphoCide
Matulane
MDX-210

Antineoplastics, Unclassified and Adjuncts (cont.)
Metastat
methoxsalen (8-methoxsalen)
metoclopramide HCl
monoclonal antibody to CD22 antigen on B-cells, radiolabeled
monoclonal antibody to CEA, humanized
MultiKine
MX-6
Neomark
9-nitrocamptothecin
Oncaspar
Onco-TCS
Oncocine-HspE7
Oncolym
Oncolysin B
Onconase
OncoRad OV103
Oncostate
Onkolox
Ontak
ONYX-015
Orzel
Ovastat
p30 protein
Pan-HER
Panorex
pegaspargase (PEG-L-asparaginase)
pemetrexed disodium
perfosfamide
Pergamid
Phosphocol P 32
Photofrin
Pivanex
porfimer sodium
prednimustine
Prevatac
procarbazine HCl
Regressin
ricin (blocked) conjugated murine MAb (anti-B4)
Rolazar
S-P-T
Sensamide
Serratia marcescens extract (polyribosomes)
sodium iodide (^{131}I)
sodium iodide I 131

Antineoplastics, Unclassified and Adjuncts (cont.)
sodium phosphate P 32
Sterecyt
Targretin
Theragyn
Thyrar
Thyrogen
thyroid
thyrotropin alfa
Tifolar
topotecan HCl
trastuzumab
treosulfan
tretinoin
Tretinoin LF
Triacana
triptorelin pamoate
uracil
Uvadex
Vesanoid
Zyloprim

Antineoplastics, Chemotherapy Protocols
5 + 2 protocol (cytarabine, daunorubicin)
5 + 2 protocol (cytarabine, mitoxantrone)
7 + 3 protocol (cytarabine, daunorubicin)
7 + 3 protocol (cytarabine, idarubicin)
7 + 3 protocol (cytarabine, mitoxantrone)
8 in 1 (Medrol, vincristine, CCNU, procarbazine, hydroxyurea, cisplatin, ara-C, cyclophosphamide)
8 in 1 (Medrol, vincristine, CCNU, procarbazine, hydroxyurea, cisplatin, ara-C, dacarbazine)
A + D (ara-C, daunorubicin)
A-DIC (Adriamycin, dacarbazine)
AA (ara-C, Adriamycin)
ABC (Adriamycin, BCNU, cyclophosphamide)
ABCM (Adriamycin, bleomycin, cyclophosphamide, mitomycin)
ABD (Adriamycin, bleomycin, DTIC)

Antineoplastics, Chemotherapy Protocols (cont.)

ABDIC (Adriamycin, bleomycin, DIC, [CCNU, prednisone])

ABDV (Adriamycin, bleomycin, DTIC, vinblastine)

ABP (Adriamycin, bleomycin, prednisone)

ABV (actimomycin D, bleomycin, vincristine)

ABV (Adriamycin, bleomycin, vinblastine)

ABVD (Adriamycin, bleomycin, vinblastine, dacarbazine)

ABVD/MOPP (alternating cycles of ABVD and MOPP)

AC (Adriamycin, carmustine)

AC (Adriamycin, CCNU)

AC (Adriamycin, cisplatin)

AC; A-C (Adriamycin, cyclophosphamide)

ACe (Adriamycin, cyclophosphamide)

ACE (Adriamycin, cyclophosphamide, etoposide)

ACFUCY (actinomycin D, fluorouracil, cyclophosphamide)

ACM (Adriamycin, cyclophosphamide, methotrexate)

ACOP (Adriamycin, cyclophosphamide, Oncovin, prednisone)

ACOPP; A-COPP (Adriamycin, cyclophosphamide, Oncovin, procarbazine, prednisone)

ADBC (Adriamycin, DTIC, bleomycin, CCNU)

ADE (ara-C, daunorubicin, etoposide)

ADOAP (Adriamycin, Oncovin, ara-C, prednisone)

ADOP (Adriamycin, Oncovin, prednisone)

Adria + BCNU (Adriamycin, BCNU)

Adria-L-PAM (Adriamycin, L-phenylalanine mustard)

AFM (Adriamycin, fluorouracil, methotrexate [with leucovorin rescue])

Antineoplastics, Chemotherapy Protocols (cont.)

ALOMAD (Adriamycin, Leukeran, Oncovin, methotrexate, actinomycin D, dacarbazine)

AOPA (ara-C, Oncovin, prednisone, asparaginase)

AOPE (Adriamycin, Oncovin, prednisone, etoposide)

AP (Adriamycin, Platinol)

APC (AMSA, prednisone, chlorambucil)

APE (Adriamycin, Platinol, etoposide)

APE (ara-C, Platinol, etoposide)

APO (Adriamycin, prednisone, Oncovin)

ara-C + 6-TG (ara-C, thioguanine)

ara-C + ADR (ara-C, Adriamycin)

ara-C + DNR + PRED + MP (ara-C, daunorubicin, prednisolone, mercaptopurine)

ara-C-HU (ara-C, hydroxyurea)

ASHAP; A-SHAP (Adriamycin, Solu-Medrol, high-dose ara-C, Platinol)

AV (Adriamycin, vincristine)

AVP (actinomycin D, vincristine, Platinol)

B-CHOP (bleomycin, Cytoxin, hydroxydaunomycin, Oncovin, prednisone)

B-DOPA (bleomycin, DTIC, Oncovin, prednisone, Adriamycin)

B-MOPP (bleomycin, nitrogen mustard, Oncovin, procarbazine, prednisone)

BAC (BCNU, ara-C, cyclophosphamide)

BACOD (bleomycin, Adriamycin, CCNU, Oncovin, dexamethasone)

BACON (bleomycin, Adriamycin, CCNU, Oncovin, nitrogen mustard)

BACOP (bleomycin, Adriamycin, cyclophosphamide, Oncovin, prednisone)

BACT (BCNU, ara-C, cyclophosphamide, thioguanine)

Antineoplastics, Chemotherapy Protocols (cont.)

BAMON (bleomycin, Adriamycin, methotrexate, Oncovin, nitrogen mustard)

BAVIP (bleomycin, Adriamycin, vinblastine, imidazole carboxamide, prednisone)

BBVP-M (BCNU, bleomycin, VePesid, prednisone, methotrexate)

BCAP (BCNU, cyclophosphamide, Adriamycin, prednisone)

BCAVe; B-CAVe (bleomycin, CCNU, Adriamycin, Velban)

BCD (bleomycin, cyclophosphamide, dactinomycin)

BCMF (bleomycin, cyclophosphamide, methotrexate, fluorouracil)

BCOP (BCNU, cyclophosphamide, Oncovin, prednisone)

BCP (BCNU, cyclophosphamide, prednisone)

BCVP (BCNU, cyclophosphamide, vincristine, prednisone)

BCVPP (BCNU, cyclophosphamide, vinblastine, procarbazine, prednisone)

BEAC (BCNU, etoposide, ara-C, cyclophosphamide)

BEAM (BCNU, etoposide, ara-C, melphalan)

BEMP (bleomycin, Eldisine, mitomycin, Platinol)

BEP (bleomycin, etoposide, Platinol)

BHD (BCNU, hydroxyurea, dacarbazine)

BHDV; BHD-V (BCNU, hydroxyurea, dacarbazine, vincristine)

BIP (bleomycin, ifosfamide [with mesna rescue], Platinol)

BLEO-COMF (bleomycin, cyclophosphamide, Oncovin, methotrexate, fluorouracil)

BMP (BCNU, methotrexate, procarbazine)

BOAP (bleomycin, Oncovin, Adriamycin, prednisone)

Antineoplastics, Chemotherapy Protocols (cont.)

BOLD (bleomycin, Oncovin, lomustine, dacarbazine)

BOMP (bleomycin, Oncovin, Matulane, prednisone)

BOMP (bleomycin, Oncovin, mitomycin, Platinol)

BOP (BCNU, Oncovin, prednisone)

BOPAM (bleomycin, Oncovin, prednisone, Adriamycin, mechlorethamine, methotrexate)

BOPP (BCNU, Oncovin, procarbazine, prednisone)

BVAP (BCNU, vincristine, Adriamycin, prednisone)

BVCPP (BCNU, vinblastine, cyclophosphamide, procarbazine, prednisone)

BVDS (bleomycin, Velban, doxorubicin, streptozocin)

BVPP (BCNU, vincristine, procarbazine, prednisone)

C-MOPP (cyclophosphamide, mechlorethamine, Oncovin, procarbazine, prednisone)-

CA (cyclophosphamide, Adriamycin)

CABOP; CA-BOP (Cytoxin, Adriamycin, bleomycin, Oncovin, prednisone)

CABS (CCNU, Adriamycin bleomycin, streptozocin)

CAC (cisplatin, ara-C, caffeine)

CAD (cyclophosphamide, Adriamycin, dacarbazine)

CAD (cytarabine [and] daunorubicin)

CAE (cyclophosphamide, Adriamycin, etoposide)

CAF (cyclophosphamide, Adriamycin, fluorouracil)

CAFP (cyclophosphamide, Adriamycin, fluorouracil, prednisone)

CAFTH (cyclophosphamide, Adriamycin, fluorouracil, tamoxifen, Halotestin)

CAFVP (cyclophosphamide, Adriamycin, fluorouracil, vincristine, prednisone)

8   Antineoplastics, Chemotherapy Protocols

Antineoplastics, Chemotherapy Protocols (cont.)

CALF (cyclophosphamide, Adriamycin, leucovorin [rescue], fluorouracil)

CALF-E (cyclophosphamide, Adriamycin, leucovorin [rescue], fluorouracil, ethinyl estradiol)

CAM (cyclophosphamide, Adriamycin, methotrexate)

CAMB (Cytoxin, Adriamycin, methotrexate, bleomycin)

CAMELEON (cytosine arabinoside, methotrexate, Leukovorin, Oncovin)

CAMEO (cyclophosphamide, Adriamycin, methotrexate, etoposide, Oncovin)

CAMF (cyclophosphamide, Adriamycin, methotrexate, folinic acid)

CAMP (cyclophosphamide, Adriamycin, methotrexate, procarbazine HCl)

CAO (cyclophosphamide, Adriamycin, Oncovin)

CAP (cyclophosphamide, Adriamycin, prednisone)

CAP; CAP-I (cyclophosphamide, Adriamycin, Platinol)

CAP-BOP (cyclophosphamide, Adriamycin, procarbazine, bleomycin, Oncovin, prednisone)

CAP-II (cyclophosphamide, Adriamycin, high-dose Platinol)

CAPPr (cyclophosphamide, Adriamycin, Platinol, prednisone)

CAT (cytarabine, Adriamycin, thioguanine)

CAV (cyclophosphamide, Adriamycin, vinblastine)

CAV (cyclophosphamide, Adriamycin, vincristine)

CAVE (cyclophosphamide, Adriamycin, vincristine, etoposide)

CAVe; CA-Ve (CCNU, Adriamycin, vinblastine)

CAVP16 (cyclophosphamide, Adriamycin, VP-16)

CBV (cyclophosphamide, BCNU, VePesid)

Antineoplastics, Chemotherapy Protocols (cont.)

CBV (cyclophosphamide, BCNU, VP-16-213)

CC (carboplatin, cyclophosphamide)

CCM (cyclophosphamide, CCNU, methotrexate)

CCV-AV (CCNU, cyclophosphamide, vincristine [alternates with] Adriamycin, vincristine)

CCVPP (CCNU, cyclophosphamide, Velban, procarbazine, prednisone)

CD (cytarabine, daunorubicin)

CDC (carboplatin, doxorubicin, cyclophosphamide)

CDDP/VP (CDDP, VePesid)

CDE (cyclophosphamide, doxorubicin, etoposide)

CEB (carboplatin, etoposide, bleomycin)

CECA (cisplatin, etoposide, cyclophosphamide, Adriamycin)

CEF (cyclophosphamide, epirubicin, fluorouracil)

CEM (cytosine arabinoside, etoposide, methotrexate)

CEP (CCNU, etoposide, prednimustine)

CEV (cyclophosphamide, etoposide, vincristine)

CF (carboplatin, fluorouracil)

CF (cisplatin, fluorouracil)

CFL (cisplatin, fluorouracil, leucovorin [rescue])

CFM (cyclophosphamide, fluorouracil, mitoxantrone)

CFP (cyclophosphamide, fluorouracil, prednisone)

CFPT (cyclophosphamide, fluorouracil, prednisone, tamoxifen)

CH1VPP; Ch1VPP (chlorambucil, vinblastine, procarbazine, prednisone)

CHAD (cyclophosphamide, hexamethylmelamine, Adriamycin, DDP)

CHAMOCA (Cytoxan, hydroxyurea, actinomycin D, methotrex-

Antineoplastics, Chemotherapy Protocols (cont.)

ate, Oncovin, calcium folinate, Adriamycin)

CHAP (cyclophosphamide, Hexalen, Adriamycin, Platinol)

CHAP (cyclophosphamide, hexamethylmelamine, Adriamycin, Platinol)

ChexUP; Chex-Up; CHEX-UP (cyclophosphamide, hexamethylmelamine, fluorouracil, Platinol)

CHF (cyclophosphamide, hexamethylmelamine, fluorouracil)

CHL + PRED (chlorambucil, prednisone)

ChlVPP (chlorambucil, vinblastine, procarbazine, prednisone)

ChlVPP/EVA (chlorambucil, vinblastine, procarbazine, prednisone, etoposide, vincristine, Adriamycin)

CHO (cyclophosphamide, hydroxydaunomycin, Oncovin)

CHOB (cyclophosphamide, hydroxydaunomycin, Oncovin, bleomycin)

CHOD (cyclophosphamide, hydroxydaunomycin, Oncovin, dexamethasone)

CHOP (cyclophosphamide, hydroxydaunomycin, Oncovin, prednisone)

CHOP-BLEO (cyclophosphamide, hydroxydaunomycin, Oncovin, prednisone, bleomycin)

CHOPE (cyclophosphamide, hydroxydaunomycin, Oncovin, prednisone, etoposide)

CHOR (cyclophosphamide, hydroxydaunomycin, Oncovin, radiation therapy)

CHVP (cyclophosphamide, hydroxydaunomycin, VM-26, prednisone)

CISCA; CisCA (cisplatin, cyclophosphamide, Adriamycin)

CISCA$_{II}$/VB$_{IV}$ (cisplatin, cyclophosphamide, Adriamycin, vinblastine, bleomycin)

Antineoplastics, Chemotherapy Protocols (cont.)

CIVPP (chlorambucil, vinblastine, procarbazine, prednisone)

CMC (cyclophosphamide, methotrexate, CCNU)

CMC-VAP (cyclophosphamide, methotrexate, CCNU, vincristine, Adriamycin, procarbazine)

CMF (cyclophosphamide, methotrexate, fluorouracil)

CMF/AV (cyclophosphamide, methotrexate, fluorouracil, Adriamycin, Oncovin)

CMFAVP (cyclophosphamide, methotrexate, fluorouracil, Adriamycin, vincristine, prednisone)

CMFP; CMF-P (cyclophosphamide, methotrexate, fluorouracil, prednisone)

CMFPT (cyclophosphamide, methotrexate, fluorouracil, prednisone, tamoxifen)

CMFPTH (cyclophosphamide, methotrexate, fluorouracil, prednisone, tamoxifen, Halotestin)

CMFT (cyclophosphamide, methotrexate, fluorouracil, tamoxifen)

CMFVAT (cyclophosphamide, methotrexate, fluorouracil, vincristine, Adriamycin, testosterone)

CMFVP (cyclophosphamide, methotrexate, fluorouracil, vincristine, prednisone)

CMH (cyclophosphamide, *m*-AMSA, hydroxyurea)

CMV (cisplatin, methotrexate, vinblastine)

CNF (cyclophosphamide, Novantrone, fluorouracil)

CNOP (cyclophosphamide, Novantrone, Oncovin, prednisone)

COAP (cyclophosphamide, Oncovin, ara-C, prednisone)

COAP-BLEO (cyclophosphamide, Oncovin, ara-C, prednisone, bleomycin)

COB (cisplatin, Oncovin, bleomycin)

Antineoplastics, Chemotherapy Protocols (cont.)

CODE (cisplatin, Oncovin, doxorubicin, etoposide)

COF/COM (cyclophosphamide, Oncovin, fluorouracil + cyclophosphamide, Oncovin, methotrexate)

COM (cyclophosphamide, Oncovin, MeCCNU)

COM (cyclophosphamide, Oncovin, methotrexate)

COMA-A (cyclophosphamide, Oncovin, methotrexate/citrovorum factor, Adriamycin, ara-C)

COMB (cyclophosphamide, Oncovin, MeCCNU, bleomycin)

COMB (Cytoxin, Oncovin, methotrexate, bleomycin)

COMe (Cytoxin, Oncovin, methotrexate)

COMF (cyclophosphamide, Oncovin, methotrexate, fluorouracil)

COMLA (cyclophosphamide, Oncovin, methotrexate, leucovorin [rescue], ara-C)

COMP (CCNU, Oncovin, methotrexate, procarbazine)

COMP (cyclophosphamide, Oncovin, methotrexate, prednisone)

CONPADRI; CONPADRI-I (cyclophosphamide, Oncovin, L-phenylalanine mustard, Adriamycin)

Cooper's regimen

COP (cyclophosphamide, Oncovin, prednisone)

COP-BLAM (cyclophosphamide, Oncovin, prednisone, bleomycin, Adriamycin, Matulane)

COP-BLEO (cyclophosphamide, Oncovin, prednisone, bleomycin)

COPA (Cytoxin, Oncovin, prednisone, Adriamycin)

COPA-BLEO (cyclophosphamide, Oncovin, prednisone, Adriamycin, bleomycin)

COPAC (CCNU, Oncovin, prednisone, Adriamycin, cyclophosphamide)

Antineoplastics, Chemotherapy Protocols (cont.)

COPB (cyclophosphamide, Oncovin, prednisone, bleomycin)

COPE (cyclophosphamide, Oncovin, Platinol, etoposide)

COPP (CCNU, Oncovin, procarbazine, prednisone)

COPP (cyclophosphamide, Oncovin, procarbazine, prednisone)

CP (chlorambucil, prednisone)

CP (cyclophosphamide, Platinol)

CP (cyclophosphamide, prednisone)

CPB (cyclophosphamide, Platinol, BCNU)

CPC (cyclophosphamide, Platinol, carboplatin)

CPM (CCNU, procarbazine, methotrexate)

CPOB (cyclophosphamide, prednisone, Oncovin, bleomycin)

CT (cisplatin, Taxol)

CT (cytarabine, thioguanine)

CTCb (cyclophosphamide, thiotepa, carboplatin)

Ctx-Plat (cyclophosphamide, Platinol)

CV (cisplatin, VePesid)

CVA (cyclophosphamide, vincristine, Adriamycin)

CVA-BMP; CVA + BMP (cyclophosphamide, vincristine, Adriamycin, BCNU, methotrexate, procarbazine)

CVAD; C-VAD (cyclophosphamide, vincristine, Adriamycin, dexamethasone)

CVB (CCNU, vinblastine, bleomycin)

CVBD (CCNU, bleomycin, vinblastine, dexamethasone)

CVD (cisplatin, vinblastine, dacarbazine)

CVEB (cisplatin, vinblastine, etoposide, bleomycin)

CVI (carboplatin, VePesid, ifosfamide [with mesna rescue])

CVM (cyclophosphamide, vincristine, methotrexate)

Antineoplastics, Chemotherapy Protocols (cont.)

CVP (cyclophosphamide, vincristine, prednisone)

CVPP (CCNU, vinblastine, procarbazine, prednisone)

CVPP (cyclophosphamide, Velban, procarbazine, prednisone)

CVPP-CCNU (cyclophosphamide, vinblastine, procarbazine, prednisone, CCNU)

CY-VA-DACT (Cytoxin, vincristine, Adriamycin, dactinomycin)

CyADIC (cyclophosphamide, Adriamycin, DIC)

CyHOP (cyclophosphamide, Halotestin, Oncovin, prednisone)

CYTABOM (cytarabine, bleomycin, Oncovin, mechlorethamine)

CYVADIC; CY-VA-DIC; CyVADIC (cyclophosphamide, vincristine, Adriamycin, DIC)

CYVMAD (cyclophosphamide, vincristine, methotrexate, Adriamycin, DTIC)

DA (daunorubicin, ara-C)

DAL (daunorubicin, ara-C, L-asparaginase)

DAT (daunorubicin, ara-C, thioguanine)

DATVP (daunorubicin, ara-C, thioguanine, vincristine, prednisone)

DAV (daunorubicin, ara-C, VePesid)

DAVH (dibromodulcitol, Adriamycin, vincristine, Halotestin)

DC (daunorubicin, cytarabine)

DCMP (daunorubicin, cytarabine, mercaptopurine, prednisone)

DCPM (daunorubicin, cytarabine, prednisone, mercaptopurine)

DCT (daunorubicin, cytarabine, thioguanine)

DCV (DTIC, CCNU, vincristine)

DECAL (dexamethasone, etoposide, cisplatin, ara-C, L-asparaginase)

DFMO-MGBG (eflornithine, mitoguazone)

DFV (DDP, fluorouracil, VePesid)

Antineoplastics, Chemotherapy Protocols (cont.)

DHAP (dexamethasone, high-dose ara-C, Platinol)

DI (doxorubicin, ifosfamide [with mesna rescue])

DMC (dactinomycin, methotrexate, cyclophosphamide)

DOAP (daunorubicin, Oncovin, ara-C, prednisone)

DTIC-ACTD; DTIC-ACT-D (DTIC, actinomycin D)

DVB (DDP, vindesine, bleomycin)

DVP (daunorubicin, vincristine, prednisone)

DVPL-ASP (daunorubicin, vincristine, prednisone, L-asparaginase)

DZAPO (daunorubicin, azacitidine, ara-C, prednisone, Oncovin)

E-VMAC (escalated methotrexate, vinblastine, Adriamycin, cisplatin)

E-VMAC (escalated methotrexate, vinblastine, Adriamycin, cyclophosphamide)

EAP (etoposide, Adriamycin, Platinol)

EC (etoposide, carboplatin)

ECHO (etoposide, cyclophosphamide, hydroxydaunomycin, Oncovin)

EDAP (etoposide, dexamethasone, ara-C, Platinol)

EFP (etoposide, fluorouracil, Platinol)

ELF (etoposide, leucovorin [rescue], fluorouracil)

EMA 86 (etoposide, mitoxantrone, ara-C)

EMACO (etoposide, methotrexate, actinomycin D, cyclophosphamide, Oncovin)

EP (etoposide, Platinol)

EPOCH (etoposide, prednisone, Oncovin, cyclophosphamide, Halotestin)

ESHAP (etoposide, Solu-Medrol, high-dose ara-C, Platinol)

ESHAP-MINE (alternating cycles of ESHAP and MINE)

Antineoplastics, Chemotherapy Protocols (cont.)

EVA (etoposide, vinblastine, Adriamycin)

F-CL (fluorouracil, leucovorin calcium [rescue])

FAC (fluorouracil, Adriamycin, cyclophosphamide)

FAC-LEV (fluorouracil, Adriamycin, Cytoxin, levamisole)

FAC-M (fluorouracil, Adriamycin, cyclophosphamide, methotrexate)

FAM (fluorouracil, Adriamycin, mitomycin)

FAM-CF (fluorouracil, Adriamycin, mitomycin, citrovorum factor)

FAM-S (fluorouracil, Adriamycin, mitomycin, streptozocin)

FAME; FAMe (fluorouracil, Adriamycin, MeCCNU)

FAMMe (fluorouracil, Adriamycin, mitomycin, MeCCNU)

FAMTX (fluorouracil, Adriamycin, methotrexate [with leucovorin rescue])

FAP (fluorouracil, Adriamycin, Platinol)

FCAP (fluorouracil, cyclophosphamide, Adriamycin, Platinol)

FCE (fluorouracil, cisplatin, etoposide)

FCP (fluorouracil, cyclophosphamide, prednisone)

FEC (fluorouracil, epirubicin, cyclophosphamide)

FED (fluorouracil, etoposide, DDP)

FIME (fluorouracil, ICRF-159, MeCCNU)

FL (flutamide, leuprolide acetate)

FLAC (fluorouracil, leucovorin [rescue], Adriamycin, cyclophosphamide)

FLAP (fluorouracil, leucovorin [rescue], Adriamycin, Platinol)

FLe (fluorouracil, levamisole)

FLEP (fluorouracil, leucovorin, etoposide, Platinol)

FMS (fluorouracil, mitomycin, streptozocin)

Antineoplastics, Chemotherapy Protocols (cont.)

FMV (fluorouracil, MeCCNU, vincristine)

FNC (fluorouracil, Novantrone, cyclophosphamide)

FNM (fluorouracil, Novantrone, methotrexate)

FOAM (fluorouracil, Oncovin, Adriamycin, mitomycin)

FOMI; FOMi (fluorouracil, Oncovin, mitomycin)

FU/LV (fluorouracil, leucovorin calcium [rescue])

FUM (fluorouracil, methotrexate)

FUVAC (5-FU, vinblastine, Adriamycin, cyclophosphamide)

FZ (flutamide, Zoladex)

H-CAP (hexamethylmelamine, cyclophosphamide, Adriamycin, Platinol)

HAD (hexamethylmelamine, Adriamycin, DDP)

HAM (hexamethylmelamine, Adriamycin, melphalan)

HAM (hexamethylmelamine, Adriamycin, methotrexate)

HD-VAC (high-dose [methotrexate], vinblastine, Adriamycin, cisplatin)

HDMTX (high-dose methotrexate [with leucovorin rescue])

HDMTX/LV (high-dose methotrexate, leucovorin [rescue])

HDMTX-CF (high-dose methotrexate, citrovorum factor)

HDPEB (high-dose PEB protocol)

HexaCAF; Hexa-CAF (hexamethylmelamine, cyclophosphamide, amethopterin, fluorouracil)

HiDAC (high-dose ara-C)

HOAP-BLEO (hydroxydaunomycin, Oncovin, ara-C, prednisone, bleomycin)

HOP (hydroxydaunomycin, Oncovin, prednisone)

ICE (ifosfamide [with mesna rescue], carboplatin, etoposide)

IE (ifosfamide [with mesna rescue], etoposide)

Antineoplastics, Chemotherapy Protocols (cont.)

IfoVP (ifosfamide [with mesna rescue], VePesid)

IMF (ifosfamide [with mesna rescue], methotrexate, fluorouracil)

L-VAM (leuprolide acetate, vinblastine, Adriamycin, mitomycin)

LAPOCA (L-asparaginase, Oncovin, cytarabine, Adriamycin)

LMF (Leukeran, methotrexate, fluorouracil)

LOMAC (leucovorin, Oncovin, methotrexate, Adriamycin, cyclophosphamide)

m-BACOD; M-BACOD (methotrexate, bleomycin, Adriamycin, cyclophosphamide, Oncovin, dexamethasone)

m-PFL (methotrexate, Platinol, fluorouracil, leucovorin [rescue])

M-2 protocol (vincristine, carmustine, cyclophosphamide, melphalan, prednisone)

M-BACOS (methotrexate, bleomycin, Adriamycin, cyclophosphamide, Oncovin, Solu-Medrol)

MABOP (Mustargen, Adriamycin, bleomycin, Oncovin, prednisone)

MAC (methotrexate, actinomycin D, chlorambucil)

MAC (mitomycin, Adriamycin, cyclophosphamide)

MAC; MAC III (methotrexate, actinomycin D, cyclophosphamide)

MACC (methotrexate, Adriamycin, cyclophosphamide, CCNU)

MACHO (methotrexate, asparaginase, cyclophosphamide, hydroxydaunomycin, Oncovin)

MACOP-B (methotrexate, Adriamycin, cyclophosphamide, Oncovin, prednisone, bleomycin)

MAD (MeCCNU, Adriamycin)

MADDOC (mechlorethamine, Adriamycin, dacarbazine, DDP, Oncovin, cyclophosphamide)

MAID (mesna [rescue], Adriamycin, ifosfamide, dacarbazine)

Antineoplastics, Chemotherapy Protocols (cont.)

MAP (mitomycin, Adriamycin, Platinol)

MAZE (m-AMSA, azacitidine, etoposide)

MBC (methotrexate, bleomycin, cisplatin)

MBD (methotrexate, bleomycin, DDP)

MC (mitoxantrone, cytarabine)

MCBP (melphalan, cyclophosphamide, BCNU, prednisone)

MCP (melphalan, cyclophosphamide, prednisone)

MCV (methotrexate, cisplatin, vinblastine)

MECY (methotrexate, cyclophosphamide)

MF (methotrexate [with leucovorin rescue], fluorouracil)

MF (mitomycin, fluorouracil)

MFP (melphalan, fluorouracil, medroxyprogesterone acetate)

MICE (mesna [rescue], ifosfamide, carboplatin, etoposide)

MIFA (mitomycin, fluorouracil, Adriamycin)

MINE (mesna [rescue], ifosfamide, Novantrone, etoposide)

MINE-ESHAP (alternating cycles of MINE and ESHAP)

mini-BEAM (BCNU, etoposide, ara-C, melphalan)

mini-COAP (cyclophosphamide, Oncovin, ara-C, prednisone)

MIV (mitoxantrone, ifosfamide, VePesid)

MM (mercaptopurine, methotrexate)

MMOPP (methotrexate, mechlorethamine, Oncovin, procarbazine, prednisone)

MOB (mechlorethamine, Oncovin, bleomycin)

MOB-III (mitomycin, Oncovin, bleomycin, cisplatin)

MOF (MeCCNU, Oncovin, fluorouracil)

Antineoplastics, Chemotherapy Protocols (cont.)

MOF-STREP; MOF-Strep (Me-CCNU, Oncovin, fluorouracil, streptozocin)

MOMP (mechlorethamine, Oncovin, methotrexate, prednisone)

MOP (mechlorethamine, Oncovin, prednisone)

MOP (mechlorethamine, Oncovin, procarbazine)

MOP-BAP (mechlorethamine, Oncovin, procarbazine, bleomycin, Adriamycin, prednisone)

MOPP (mechlorethamine, Oncovin, procarbazine, prednisone)

MOPP (mustine HCl, Oncovin, procarbazine, prednisone)

MOPP/ABV (mechlorethamine, Oncovin, procarbazine, prednisone, Adriamycin, bleomycin, vinblastine)

MOPP/ABVD (alternating cycles of MOPP and ABVD)

MOPP-BLEO; MOPP-Bleo (mechlorethamine, Oncovin, procarbazine, prednisone, bleomycin)

MOPPHDB (mechlorethamine, Oncovin, procarbazine, prednisone, high-dose bleomycin)

MOPPLDB (mechlorethamine, Oncovin, procarbazine, prednisone, low-dose bleomycin)

MOPr (mechlorethamine, Oncovin, procarbazine)

MP (melphalan, prednisone)

MPL + PRED (melphalan, prednisone)

MTX + MP (methotrexate, mercaptopurine)

MTX + MP + CTX (methotrexate, mercaptopurine, cyclophosphamide)

MTXCP-PDAdr (methotrexate [with leucovorin rescue], cisplatin, doxorubicin)

MV (mitomycin, vinblastine)

MV (mitoxantrone, VePesid)

Antineoplastics, Chemotherapy Protocols (cont.)

MVAC; M-VAC (methotrexate, vinblastine, Adriamycin, cisplatin)

MVF (mitoxantrone, vincristine, fluorouracil)

MVP (mitomycin, vinblastine, Platinol)

MVPP (mechlorethamine, vinblastine, procarbazine, prednisone)

MVT (mitoxantrone, VePesid, thiotepa)

MVVPP (mechlorethamine, vincristine, vinblastine, procarbazine, prednisone)

NAC (nitrogen mustard, Adriamycin, CCNU)

NFL (Novantrone, fluorouracil, leucovorin [rescue])

NOVP (Novantrone, Oncovin, vinblastine, prednisone)

OAP (Oncovin, ara-C, prednisone)

OMAD (Oncovin, methotrexate/citrovorum factor, Adriamycin, dactinomycin)

OPA (Oncovin, prednisone, Adriamycin)

OPAL (Oncovin, prednisone, L-asparaginase)

OPEN (Oncovin, prednisone, etoposide, Novantrone)

OPP (Oncovin, procarbazine, prednisone)

OPPA (Oncovin, prednisone, procarbazine, Adriamycin)

P-MVAC (Platinol, methotrexate, vinblastine, Adriamycin, carboplatin)

PAB-Esc-C (Platinol, Adriamycin, bleomycin, escalating doses of cyclophosphamide)

PAC; PAC-I (Platinol, Adriamycin, cyclophosphamide)

PACE (Platinol, Adriamycin, cyclophosphamide, etoposide)

PATCO (prednisone, ara-C, thioguanine, cyclophosphamide, Oncovin)

Antineoplastics, Chemotherapy Protocols (cont.)

PAVe (procarbazine, Alkeran, Velban)

PBV (Platinol, bleomycin, vinblastine)

PC (paclitaxel, carboplatin)

PCE (Platinol, cyclophosphamide, etoposide)

PCV (procarbazine, CCNU, vincristine)

PEB (Platinol, etoposide, bleomycin)

PFL (Platinol, fluorouracil, leucovorin [rescue])

PFT (L-phenylalanine mustard, fluorouracil, tamoxifen)

PHRT (procarbazine, hydroxyurea, radiotherapy)

PIA (Platinol, ifosfamide, Adriamycin)

POC (procarbazine, Oncovin, CCNU)

POCA (prednisone, Oncovin, cytarabine, Adriamycin)

POCC (procarbazine, Oncovin, cyclophosphamide, CCNU)

POMP (prednisone, Oncovin, methotrexate, Purinethol)

ProMACE (prednisone, methotrexate [with leucovorin rescue], Adriamycin, cyclophosphamide, etoposide)

ProMACE/cytaBOM (ProMACE [above], cytarabine, bleomycin, Oncovin, mitoxantrone)

ProMACE/MOPP (full course of ProMACE, followed by MOPP)

pulse VAC (vincristine, actinomycin D, cyclophosphamide)

pulse VAC (vincristine, Adriamycin, cyclophosphamide)

PVB (Platinol, vinblastine, bleomycin)

PVDA (prednisone, vincristine, daunorubicin, asparaginase)

PVP; PVP-16 (Platinol, VP-16)

RIDD (recombinant interleukin-2, dacarbazine, DDP)

Antineoplastics, Chemotherapy Protocols (cont.)

SMF (streptozocin, mitomycin, fluorouracil)

standard VAC

Stanford V (mechlorethamine, doxorubicin, vinblastine, vincristine, bleomycin, VePesid, prednisone)

STEAM (streptonigrin, thioguanine, cyclophosphamide, actinomycin, mitomycin)

T-2 protocol (dactinomycin, doxorubicin, vincristine, cyclophosphamide, radiation)

T-10 protocol (methotrexate, doxorubicin, cisplatin, bleomycin, cyclophosphamide, dactinomycin)

TAD (thioguanine, ara-C, daunorubicin)

TC (thioguanine, cytarabine)

TEC (thiotepa, etoposide, carboplatin)

TEMP (tamoxifen, etoposide, mitoxantrone, Platinol)

TOAP (thioguanine, Oncovin, [cytosine] arabinoside, prednisone)

TPCH (thioguanine, procarbazine, CCNU, hydroxyurea)

TPDCV (thioguanine, procarbazine, DCD, CCNU, vincristine)

V-CAP III (VP-16-213, cyclophosphamide, Adriamycin, Platinol)

V-TAD (VePesid, thioguanine, ara-C, daunorubicin)

VA (vincristine, actinomycin D)

VAAP (vincristine, asparaginase, Adriamycin, prednisone)

VAB; VAB-I (vinblastine, actinomycin D, bleomycin)

VAB-6 (vinblastine, actinomycin D, bleomycin, cyclophosphamide, cisplatin)

VAB-II (vinblastine, actinomycin D, bleomycin, cisplatin)

VAB-III (vinblastine, actinomycin D, bleomycin, cisplatin, chlorambucil, cyclophosphamide)

Antineoplastics, Chemotherapy Protocols (cont.)

VAB-V (vinblastine, actinomycin D, bleomycin, cyclophosphamide, cisplatin)

VABCD (vinblastine, Adriamycin, bleomycin, CCNU, DTIC)

VAC (vincristine, Adriamycin, cisplatin)

VAC; VAC pulse; VAC standard (vincristine, actinomycin D, cyclophosphamide)

VAC; VAC pulse; VAC standard (vincristine, Adriamycin, cyclophosphamide)

VACA (vincristine, actinomycin D, cyclophosphamide, Adriamycin)

VACAD (vincristine, actinomycin D, cyclophosphamide, Adriamycin, dacarbazine)

VACAdr-IfoVP (vincristine, actinomycin D, cyclophosphamide, Adriamycin, ifosfamide, VePesid)

VACP (VePesid, Adriamycin, cyclophosphamide, Platinol)

VAD (vincristine, Adriamycin, dactinomycin)

VAD (vincristine, Adriamycin, dexamethasone)

VAD/V (vincristine, Adriamycin, dexamethasone, verapamil)

VAdrC (vincristine, Adriamycin, cyclophosphamide)

VAFAC (vincristine, amethopterin, fluorouracil, Adriamycin, cyclophosphamide)

VAI (vincristine, actinomycin D, ifosfamide)

VAM (vinblastine, Adriamycin, mitomycin)

VAM (VP-16-213, Adriamycin, methotrexate)

VAMP (vincristine, actinomycin, methotrexate, prednisone)

VAMP (vincristine, Adriamycin, methylprednisolone)

VAMP (vincristine, amethopterin, mercaptopurine, prednisone)

VAP (vinblastine, actinomycin D, Platinol)

Antineoplastics, Chemotherapy Protocols (cont.)

VAP (vincristine, Adriamycin, prednisone)

VAP (vincristine, Adriamycin, procarbazine)

VAP (vincristine, asparaginase, prednisone)

VAT (vinblastine, Adriamycin, thiotepa)

VATD; VAT-D (vincristine, ara-C, thioguanine, daunorubicin)

VATH (vinblastine, Adriamycin, thiotepa, Halotestin)

VAV (VP-16-213, Adriamycin, vincristine)

VB (vinblastine, bleomycin)

VBA (vincristine, BCNU, Adriamycin)

VBAP (vincristine, BCNU, Adriamycin, prednisone)

VBC (VePesid, BCNU, cyclophosphamide)

VBC (vinblastine, bleomycin, cisplatin)

VBD (vinblastine, bleomycin, DDP)

VBM (vincristine, bleomycin, methotrexate)

VBMCP (vincristine, BCNU, melphalan, cyclophosphamide, prednisone)

VBMF (vincristine, bleomycin, methotrexate, fluorouracil)

VBP (vinblastine, bleomycin, Platinol)

VC (VePesid, carboplatin)

VC (vinorelbine, cisplatin)

VCAP (vincristine, cyclophosphamide, Adriamycin, prednisone)

VCF (vincristine, cyclophosphamide, fluorouracil)

VCMP (vincristine, cyclophosphamide, melphalan, prednisone)

VCP (vincristine, cyclophosphamide, prednisone)

VDA (vincristine, daunorubicin, asparaginase)

VDP (vinblastine, dacarbazine, Platinol)

Antineoplastics, Chemotherapy Protocols (cont.)

VDP (vincristine, daunorubicin, prednisone)

VeIP (Velban, ifosfamide, Platinol)

VIC (VePesid, ifosfamide [with mesna rescue], carboplatin)

VIC (vinblastine, ifosfamide, CCNU)

VIE (vincristine, ifosfamide, etoposide)

VIP (vinblastine, ifosfamide [with mesna rescue], Platinol)

VIP; VIP-1; VIP-2 (VePesid, ifosfamide [with mesna rescue], Platinol)

VIP-B (VP-16, ifosfamide, Platinol, bleomycin)

VLP (vincristine, L-asparaginase, prednisone)

VM (vinblastine, mitomycin)

VM-26PP (teniposide, procarbazine, prednisone)

VMAD (vincristine, methotrexate, Adriamycin, actinomycin D)

VMCP (vincristine, melphalan, cyclophosphamide, prednisone)

VMP (VePesid, mitoxantrone, prednimustine)

VOCAP (VP-16-213, Oncovin, cyclophosphamide, Adriamycin, Platinol)

VP (vincristine, prednisone)

VP + A (vincristine, prednisone, asparaginase)

VP-L-asparaginase (vincristine, prednisone, L-asparaginase)

VPB (vinblastine, Platinol, bleomycin)

VPBCPr (vincristine, prednisone, vinblastine, chlorambucil, procarbazine)

VPCA (vincristine, prednisone, cyclophosphamide, ara-C)

VPCMF (vincristine, prednisone, cyclophosphamide, methotrexate, fluorouracil)

VPP (VePesid, Platinol)

Contrast Media
Contrast Media, Paramagnetic

AngioMark

Combidex

Dynospheres M-035

Feridex

ferristene

ferucarbotran

ferumoxides

ferumoxsil

ferumoxtran-10

gadodiamide

gadopentetate dimeglumine

gadoteridol

GastroMARK

Imagent GI

Magnevist

mangafodipir trisodium

mangofodipir trisodium

MS-325

Omniscan

Optimark

perflubron

ProHance

Resovist

Teslascan

Contrast Media, Radiopaque

Amipaque

Anatrast

Angio-Conray

Angiovist 282

Angiovist 292; Angiovist 370

arcitumomab

Baricon

barium sulfate

Baro-cat

Barobag

Baroflave

Barosperse

Barosperse, Liquid

Bear-E-Bag Pediatric

Bear-E-Yum CT

Bear-E-Yum GI

Bilivist

Bilopaque

CEA-Scan

Cholebrine

Cholografin Meglumine

Conray 325

Conray 400

Contrast Media, Radiopaque (cont.)
Conray; Conray 30; Conray 43
Cysto-Conray; Cysto-Conray II
Cystografin; Cystografin Dilute
diatrizoate meglumine
diatrizoate sodium
Dionosil Oily
Enecat
Enhancer
Entrobar
Epi-C
ethiodized oil
Ethiodol
Flo-Coat
Gastrografin
HD 200 Plus
HD 85
Hexabrix
Hypaque-76
Hypaque-Cysto
Hypaque-M 75; Hypaque-M 90
Hypaque Meglumine 30%; Hypaque
   Meglumine 60%
Hypaque Sodium
Hypaque Sodium 20%
Hypaque Sodium 25%; Hypaque
   Sodium 50%
Imager ac
Intropaste
iocetamic acid
iodamide meglumine
iodipamide meglumine
iodixanol
iohexol
iopamidol
iopanoic acid
iopromide
iosulfan blue
iothalamate meglumine
iothalamate sodium
iotrolan
ioversol
ioxaglate meglumine
ioxaglate sodium
ipodate calcium
ipodate sodium
Isovue-M 200; Isovue-M 300
Isovue-128; Isovue-200; Isovue-250;
   Isovue-300; Isovue-370
Liqui-Coat HD

Contrast Media, Radiopaque (cont.)
Liquipake
Lymphazurin 1%
MD-60; MD-76
MD-76 R
MD-Gastroview
Medebar Plus
Medescan
metrizamide
Novopaque
OctreoScan
Omnipaque
Optiray 160; Optiray 240; Optiray
   300; Optiray 320; Optiray 350
Oragrafin Calcium
Oragrafin Sodium
Osmovist
oxidronate sodium
polyvinyl chloride, radiopaque
Prepcat
propyliodone
Quick AC Enema Kit
Reno-30
Reno-Dip; Reno-60
RenoCal-76
Renografin-60
Renografin-76
Renovist; Renovist II
Renovue-Dip; Renovue-65
Sinografin
Sitzmarks
Telepaque
Tomocat
Tonopaque
tyropanoate sodium
Ultravist
Urovist Cysto
Urovist Meglumine DIU/CT
Urovist Sodium 300
Vascoray
Visipaque
Contrast Media, Ultrasound
albumin, human (sonicated with
   chlorofluorocarbons)
Albunex
Definity
EchoGen
Echovist ⊛
Filmix
galactose

Contrast Media, Ultrasound (cont.)
Imagent US
Levovist 🌑
microbubble contrast agent
Optison
perflenapent
perflisopent
perflutren

Immunostimulants
acetylcysteine (N-acetylcysteine)
Actimmune
Aldara
Aliminase
Ampligen
Betafectin
cilmostim
Copaxone
disaccharide tripeptide glycerol
  dipalmitoyl
Ergamisol
Fluimucil
glatiramer acetate
Iamin
ImmTher
imiquimod
Imreg-1
Imuthiol
interleukin-4 receptor (IL-4R)
Leucomax
Leucotropin
Leukine
Linomide
lisofylline (LSF)
Macstim
Megagen
megakaryocyte growth and develop-
  ment factor, pegylated, recombi-
  nant human
milodistim
molgramostim
Neumega
Nuvance
oprelvekin
oxothiazolidine carboxylate (L-2-
  oxothiazolidine-4-carboxylic acid)
PGG glucan
Pixykine
poly I: poly C12U

Immunostimulants (cont.)
prezatide copper acetate
Procysteine
ProTec
regramostim
Remune
roquinimex
sargramostim
Stimulon
Sulfasim
T-cell gene therapy
thalidomide
Thalomid
thymopentin
Timunox
Vendona

Immunosuppressants
[see also: Antineoplastics]
anti-human thymocyte immuno-
  globulin, rabbit
Atgam
azathioprine
azathioprine sodium
Campath 1H
CellCept
Centara
cyclosporine
dacliximab
Imuran
LJP-394
lymphocyte immune globulin, anti-
  thymocyte
muromonab-CD3
mycophenolate mofetil
mycophenolate mofetil HCl
Nashville Rabbit Antithymocyte
  Serum
Neoral
Orthoclone OKT3
priliximab
Prograf
Rapamune
Sandimmune
Sandimmune Neoral 🌑
SangCya
sirolimus
tacrolimus
Thymoglobulin

Immunosuppressants (cont.)
Zenapax

Radiopharmaceuticals
AcuTect
Bexxar
Cardiolite
chromic phosphate P 32
depreotide
ImmuRAID-AFP
ImmuRAID-hCG
ImmuRAIT-LL2
indium In 111 IGIV pentetate
indium In 111 pentetreotide
indium In 111 satumomab pendetide
iodine I 123 murine MAb to alpha-fetoprotein (AFP)
iodine I 123 murine MAb to human chorionic gonadotropin (hCG)
iodine I 131 6B-iodomethyl-19-nor-cholesterol
iodine I 131 Lym-1 MAb
iodine I 131 murine MAb IgG$_2$a to B cell
iodine I 131 murine MAb to alpha-fetoprotein (AFP)
iodine I 131 murine MAb to human chorionic gonadotropin (hCG)
iodine I 131 radiolabeled B1 MAb
iodine I 131 tositumomab
Iodotope
LeuTech
LeukoScan
LymphoScan
Macroscint
mespiperone C 11
Metastron
Miraluma
NeoTect
Neurolite
nofetumomab merpentan
OctreoScan 111

Radiopharmaceuticals (cont.)
OncoTrac
Oncolym
OncoScint CR/OV
Phosphocol P 32
Quadramet
samarium Sm 153 lexidronam
sodium iodide (^{131}I)
sodium iodide I 123
sodium iodide I 131
sodium phosphate P 32
strontium chloride Sr 89
technetium (^{99m}Tc) dimercaptosuc-cinic acid
technetium (^{99m}Tc) methylenedi-phosphonate
technetium Tc 99m albumin aggre-gated
technetium Tc 99m antimelanoma murine MAb
technetium Tc 99m apcitide
technetium Tc 99m arcitumomab
technetium Tc 99m bectumomab
technetium Tc 99m biciromab
technetium Tc 99m bicisate
technetium Tc 99m disofenin
technetium Tc 99m furifosmin
technetium Tc 99m medronate
technetium Tc 99m mertiatide
technetium Tc 99m murine MAb to human alpha-fetoprotein (AFP)
technetium Tc 99m murine MAb to human chorionic gonadotropin (hCG)
technetium Tc 99m oxidronate
technetium Tc 99m sestamibi
technetium Tc 99m siboroxime
technetium Tc 99m succimer
technetium Tc 99m sulesomab
technetium Tc 99m teboroxime
technetium Tc 99m tetrofosmin
Verluma